Principles
& Protocols

Be ON CALL with confidence!

Successfully managing on-call situations requires a masterful combination of speed, skills, and knowledge. Rise to the occasion with **ELSEVIER's On Call Series!** These pocket-size resources provide you with immediate access to the vital, step-by-step information you need to succeed!

Other Titles in the ON CALL Series

Principles
& Protocols

SHANE A. MARSHALL, MD, FRCPC
Director of Cardiac Care
Chief of Medicine
King Edward VIIth Memorial Hospital
Paget, Bermuda

JOHN RUEDY, MDCM, FRCPC, LLD (hon)
Professor (Emeritus) of Pharmacology
Faculty of Medicine
Dalhousie University
Halifax, Nova Scotia
Canada

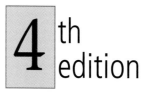

4th edition

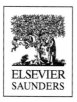

ELSEVIER
SAUNDERS

ELSEVIER
SAUNDERS

The Curtis Center
170 S Independence Mall W 300E
Philadelphia, Pennsylvania 19106

ON CALL PRINCIPLES & PROTOCOLS   0-7216-3902-X
Copyright © 2004, 2000, 1993, 1989, Elsevier Inc.

Library of Congress Cataloging-in-Publication Data

Marshall, Shane A.
    On call: principles and protocols / Shane A. Marshall, John Ruedy. –4th ed.
        p. ; cm.
    Includes bibliographical references and index.
    ISBN 0-7216-3902-X
        1. Medical emergencies–Handbooks, manuals, etc. 2. Medical
        consultation–Handbooks, manuals, etc. I.Ruedy, John. II. Title.
    [DNLM: 1. Emergencies–Handbooks. 2. Emergency Medicine–Handbooks.
WB 39 M369o 2004]
RC86.7.G55 2004
616.02'5–dc22   2004046717

Acquisitions Editor: William Schmitt
Publishing Services Manager: Tina Rebane
Project Manager: Amy Norwitz
Designer: Ellen Zanolle

Printed in the United States of America.

Last digit is the print number: 9   8   7   6   5   4   3   2   1

To our families in
Bermuda and Canada

Preface

Taking calls at night is one of the traditional duties of medical students and residents in teaching hospitals. *On Call Principles and Protocols* is designed to facilitate the transition of medical students and residents from the classroom to the hospital setting. We believe that the initiation of the medical student to hospital practice need not be one of trial and error and need not be recalled as a time of stress and uncertainty.

The fourth edition of *On Call Principles and Protocols* provides referenced updates for the assessment and management of the common problems for which medical students and residents are called at night. The popular On Call Formulary, a quick reference of commonly prescribed medications, has also been expanded and updated.

We have been careful to maintain an approach that provides both instruction and reference while emphasizing the rational thought processes required for optimal patient care in specific clinical situations. In this edition of *On Call Principles and Protocols* medications are in blue type, and where appropriate the thought processes behind management decisions and instructions are indented. We hope readers will find this new, two-color edition helpful in managing patients while on call. It is our belief that this structured approach deserves greater emphasis in the undergraduate years, and we are hopeful that it will help in the introduction of students to clinical medicine.

Shane A. Marshall

John Ruedy

Acknowledgments

We are grateful to the physicians and allied health care workers who provided helpful and detailed comments on individual chapters, particularly Dr. J. T. Heir, Mrs. Linda Rothwell, and Mrs. Debbie Jones. We would also like to thank Dr. J. Gillies for her major contribution to the first edition of *On Call Principles and Protocols* and to Mr. William Schmitt for his patience and encouragement during the preparation of the fourth edition of this book.

Structure of the Book

The book is divided into three main sections.

The first section covers introductory material in four separate chapters: Chapter 1, Approach to the Diagnosis and Management of On-Call Problems; Chapter 2, Documentation of On-Call Problems; Chapter 3, Assessment and Management of Volume Status; and Chapter 4, AIDS, HBV, HCV, and the House Officer. Volume status is discussed in the introductory section because its assessment is essential for the proper management of many problems in hospitalized patients. A statement on AIDS is included because of the small risk that caring for HIV-infected patients poses to health care workers.

The second section contains the common calls associated with patient-related problems. Each problem is approached from its inception, beginning with the relevant questions that should be asked over the phone, the temporary orders that should be given, and the major life-threatening problems to be considered as one approaches the bedside. The names and doses of medications are in blue for easy location and reference. The rationales behind questions that are asked are indented, and the thoughts behind management decisions that are recommended are set off with a blue line.

Each chapter in the second section is divided as follows:

PHONE CALL

Questions

Pertinent questions that should be asked to assess the urgency of the situation.

Orders

Urgent orders to be carried out before you arrive at the bedside.

Inform RN

The time you anticipate arriving at the bedside.

ELEVATOR THOUGHTS

The differential diagnosis that should be considered while you are on the way to assess the patient (i.e., while in the elevator).

MAJOR THREAT TO LIFE

Identification of the major threat to life is essential in providing a focus for the effective management of the patient.

BEDSIDE

Quick-Look Test

A rapid visual assessment to place the patient in one of three categories: well, sick, or critical. This helps determine the necessity for immediate intervention.

Airway and Vital Signs

Selective History

Selective Physical Examination

Management

The third section contains the common calls associated with laboratory-related problems.

The appendices consist of reference items that are useful in managing calls.

The On-Call Formulary is a compendium of commonly used medications that are likely to be prescribed by the student or resident on call. The alphabetically arranged formulary serves as a quick reference for drug dosages, routes of administration, side effects, contraindications, and modes of action.

Commonly Used Abbreviations

ABD	Abdomen
ABG	Arterial blood gas
AC	*Ante cibum* (before meals)
ACE	Angiotensin-converting enzyme
ACS	Acute coronary syndrome
ACTH	Adrenocorticotropic hormone
ADH	Antidiuretic hormone
AFB	Acid-fast bacillus
AIDS	Acquired immunodeficiency syndrome
AMI	Acute myocardial infarction
AMP	Adenosine monophosphate
ANA	Antinuclear antibody
AP	Anteroposterior
aPTT	Activated partial thromboplastin time
ARDS	Adult respiratory distress syndrome
ASD	Atrial septal defect
AV	Atrioventricular
BBB	Bundle branch block
BID	Twice a day
BLS	Basic life support
BP	Blood pressure
BPH	Benign prostatic hypertrophy
C+S	Culture and sensitivity
Ca	Calcium

CBC	Complete blood (cell) count
CCU	Cardiac care unit
CGL	Chronic granulocytic leukemia
CHF	Congestive heart failure
CLL	Chronic lymphocytic leukemia
CMV	Cytomegalovirus
CNS	Central nervous system
CO	Cardiac output
CO$_2$	Carbon dioxide
COPD	Chronic obstructive pulmonary disease
CPK	Creatine phosphokinase
CPR	Cardiopulmonary resuscitation
CrCl	Creatinine clearance
CSF	Cerebrospinal fluid
CT	Computed tomography
CVS	Cardiovascular system
CXR	Chest x-ray
D5NS	5% dextrose in normal saline
D5W	5% dextrose in water
D10W	10% dextrose in water
D20W	20% dextrose in water
D50W	50% dextrose in water
DC	Direct current
DIC	Disseminated intravascular coagulation
DKA	Diabetic ketoacidosis
DVT	Deep venous (vein) thrombosis
ECF	Extracellular fluid
ECG	Electrocardiogram
ED	Emergency department
EDTA	Edetate disodium
EF	Ejection fraction
ELISA	Enzyme-linked immunosorbent assay

EMT	Emergency medical technician
ENDO	Endocrine
ENT	Ears, nose, and throat
ESR	Erythrocyte sedimentation rate
ET	Endotracheal
Ext	Extremities
FDA	Food and Drug Administration
FDP	Fibrin degradation product
FEV$_1$	Forced expiratory volume in 1 second
FFP	Fresh frozen plasma
FIO$_2$	Fraction of inspired oxygen
FPBG	Finger-prick blood glucose
FTA-ABS	Fluorescent treponemal antibody absorption
FUO	Fever of unknown origin
G-6-PD	Glucose-6-phosphate dehydrogenase
GERD	Gastroesophageal reflux disease
GI	Gastrointestinal
GTT	Glucose tolerance test
GU	Genitourinary
HAART	Highly active antiretroviral therapy
Hb	Hemoglobin
HBV	Hepatitis B virus
HCV	Hepatitis C virus
HEENT	Head, eyes, ears, nose, and throat
HIV	Human immunodeficiency virus
HJR	Hepatojugular reflux
HPI	History of present illness
HR	Heart rate
HS	*Hora somni* (at bedtime)
IBW	Ideal body weight
ICF	Intracellular fluid
ICU	Intensive care unit

ICU/CCU	Intensive care unit/cardiac care unit
Ig	Immunoglobulin
IM	Intramuscular
INR	International normalized ratio
IP	Intraperitoneally
ISI	International Sensitivity Index
ITP	Idiopathic thrombocytopenic purpura
IV	Intravenous
IVP	Intravenous pyelogram
J	Joule
JVP	Jugular venous pressure
K	Potassium
L	Liter
LDH	Lactate dehydrogenase
LLL	Left lower lobe
LLQ	Left lower quadrant
LMWH	Low-molecular-weight heparin
LOC	Level of consciousness
LP	Lumbar puncture
LUQ	Left upper quadrant
LV	Left ventricle (ventricular)
LVH	Left ventricular hypertrophy
MAO	Monoamine oxidase
MAOI	Monoamine oxidase inhibitor
MCV	Mean corpuscular volume
MD	Doctor of medicine
MHA-TP	Microhemagglutinin assay—*Treponema pallidum*
MI	Myocardial infarction
Misc	Miscellaneous
MRI	Magnetic resonance imaging
MSS	Musculoskeletal system
MVP	Mitral valve prolapse

NA	Sodium
Neuro	Neurologic system
NG	Nasogastric
NMR	Nuclear magnetic resonance (scan)
NNRTI	Non-nucleoside reverse transcriptase inhibitor
NPH	Neutral protamine Hagedorn (insulin)
NPO	*Nil per os* (nothing by mouth)
NRTI	Nucleoside/nucleotide reverse transcriptase inhibitor
NS	Normal saline (0.9% saline in water)
NSAID	Nonsteroidal anti-inflammatory drug
NYD	Not yet diagnosed
OD	Overdose
P_2	Pulmonic second sound
PA	Posteroanterior
PAC	Premature atrial contraction
PAT	Paroxysmal atrial tachycardia
PC	*Post cibum* (after meals)
P_{CO_2}	Partial pressure of carbon dioxide
PEA	Pulseless electrical activity
PEEP	Positive end-expiratory pressure
PEFR	Peak expiratory flow rate
PI	Protease inhibitor
PMN	Polymorphonuclear cell
PND	Paroxysmal nocturnal dyspnea
PO	*Per os* (by mouth)
P_{O_2}	Partial pressure of oxygen
PR	Per rectum
PRN	*Pro re nata* (as needed)
PSVT	Paroxysmal Supraventricular tachycardia
Psych	Psychiatric
PT	Prothrombin time+
PTH	Parathyroid hormone

PUD	Peptic ulcer disease
PVC	Premature ventricular contraction
QD	Every day
QHS	*Quaque hora somnia* (every hour of sleep)
QID	Four times a day
RA	Rheumatoid arthritis
RAD	Right axis deviation
RBBB	Right bundle branch block
RBC	Red blood cell (count)
Resp	Respiratory system
RLL	Right lower lobe
RLQ	Right lower quadrant
RN	Registered nurse
ROM	Range of motion
RR	Respiratory rate
RTA	Renal tubular acidosis
RUQ	Right upper quadrant
RV	Right ventricle (ventricular)
S$_3$	Third heart sound
SA	Sternal angle
SAH	Subarachnoid hemorrhage
SBE	Subacute bacterial endocarditis
SC	Subcutaneous
SI	International System of Units
SIADH	Syndrome of inappropriate antidiuretic hormone (secretion)
SL	Sublingual
SLE	Systemic lupus erythematosus
SOB	Shortness of breath
SSRI	Selective serotonin reuptake inhibitor
SSS	Sick sinus syndrome
stat	*Statim* (immediately)

STS	Serological test for syphilis
SV	Stroke volume
SVT	Supraventricular tachycardia
T_3	Triiodothyronine
T_4	Thyroxine
TB	Tuberculosis
TBW	Total body water
TEMP	Temperature
TIA	Transient ischemic attack
TID	Three times a day
TKVO	To keep the vein open
tPA	Tissue plasminogen activator
TPN	Total parenteral nutrition
TPR	Total peripheral resistance
TSH	Thyroid-stimulating hormone
TTP	Thrombotic thrombocytopenic purpura
URTI	Upper respiratory tract infection
UTI	Urinary tract infection
$\dot{V}/\dot{Q}$	Ventilation-perfusion
VF	Ventricular fibrillation
VIPoma	Vasoactive intestinal polypeptide-secreting tumor
VP	Ventriculoperitoneal
VSD	Ventricular septal defect
VT	Ventricular tachycardia
WBC	White blood cell (count)
WPW	Wolff-Parkinson-White
ZN	Ziehl-Neelsen

Contents

Introduction

Patient-Related Problems: The Common Calls

Laboratory-Related Problems: The Common Calls

Appendices

Introduction

1

Approach to the Diagnosis and Management of On-Call Problems

Clinical problem solving is an important skill for the physician on call. Traditionally, a physician approaches the diagnosis and management of a patient's problems with an ordered, structured system (e.g., history taking, physical examination, and review of available investigations) before formulating the provisional and differential diagnoses and the management plan. The history and physical examination may take 30 to 40 minutes for a patient with a single problem visiting a family physician for the first time, or they may take 60 to 90 minutes for a geriatric patient with multiple complaints. Clearly, if the patient arrives at the emergency department unconscious, having been found on the street, the chief complaint is coma, and the history of present illness is limited to the minimal information provided by the ambulance attendants or by the contents of the patient's wallet. In this situation, physicians are trained to proceed concurrently with examination, investigation, and treatment. How this should be achieved is not always clear, although there is agreement on the steps that should be completed within the initial 5 to 10 minutes.

The physician first confronts on-call problem solving in the final years of medical school. It is at this stage that the structured history taking and physical examination direct the student's approach in evaluating a patient. When on call, the medical student is faced with well-defined problems (e.g., fall out of bed, fever, chest pain) yet may feel ill-equipped to begin clinical problem solving unless the "complete history and physical examination" have been obtained. Anything less engenders guilt over a task only partially completed; however, not every on-call problem can involve 60 minutes or more of the physician's time, because unnecessary time spent on patients with relatively minor complaints may deny adequate treatment time to patients who are very ill.

The approach recommended in this book is based on a structured system, but one that can be logically adapted to most situations. It is intended as a practical guide to assist in efficient clinical problem solving when on call. The clinical chapters are divided into four parts:

1. Phone call
2. Elevator thoughts
3. Major threat to life
4. Bedside

PHONE CALL

Most problems confronting the physician on call are first communicated by telephone. The physician must be able to determine the severity of the problem based on this information because it is not always possible to immediately assess the patient at the bedside. Patients must be evaluated in order of priority. The phone call section of each chapter is divided into three parts:

1. Questions
2. Orders
3. Inform RN

The questions are intended to assist in determining the urgency of the problem. Orders that will expedite the investigation and management of urgent situations are suggested. Finally, the registered nurse (RN) is informed of the physician's anticipated time of arrival at the bedside and the responsibilities of the RN in the interim.

ELEVATOR THOUGHTS

The physician on call is usually not in the immediate vicinity when he or she is informed of a problem that requires assessment, but the time spent traveling to the ward (up to 10 minutes in some large hospitals) can be used efficiently to consider the differential diagnosis of the problem at hand. Because this time is often spent in the elevator, the term "elevator thoughts" has been coined to summarize the directed differential diagnosis. It should be emphasized that the differential diagnosis lists presented are not exhaustive; rather, they focus on the most common or most serious (life-threatening) causes that should be considered in hospitalized patients.

MAJOR THREAT TO LIFE

Identifying each problem's major threat to life follows logically from a consideration of the differential diagnosis, and it provides a focus for the subsequent investigation and management of the patient. Rather than arriving at the bedside with a memorized list of possible diagnoses, it is more useful and relevant to appreciate the one or two most likely threats to life and use them to direct one's questions and physical examination. This process ensures that the most serious life-threatening possibility in each clinical scenario is both considered and sought in the initial evaluation of the patient.

BEDSIDE

The protocols for what to do on arrival at the bedside are divided into the following parts:
- Quick-look test
- Airway and vital signs
- Selective history
- Selective physical examination
- Selective chart review
- Management

The bedside assessment begins with the quick-look test, which is a rapid visual assessment that may enable the physician to categorize the patient's condition in terms of severity: well (comfortable), sick (uncomfortable or distressed), or critical (about to die). Next is an assessment of the airway and vital signs, which is important in the evaluation of any potentially sick patient. Because of the nature of the various problems that require assessment when on call, the order of the remaining parts is not uniform. For example, the selective physical examination may either precede or follow the selective history and chart review, and either of these may be superseded by management if the clinical situation dictates.

Occasionally, the Selective Physical Examination and Management sections are subdivided, allowing one to focus on urgent, life-threatening problems, and leaving the less urgent problems to be reviewed later.

It is hoped that the principles and protocols offered will provide a logical, efficient system for the assessment and management of common on-call problems.

Documentation of On-Call Problems

Accurate, concise documentation of on-call problems is essential for the continued efficient care of hospitalized patients. In many instances, you will not know the patient you are asked to see, and you may not be involved in his or her continuing care after your night on call. Some problems can be handled safely over the telephone, but in the majority of situations, a selective history and physical examination are required to correctly diagnose and treat the problem. Documentation is recommended for every patient you examine. If the problem is straightforward, a brief note is sufficient; however, if the problem is complicated, your note should be concise but complete.

Begin by recording the date, time, and who you are. For example:

Aug. 10, 2004, 0200H. "Medical student on-call note" or "Resident on-call note."

State who called you and at what time you were called. For example:

"Called to see patient by RN at 0130H because the patient 'fell out of bed.'"

If your assessment was delayed by more urgent problems, say so. A brief one- or two-sentence summary of the patient's admission diagnosis and major medical problems should follow. For example:

This 74-year-old woman with a history of chronic renal failure, type 2 diabetes mellitus, and rheumatoid arthritis was admitted 10 days ago with increasing joint pain.

Next, describe the history of present illness (HPI)—the "fall out of bed"—from the viewpoint of both the patient and any witnesses. This HPI is no different from the HPI you would document in an admission history. For example:

HPI. The patient was on the way to the bathroom to void, tripped on her bathrobe, and fell to the floor, landing on her left side. She denied palpitations, chest pain, lightheadedness, nausea, and hip pain. There was no difficulty walking unaided and no pain afterward. The fall was not witnessed. The RN found the patient lying on the floor. Vital signs were normal.

If your chart review has relevant findings, include these in your HPI. For example:

Three previous "falls out of bed" on this admission. Patient has no recall of these events.

Documentation of your examination should be *selective*. For example, a call regarding a fall out of bed requires you to examine relevant components of the vital signs, head and neck, and cardiovascular, musculoskeletal, and neurologic systems. It is not necessary to examine the respiratory system or the abdomen unless there is a second separate problem (e.g., you arrive at the bedside and find the patient febrile).

On-call problems should not require a complete history and complete physical examination. These were done when the patient was admitted. Your history, physical examination, and chart documentation should be *directed* (i.e., problem oriented). *It may be useful to <u>underline</u> the positive physical findings both for yourself (it aids your summary) and for the house staff who will be reviewing the patient in the morning.*

Vitals	BP: 140/85
	HR: <u>104</u>/min
	RR: <u>36</u>/min
	Temp: <u>38.9</u> PO
HEENT	No tongue or cheek lacerations
	No hemotympanum
CVS	Pulse rhythm normal; JVP 2 cm > SA
MSS	No skull or face lacerations or hematomas
	Spine and ribs normal
	Full, painless ROM of all 4 limbs
	7- × 9-cm hematoma left thigh
Reflexes	
Motor	Normal
Sensory	
Neuro	Alert; oriented to time, place, and person

Relevant laboratory, electrocardiographic, or x-ray findings should be documented. Again, it is useful to underline abnormal findings. For example:

Glucose	6.1 mmol/L
Sodium	141 mmol/L
Potassium	3.9 mmol/L
Calcium	Not available
Urea	<u>12 mmol/L</u>
Creatinine	<u>180 mmol/L</u>

Your diagnostic conclusion regarding the problem for which you were called must be clearly stated. It is not enough to write "patient fell out of bed." The RN could have written that without consulting you. The information gathered must be synthesized to achieve the highest level of diagnostic integration possible. This provisional diagnosis should be followed by a differential diagnosis, listing the most likely alternative explanations in order. For a patient who fell out of bed, your diagnostic conclusion might be as follows:

1. "Fall out of bed" due to difficulty reaching the bathroom to void (?diuretic-induced nocturia, ?contribution of sedation)
2. Large hematoma (7 × 9 cm) left thigh

Your plan must be clearly stated—both the measures taken during the night and the investigations or treatment you have organized for the morning. Avoid writing "Plan—see orders." It is not always obvious to the staff handling the patient's care the next day why certain measures were taken. If you informed the intern, resident, or attending physician of the problem, document with whom you spoke and the recommendations given. Record whether any of the patient's family members were informed of the problem and what they were told. Finally, sign or print your name clearly so the staff knows whom to contact should there be any questions about the management of this patient the following day.

Assessment and Management of Volume Status

The assessment of volume status is an integral part of the physical examination. As a medical student and intern, and later as a practicing physician, you will find that this skill plays a key role in choosing the appropriate investigation and management in many clinical situations.

Ideally, this skill is learned at the bedside. However, some background knowledge will help you in the accurate assessment and interpretation of a patient's volume status.

First, terminology must be clarified. The human body is composed mostly of water (Fig. 3–1). In fact, *total body water* (TBW) makes up 60% of the weight of the adult male. Of this, two thirds is *intracellular fluid* (ICF) and one third is *extracellular fluid* (ECF) (i.e., water that is outside of cells). Of the ECF, two thirds is *interstitial fluid*, such as fluid bathing the cells, cerebrospinal fluid, and intraocular fluid. Only 7% of total body weight is *intravascular fluid* (plasma). Clinically, it is the ECF, consisting of intravascular and interstitial fluids, that one assesses when determining the volume status of a patient.

ASSESSMENT OF VOLUME STATUS

There are only three basic states of volume status that a patient can have: volume depleted, normovolemic (euvolemic), and volume overloaded. On approaching the bedside, ask yourself whether the patient is volume depleted, normovolemic, or volume overloaded.

Quick-Look Test

Does the patient look well (comfortable), sick (uncomfortable or distressed), or critical (about to die)?

In most instances, when you first enter the room and see the patient, it will be apparent whether there is a serious fluid balance abnormality. Patients who are seriously volume depleted look wan, drawn, and tired, whereas patients who are volume

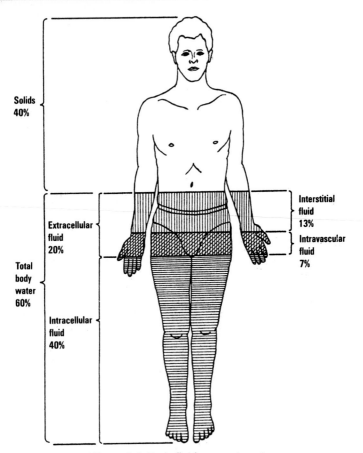

Solids
40%

Extracellular
fluid
20%

Interstitial
fluid
13%

Intravascular
fluid
7%

Total
body
water
60%

Intracellular
fluid
40%

Figure 3–1 Body fluid compartments.

overloaded look uncomfortable, anxious, and restless. Of course, these are only general guidelines, and a more detailed physical examination is required.

Vital Signs

In most cases, simply taking the patient's vital signs will help you determine whether there is significant volume depletion.

Measure the heart rate (HR) and blood pressure (BP) first with the patient supine and then after the patient stands for 1 minute. If the patient is unable to stand alone, ask for assistance or have the patient sit up and dangle his or her legs over the side of the bed. If the patient is hypotensive in the supine position, this maneuver is not necessary.

An increase in HR of >15 beats/min, a fall in systolic BP of >15 mm Hg, or any fall in diastolic BP signifies the presence of postural hypotension, which may indicate *intravascular volume depletion.*

A patient with autonomic dysfunction (e.g., due to beta blockers, diabetic neuropathy, Shy-Drager syndrome) may also have a pronounced postural fall in BP but without the expected degree of compensatory tachycardia. Also, unlike in a volume-depleted patient, there should be no other features of ECF deficit in a patient with uncomplicated autonomic dysfunction.

A *resting tachycardia* may be seen with either volume depletion or volume overload. Volume depletion results in a low stroke volume. As can be seen from the following formula, the patient must therefore generate a tachycardia to maintain cardiac output.

Cardiac output (CO) = Heart rate (HR) × Stroke volume (SV)

A volume-overloaded patient also generates a tachycardia in an effort to increase forward flow and thereby relieve the lungs of venous congestion. A normovolemic patient without other complicating features will have a normal HR.

Measure the respiratory rate. The most important feature to look for when measuring the respiratory rate is tachypnea, which may be seen in a volume-overloaded patient in whom pulmonary edema has developed.

Selective Physical Examination

HEENT   *Look at the oral mucous membranes.* An adequately hydrated patient has moist mucous membranes. It is normal for a small pool of saliva to collect at the undersurface of the tongue in the area of the frenulum, and this should be looked for.

Resp   *Listen for crackles.* Pulmonary edema with bilateral basilar crackles and, occasionally, wheezes or pleural effusions may be a manifestation of volume overload.

CVS   *Look at the neck veins.* Examination of the internal jugular veins is one of the most helpful components of the volume status examination. The JVP can be assessed with the patient at any inclination from 0 to 90 degrees, but it is easiest to begin looking for the JVP pulsation with the patient at a 45-degree inclination. If you are unable to visualize the neck veins at 45 degrees, this usually signifies that the JVP is either very low (in which case you need to lower the head of the bed) or very high (in which case you may need to sit the patient upright to see the top of the column of blood in the internal jugular vein). Once the internal jugular vein pulsation is identified,

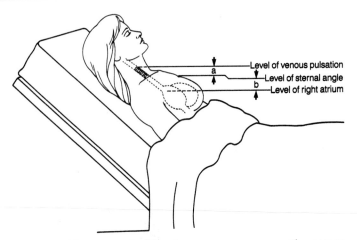

Figure 3–2 Measurement of jugular venous pressure. a, The perpendicular distance from the sternal angle to the top of the column of blood. b, The distance from the center of the right atrium to the sternal angle, commonly accepted as measuring 5 cm, regardless of inclination.

measure the perpendicular distance from the sternal angle to the top of the column of blood (Fig. 3–2). This distance represents the patient's JVP in cm of H_2O above the sternal angle. Its value represents a composite of the volume of venous return to the heart, the central venous pressure, and the efficiency of right atrial and right ventricular emptying. A JVP of 2 to 3 cm above the sternal angle is normal in adult patients. A significantly volume-depleted patient has flat neck veins, which may fill only when the patient is placed in the Trendelenburg position. A volume-overloaded patient usually has an elevated JVP of >3 cm above the sternal angle.

Listen for an S_3. An S_3 is most often associated with the volume-overloaded state and is best heard with the patient in the left lateral position.

ABD   *Examine the liver*. An enlarged, tender liver and a positive hepatojugular reflux may be manifestations of volume overload.

Skin   *Check the skin turgor*. This is best evaluated in an adult by raising a fold of skin from the anterior chest area over the sternal angle. In a normovolemic patient, the skin should return promptly to its usual position. A sluggish return suggests an interstitial fluid deficit. Taut, nonpliable skin that cannot be raised in a fold suggests interstitial fluid excess.

Look at the skin creases and check for edema. Accentuated skin creases from bed sheets pressing against the posterior thorax and sacral or pedal edema indicate interstitial fluid excess.

Selective Chart Review

Sometimes, it is difficult to decide at the bedside whether a patient's volume status is normal. There are a few items in the chart that may guide you in a difficult case.

1. Look at the creatinine-to-urea ratio. A ratio of <12 (calculated in SI units) is suggestive of volume depletion.
2. Examine the fluid balance records. Unfortunately, fluid balance records are notoriously inaccurate. However, if well-kept records are present, a number of clues may be found. A patient who is taking in very little fluid (whether orally or intravenously) may well be volume depleted. A patient whose urine output is >20 mL/hr probably is not volume depleted. A net positive intake of several liters over a few days may be indicative of fluid retention with concomitant volume overload.
3. Look for a change in weight. A gain or loss of several pounds since admission may indicate a significant fluid gain or loss, respectively.
4. In the volume-depleted patient, look at the chart for contributing causes:

GI losses	Vomiting
	Nasogastric suction
	Diarrhea
Urinary losses	Diuretics
	Osmotic diuresis (hyperglycemia, mannitol administration, hypertonic IV contrast material)
	Postobstructive diuresis
	Diabetes insipidus
	Recovery phase of acute tubular necrosis
	Adrenal insufficiency
Surface losses	Skin (increased sweating due to fever, evaporation in burn patients)
	Respiratory tract (hyperventilation, nonhumidified inhalation therapy)
Fluid sequestration	Pancreatitis
	Ileus
	Burns
Blood losses	GI tract
	Surgical
	Trauma
	Iatrogenic (laboratory sampling)
Other	Inadequate oral or parenteral intake

CLASSIC STATES OF VOLUME STATUS

Only rarely does a patient have every feature of volume depletion or volume overload. Still, it is useful when examining a patient to carry a mental picture of the three "classic" states of volume status.

The Classic Volume-Depleted Patient

Quick-Look Test

The patient looks wan, tired, and drawn.

Vital Signs

HR	Resting tachycardia
	Postural rise in HR of >15 beats/min
BP	Normal or low resting BP
	Postural drop in systolic BP of >15 mm Hg or any drop in diastolic BP
RR	Normal
HEENT	Dry oral mucous membranes
Resp	Clear
CVS	JVP flat
	No S_3
ABD	Normal
Skin	Poor turgor
	No edema

The Classic Volume-Overloaded Patient

Quick-Look Test

The patient looks sick and is short of breath. Often, he or she is sitting upright and appears uncomfortable, anxious, and restless.

Vital Signs

HR	Resting tachycardia
	Postural rise in HR of <15 beats/min
BP	May be low, normal, or high
	No postural fall in systolic or diastolic BP
RR	Tachypnea
Resp	Crackles bilaterally at bases
	± Wheezing
	± Pleural effusions
CVS	JVP >3 cm above the sternal angle
	S_3 present
ABD	Positive hepatojugular reflux
	± Enlarged tender liver
Ext	Accentuated skin creases on posterior thorax
	Sacral or pedal edema

The Classic Patient with Normal Volume Status

Quick-Look Test

The patient looks well.

Vital Signs

HR	Normal
	Postural rise in HR of <15 beats/min
BP	Normal
	Postural fall in systolic BP of <15 mm Hg and no fall in diastolic BP
RR	Normal
HEENT	Moist oral mucous membranes
Resp	Clear
CVS	JVP 2 to 3 cm above the sternal angle
	No S_3
ABD	Normal
Ext	No edema

CHOOSING THE CORRECT INTRAVENOUS FLUID

Selection of an appropriate intravenous (IV) fluid for a particular clinical situation need not be a guessing game. A basic understanding of physiology will help you make rational and effective fluid management decisions.

Water is important in the body because it serves as a *solvent* for a variety of solutes. *Solutes* can be either electrolytes or nonelectrolytes.

Electrolytes are substances that dissociate into charged components (ions) when placed in water, and they include the following commonly measured substances:

Sodium	
Potassium	Cations
Calcium	
Magnesium	
Chloride	Anions
Bicarbonate	

In physiologic solutions, the total number of cations always equals the total number of anions.

Nonelectrolytes are solutes that have no electrical charges, and they include such substances as glucose and urea.

As mentioned previously, intravascular volume is made up mostly of *water*, which acts as a solvent to dissolve and transport electrolytes and nonelectrolytes. Water is able to move from one

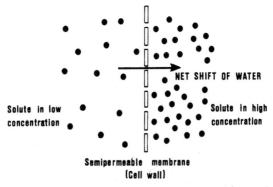

Figure 3–3 Osmosis. Water flows across a semipermeable membrane to equalize solute concentrations on each side of the membrane.

body compartment to the next by the process of *osmosis*. When two solutes are separated by a semipermeable membrane, such as a cell membrane, water tends to flow across the membrane from the solution of lower concentration to that of higher concentration, with the net effect being to equalize the solute concentration on each side of the membrane (Fig. 3–3).

Suppose you decided to infuse a liter of pure water into a patient without any solutes. What would happen to the patient's red blood cells (RBCs)? Understanding the process of osmosis allows you to reason that because the solute concentration inside the RBCs is vastly higher than that in the water infused, water would move across the cell membrane into the RBCs (Fig. 3–4). There is a limit to how much the RBC membrane can stretch, and eventually the RBCs would burst. Similarly, you can see that if a hypertonic solution was infused directly into the patient's vein, the RBCs would shrink (crenate) as water moved out of the RBCs and into the surrounding solution.

For these reasons, most IV solutions that are prepared for hospital use are usually close to isotonic—that is, they have the same solute concentration as blood—to minimize such fluid shifts. Although cell membranes allow water to pass freely by the process of osmosis, they limit the passage of solutes to varying degrees. Some solute molecules cross membranes more readily than others, depending on their size and physical properties.

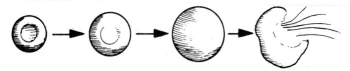

Figure 3–4 Osmosis. Effect of infusion of pure water on red blood cell volume.

In hospitalized patients, there are only three solutes that you need to consider to effectively diagnose and treat disorders of fluid balance. *Glucose* distributes widely throughout both intracellular and extracellular spaces, whereas *sodium* is limited primarily to the extracellular space. *Albumin* remains largely within the intravascular space. The distribution of these three solutes is a fundamental principle that will be useful in guiding your choices of fluid therapy.

D5W consists of 50 g of dextrose dissolved in 1 L of water. It has an osmolality of 252 mOsm/L, which prevents the patient's RBCs from shrinking or swelling. Dextrose can be expected to equilibrate rapidly among the intravascular, interstitial, and intracellular spaces, and water follows along quickly by osmosis.

Normal saline (NS) is another commonly used IV solution. It has an osmolality of 308 mOsm/L, and although it is slightly hypertonic, it is not sufficiently different from blood tonicity to cause cell shrinkage. NS stays predominantly in the extracellular space longer than a glucose infusion does, because sodium does not readily move intracellularly.

Albumin and *plasma* stay in the intravascular space for many hours, because albumin is a large molecule that does not easily traverse the endothelial pores of the blood vessels. The half-life of albumin within the intravascular space is 17 to 20 hours.

With this knowledge of solutes and their membrane permeability, you can make logical choices regarding fluid management.

In patients with *intravascular volume depletion*, the goal of treatment is to correct and maintain adequate intravascular volume and tissue perfusion. Hence, a volume-depleted patient could be treated with IV NS, albumin, or plasma. Because NS is more readily available and much less expensive, it is the treatment of choice for the initial resuscitation of a volume-depleted patient. Infusion of D5W would be of little benefit, because the glucose and water would rapidly distribute throughout the intravascular, interstitial, and extravascular spaces.

In patients with *intravascular volume excess*, the goal of treatment is to improve and maintain adequate cardiac function and tissue perfusion. This usually requires the use of preload reducing measures, as outlined in Chapter 24, pages 271 to 272. However, because these patients are often critically ill, IV access is required for the administration of medication. The best fluid to give, usually at a TKVO (to keep the vein open) rate, is D5W, which quickly leaves the intravascular space. Infusion of NS or albumin could worsen the patient's condition by further increasing intravascular volume. This is why cardiac patients, who are at risk for volume overload, are usually given an IV infusion of D5W when IV access is required for the administration of medication. An alternative is to use a Heplock at the IV site.

Another IV solution, $^2/_3$–$^1/_3$, contains 33 g/L glucose and 51 mmol/L each sodium and chloride and is approximately isotonic at 269 mOsm/L. Although there is no particular physiologic basis for its use, it has become a popular maintenance IV solution for patients in whom oral intake cannot be accomplished.

REMEMBER

1. Volume status abnormalities should be corrected at a rate similar to that at which they developed. Biologic systems are more responsive to rates of change than to absolute amounts of change. It is safest to correct half the deficit and then reevaluate. There is no substitute for frequent repeated examination of the patient when trying to effect changes in volume status.
2. Occasionally, you will be faced with a patient in whom there is a discrepancy between the two compartments of the ECF, such as a patient with a decreased intravascular volume but an excess of interstitial fluid (i.e., edema). This discrepancy is most commonly seen in states of marked hypoalbuminemia.

Fluid transfer from the intravascular space to the interstitial space depends on the permeability of the capillary bed, how much hydrostatic pressure is being exerted to force fluid out of the intravascular space, and the difference in *oncotic pressure* between the intravascular and interstitial spaces (Fig. 3–5).

Oncotic pressure is exerted by *plasma protein* (i.e., albumin). There is little, if any, protein in the interstitium; hence the intravascular oncotic pressure exerted by albumin tends to

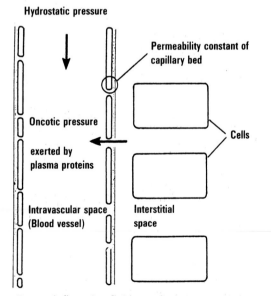

Figure 3–5 Factors influencing fluid transfer between the intravascular and extravascular spaces.

draw water out of the interstitium and into the intravascular space. This knowledge is important when treating the occasional patient with intravascular volume depletion, as assessed by your clinical examination, together with interstitial fluid excess (i.e., edema). To help shift fluid from the interstitium to the intravascular space in such a patient, a logical choice is to administer IV albumin. Artificial plasma expanders (e.g., gelofusine, polygeline, dextran, hetastarch) also may be used. These are high-molecular-weight glucose polymers that remain in the intravascular space because of their large size.

Remember that oncotic pull comes from albumin. It does not come from sodium, so NS is not an appropriate fluid to give in this situation. It does not come from RBCs, so a blood transfusion is an equally inappropriate choice. Note that albumin is available in two concentrations—5% and 25%. The 25% albumin is preferred when trying to effect a shift in fluid from the interstitial space to the intravascular space.

Unfortunately, albumin, plasma, and artificial plasma expanders are expensive, and their effect in removing edema fluid is transient. Hence, their continued use for this indication is controversial. Certainly, the best way to correct edema in a patient with a decreased intravascular volume but an excess of interstitial fluid is to correct the underlying cause of interstitial volume excess. In most cases, the cause is hypoproteinemia (e.g., malabsorption, liver disease, nephrotic syndrome, protein-losing enteropathy).

In summary, most disorders of fluid balance can be treated logically and successfully with the simple principles of water and solute transfer across cell membranes. Table 3–1 provides a listing of the commonly used IV fluids.

TABLE 3–1 Commonly Used Intravenous Fluids

Fluid	Glucose (g/L)	Na (mmol/L)	Cl (mmol/L)	K (mmol/L)	Ca (mmol/L)	Lactate (mmol/L)	Approximate Osmolality (mOsm/L)
D5W	50	—	—	—	—	—	252
D10W	100	—	—	—	—	—	505
D20W	200	—	—	—	—	—	1010
D50W	500	—	—	—	—	—	2525
"{2/3} {1/3}"	33	51	51	—	—	—	269
0.45% NaCl ({1/2} NS)	—	77	77	—	—	—	154
0.9% NaCl (NS)	—	154	154	—	—	—	308
D5NS	50	154	154	—	—	—	560
D5/0.2% NS	50	34	34	—	—	—	321
Ringer's lactate	—	130	109	4	3	28	272
Albumin*	—	145	145	—	—	—	—
Fresh frozen plasma[†]							
Stored plasma[‡]							

*Available in 5% concentrations (50, 250, or 500 mL) or 25% concentrations (20, 50, or 100 mL).
[†]200–250 mL of plasma that has been separated from whole blood and frozen within 8 hr of collection; it contains all coagulation factors.
[‡]200–250 mL of plasma that has been separated from whole blood and frozen 8–72 hr after collection; it contains all coagulation factors but has reduced levels of factors V and VIII.

AIDS, HBV, HCV, and the House Officer

The risk of transmission of human immunodeficiency virus (HIV) from patient to health care worker is extremely low. The rate of transmission is <0.5% after direct inoculation of infected blood through a needlestick puncture and even lower after other types of exposure.[1] Circumstances that may increase the risk of seroconversion include procedures involving a needle placed directly in a vein or artery, a deep injury, the presence of visible blood on the device, or a high viral load in the source patient (e.g., at the time of seroconversion or in the terminal stages of acquired immunodeficiency syndrome [AIDS]).[2]

The risk of transmission of hepatitis B virus (HBV) is many times that of HIV. In the United States, thousands of health care workers become infected with HBV each year.[3] Hepatitis B vaccination is strongly recommended for all staff.

The risk of seroconversion following percutaneous exposure to hepatitis C virus (HCV) is very low, in the range of 1.8%.[4]

Strict adherence to standard precautions will minimize these risks (Box 4-1).

Despite attention to safe practices, you may, in the course of your training, be accidentally exposed to potentially infectious blood or body fluids. The hospital should have an established policy for helping you, and you should contact the appropriate individual if you have been exposed. Exposures that might place you at risk for HBV, HCV, or HIV infection include a needlestick injury, a cut from a sharp object, or contact of your mucous membranes or nonintact (cut, scraped, chapped, or inflamed) skin with blood, tissue, or other potentially infectious secretions from an individual infected with one of these agents.

The following general guidelines are recommended if you have been exposed to blood or body fluids.

FIRST AID

1. Seek assistance from a more senior staff member.
2. Immediately cleanse the contaminated site.
   a. Needlestick

BOX 4–1 Standard Precautions to Prevent Transmission of HIV, HBV, HCV, and Other Blood-borne Pathogens

Standard precautions are now recommended for the care of all patients in hospitals, regardless of their diagnosis or presumed infection status. Standard precautions apply to (1) blood; (2) all body fluids, secretions, and excretions *except sweat*, regardless of whether they contain visible blood; (3) nonintact skin; and (4) mucous membranes. Standard precautions are designed to reduce the risk of transmission of microorganisms from both recognized and unrecognized sources of infection in hospitals.

Standard precautions include the following:

Hand Washing

1. Wash hands after touching blood, body fluids, secretions, excretions, and contaminated items, whether or not gloves are worn. Wash hands immediately after gloves are removed, between patient contacts, and when otherwise indicated to avoid the transfer of microorganisms to other patients or environments. It may be necessary to wash hands between tasks and procedures performed on the same patient to prevent cross-contamination of different body sites.
2. Use a plain (nonantimicrobial) soap for routine hand washing.
3. Use an antimicrobial agent or a waterless antiseptic agent for specific circumstances (e.g., control of outbreaks or hyperendemic infections), as defined by the infection control program.

Gloves

Wear gloves (clean, nonsterile gloves are adequate) when touching blood, body fluids, secretions, excretions, and contaminated items. Put on clean gloves just before touching mucous membranes and nonintact skin. Change gloves between tasks and procedures performed on the same patient after contact with material that may contain a high concentration of microorganisms. Remove gloves promptly after use, before touching noncontaminated items and environmental surfaces, and before going to another patient, and wash hands immediately to avoid the transfer of microorganisms to other patients or environments.

Mask, Eye Protection, Face Shield

Wear a mask and eye protection or a face shield to protect mucous membranes of the eyes, nose, and mouth during procedures and patient care activities that are likely to generate splashes or sprays of blood, body fluids, secretions, or excretions.

Gown

Wear a gown (a clean, nonsterile gown is adequate) to protect skin and to prevent soiling of clothing during procedures and patient care activities that are likely to generate splashes or sprays of blood, body fluids,

Continued

BOX 4–1 Standard Precautions to Prevent Transmission of HIV, HBV, HCV, and Other Blood-borne Pathogens—cont'd

secretions, or excretions. Select a gown that is appropriate for the activity and the amount of fluid likely to be encountered. Remove a soiled gown as promptly as possible, and wash hands to avoid the transfer of microorganisms to other patients or environments.

Patient Care Equipment

Handle used patient care equipment soiled with blood, body fluids, secretions, or excretions in a manner that prevents skin and mucous membrane exposure, contamination of clothing, and transfer of microorganisms to other patients and environments. Ensure that reusable equipment is not used for the care of another patient until it has been cleaned and processed appropriately. Ensure that single-use items are discarded properly.

Linen

Handle, transport, and process used linen soiled with blood, body fluids, secretions, or excretions in a manner that prevents skin and mucous membrane exposure, contamination of clothing, and transfer of microorganisms to other patients and environments.

Occupational Health and Blood-borne Pathogens

1. Take care to prevent injuries when using needles, scalpels, and other sharp instruments or devices; when handling sharp instruments after procedures; when cleaning used instruments; and when disposing of used needles. Never recap used needles or otherwise manipulate them using both hands, and never use any technique that involves directing the point of the needle toward any part of the body; rather, use either a one-handed "scoop" technique or a mechanical device designed for holding the needle sheath. Do not remove used needles from disposable syringes by hand, and do not bend, break, or otherwise manipulate used needles by hand. Place used disposable syringes and needles, scalpel blades, and other sharp items in appropriate puncture-resistant containers, which should be located as close as practical to the area in which the items were used, and place reusable syringes and needles in a puncture-resistant container for transport to their reprocessing area.
2. Use mouthpieces, resuscitation bags, or other ventilation devices as an alternative to mouth-to-mouth resuscitation methods in areas where the need for resuscitation is predictable.

Modified from Garner JS: Guideline for isolation precautions in hospitals. Infect Control Hosp Epidemiol 1996;17:68-69.

        (1) Allow the puncture site to bleed
        (2) Thoroughly wash the site for 2 to 4 minutes with soap and water
    b. Skin contamination
        (2) Open wound: flush the area with water or saline
    c. Mucous membrane or eye contact
        (1) Mouth: rinse with water; repeat several times
        (2) Eyes: rinse well with water for 3 to 5 minutes
3. Save the instrument, without washing, in a sharps container.
4. Report immediately to the designated officer responsible for helping you.

IMMEDIATE MANAGEMENT

Treatment of parenteral exposure (i.e., nonintact skin, mucous membrane, or skin puncture) may include the following:

1. Tetanus prophylaxis—*tetanus toxoid* 0.5 mL, if indicated.
2. HBV prophylaxis after exposure (Table 4–1).
3. HIV prophylaxis after exposure.

    Procedures for assessing the source person vary among institutions. Current recommendations differ slightly, depending on whether the exposure involves a percutaneous injury (Table 4–2) or mucous membranes or nonintact skin (Table 4–3). A case-control study suggests that the risk of HIV conversion after percutaneous exposure can be reduced with zidovudine (AZT) prophylaxis.[2] Because combination therapy has been shown to reduce viral load more effectively than AZT alone, combination therapy may provide more effective prophylaxis.[5] Therapy should be initiated as soon as possible, preferably within 1 to 2 hours after exposure, and should involve either a basic two-drug regimen or an expanded three-drug regimen, based on the likelihood of the source's HIV positivity and the nature and severity of exposure.

    One basic two-drug regimen recommended for adults is *zidovudine* 600 mg PO per day in two or three divided doses and *lamivudine (3TC)* 150 mg PO twice a day. An alternative two-drug regimen is *lamivudine* 150 mg PO twice a day and *stavudine (d4T)* 40 mg PO twice a day. *Didanosine (ddI)* 400 mg PO daily and *stavudine* 40 mg PO twice a day may also be used. The expanded three-drug regimen includes one of the basic two-drug regimens plus *indinavir* 800 mg PO every 8 hours or *nelfinavir* 1250 mg PO twice a day, or *efavirenz (EFV)* 600 mg PO daily or *abacavir (ABC)* 300 mg PO twice a day. Other antiretrovirals are available but should be used only after consulting an expert in this field.[4] One month of

TABLE 4–1 **Prophylaxis after Parenteral Exposure to HBV**

Vaccination and Antibody Response Status of Exposed Worker	Prophylactic Treatment*		
	Source HbsAg Positive	Source HBsAg Negative	Source Unknown or Unavailable for Testing
Unvaccinated	HBIG[†] × 1 and initiate HB vaccine series	Initiate HB vaccine series	Initiate HB vaccine series
Previously Vaccinated			
Known responder[‡]	No treatment	No treatment	No treatment
Known non-responder[§]	HBIG × 1 and initiate revaccination or HBIG × 2[¶]	No treatment	If suspected high-risk source, treat as if source were HBsAg positive
Antibody response unknown	Test exposed person for anti-HBs 1. If adequate,[‡] no treatment is necessary 2. If inadequate,[§] administer HBIG × 1 and vaccine booster	No treatment	Test exposed person for anti-HBs 1. If adequate,[‡] no treatment is necessary 2. If inadequate,[§] administer vaccine booster and recheck titer in 1–2 mos

*Persons who have previously been infected with HBV are immune to reinfection and do not require postexposure prophylaxis.
[†]Dose is 0.06 mL/kg IM.
[‡]A responder is a person with adequate levels of serum antibody to HBsAg (i.e., anti-HBs ≥10 mIU/mL).
[§]A nonresponder is a person with inadequate response to vaccination (i.e., serum anti-HBs <10 mIU/mL).
[¶]The option of giving one dose of HBIG and reinitiating the vaccine series is preferred for nonresponders who have not completed a second three-dose vaccine series. For persons who previously completed a second vaccine series but failed to respond, two doses of HBIG are preferred.
anti-HBs, antibody to HBsAg; HB, hepatitis B; HBIG, hepatitis B immune globulin; HBsAg, hepatitis B surface antigen.
From Updated U.S. Public Health Service guidelines for the management of occupational exposures to HBV, HCV, and HIV and recommendations for postexposure prophylaxis. MMWR Morb Mortal Wkly Rep 2001;50:1-52.

TABLE 4-2 HIV Prophylaxis after Percutaneous Injury

	Infection Status of Source*				
Exposure Type	HIV Positive Class 1[†]	HIV Positive Class 2[‡]	Source of Unknown HIV Status[§]	Unknown Source[¶ǁ]	HIV Negative
Less severe[¶]	Recommend basic 2-drug regimen	Recommend expanded 3-drug regimen	Generally, no postexposure prophylaxis warranted; however, consider basic 2-drug regimen** for source with HIV risk factors[††]	Generally, no postexposure prophylaxis warranted; however, consider basic 2-drug regimen** in settings where exposure to HIV-infected persons is likely	No postexposure prophylaxis warranted
More severe[‡‡]	Recommend expanded 3-drug regimen	Recommend expanded 3-drug regimen	Generally, no postexposure prophylaxis warranted; however, consider basic 2-drug regimen** for source with HIV risk factors[††]	Generally, no postexposure prophylaxis warranted; however, consider basic 2-drug regimen** in settings where exposure to HIV-infected persons is likely	No postexposure prophylaxis warranted

*Local policies and laws regarding informed consent for testing source blood should be followed.
[†]Asymptomatic HIV infection or known low viral load (e.g., <1500 RNA copies/mL). If drug resistance is a concern, obtain expert consultation, but do not delay initiation of postexposure prophylaxis pending such consultation.
[‡]Symptomatic HIV infection, AIDS, acute seroconversion, or known high viral load. If drug resistance is a concern, obtain expert consultation, but do not delay initiation of postexposure prophylaxis pending such consultation.
[§]For example, a deceased source person with no samples available for HIV testing.
[¶ǁ]For example, a needle from a sharps disposal container.
[¶]For example, solid needle and superficial injury.
**In this case, postexposure prophylaxis is optional and should be based on an individual decision between the exposed person and the treating clinician.
[††]If postexposure prophylaxis is taken and the source is later determined to be HIV negative, postexposure prophylaxis should be discontinued.
[‡‡]For example, large-bore hollow needle, deep puncture, visible blood on device, or needle used in patient's artery or vein.

From Updated U.S. Public Health Service guidelines for the management of occupational exposures to HBV, HCV, and HIV and recommendations for postexposure prophylaxis. MMWR Morb Mortal Wkly Rep 2001;50:1-52.

TABLE 4–3 HIV Prophylaxis after Mucous Membrane or Nonintact Skin* Exposure

Exposure Type	Infection Status of Source[†]				
	HIV Positive Class 1[‡]	HIV Positive Class 2[§]	Source of Unknown HIV Status[¶‖]	Unknown Source[¶]	HIV Negative
Small volume**	Consider basic 2-drug regimen	Recommend basic 2-drug regimen	Generally, no postexposure prophylaxis warranted; however, consider basic 2-drug regimen[††] for source with HIV risk factors[‡‡]	Generally, no postexposure prophylaxis warranted; however, consider basic 2-drug regimen[††] in settings where exposure to HIV-infected persons is likely	No postexposure prophylaxis warranted
Large volume[§§]	Recommend basic 2-drug regimen	Recommend expanded 3-drug regimen	Generally, no postexposure prophylaxis warranted; however, consider basic 2-drug regimen[††] in settings where exposure to HIV-infected persons is likely	Generally, no postexposure prophylaxis warranted; however, consider basic 2-drug regimen[††] in settings where exposure to HIV-infected persons is likely	No postexposure prophylaxis warranted

*For skin exposure, follow-up is indicated only if there is evidence of compromised skin integrity (e.g., dermatitis, abrasion, open wound).

[†]Local policies and laws regarding informed consent for testing source blood should be followed.

[‡]Asymptomatic HIV infection or known low viral load (e.g., <1500 RNA copies/mL). If drug resistance is a concern, obtain expert consultation, but do not delay initiation of postexposure prophylaxis pending such consultation.

[§]Symptomatic HIV infection, AIDS, acute seroconversion, or known high viral load. If drug resistance is a concern, obtain expert consultation, but do not delay initiation of postexposure prophylaxis pending such consultation.

[¶‖]For example, a deceased source person with no samples available for HIV testing.

[¶]For example, a needle from a sharps disposal container.

**For example, a few drops.

[††]In this case, postexposure prophylaxis is optional and should be based on an individual decision between the exposed person and the treating clinician.

[‡‡]If postexposure prophylaxis is taken and the source is later determined to be HIV negative, postexposure prophylaxis should be discontinued.

[§§]For example, a major blood splash.

From Updated U.S. Public Health Service guidelines for the management of occupational exposures to HBV, HCV, and HIV and recommendations for postexposure prophylaxis. MMWR Morb Mortal Wkly Rep 2001;50:1-52.

therapy is recommended. A reversible decrease in white blood cell count is the most common side effect of lamivudine. The main adverse effect of stavudine is peripheral neuropathy, but this is uncommon with 1 month's therapy. Diarrhea is common with didanosine, and serious toxicities may include neuropathy, pancreatitis, or hepatitis. The main serious toxicity with indinavir is nephrolithiasis, and patients should be encouraged to take 8 glasses of fluid per day. Side effects are common with nelfinavir, particularly diarrhea, gas, nausea, and rash.

4. HCV prophylaxis after exposure.

    Current guidelines do not support the use of antiviral agents in the postexposure prophylaxis of HCV. Follow-up to determine seroconversion and the presence of infection is recommended, allowing early referral for treatment.

References

1. Gerberding JL: Management of occupational exposures to blood-borne viruses. N Engl J Med 1995;332:444-451.
2. Centers for Disease Control and Prevention: Case control study of HIV seroconversion in health-care workers after percutaneous exposure to HIV-infected blood—France, United Kingdom, and United States, January 1988–August 1994. MMWR Morb Mortal Wkly Rep 1995;44:929-933.
3. Alter MJ, Hadler SC, Margolis HS, et al: The changing epidemiology of hepatitis B in the United States. JAMA 1990;263:1218-1222.
4. Updated US Public Health Service guidelines for the management of occupational exposures to HBV, HCV, and HIV and recommendations for postexposure prophylaxis. MMWR Morb Mortal Wkly Rep 2001;50:1-52.
5. Gerberding JL, Henderson DK: Management of occupational exposures to bloodborne pathogens: Hepatitis B virus, hepatitis C virus, and human immunodeficiency virus. Clin Infect Dis 1992;14:1179-1185.

Patient-Related Problems: The Common Calls

Abdominal Pain

Many patients complain of abdominal pain during their hospital stays. It is essential to distinguish the acute abdominal emergency from the recurrent nonemergency. The former requires urgent medical or surgical intervention, whereas the latter requires thorough but less urgent investigation. Avoid ordering analgesic agents until a preliminary diagnosis has been made. Narcotic analgesic agents may mask the physical findings of an acute abdomen, thereby delaying recognition and treatment of a serious intra-abdominal disorder.

PHONE CALL

Questions

1. **How severe is the pain?**
2. **Is the pain localized or generalized?**
3. **What are the vital signs?**
   Fever and abdominal pain are suggestive of intra-abdominal infection or inflammation.
4. **Is this a new problem?**
5. **What was the reason for admission?**
6. **Is the patient on steroids or other anti-inflammatory drugs?**
   Steroids may mask the pain and fever of an inflammatory process, leading you to underestimate the nature or severity of a patient's abdominal pain. If the patient is on steroids, even mild abdominal pain should be assessed soon.

Orders

If the abdominal pain is mild and the vital signs are normal, ask the RN to call immediately if the pain becomes worse before you are able to assess the patient.

Inform RN

"I will arrive at the bedside in . . . minutes."
   Abdominal pain of acute onset, severe abdominal pain, or pain associated with fever or hypotension requires you to see the patient immediately. Mild recurrent abdominal pain is a less urgent

problem and may be attended to in an hour or two if there are other patients with higher-priority problems.

ELEVATOR THOUGHTS

What causes abdominal pain?

The causes of *localized abdominal pain* are numerous. A useful system for approaching the problem is "diagnosis by location." Figure 5–1 illustrates a differential diagnosis by location.

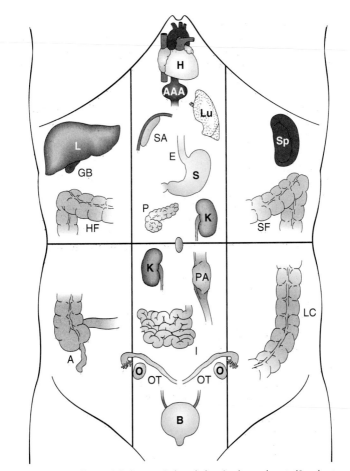

Figure 5–1 Differential diagnosis by abdominal quadrant. (See key on opposite page.)

Key to Figure 5–1
Right upper quadrant
  L, liver (hepatitis, abscess, perihepatitis)
  GB, gallbladder (cholecystitis, steatosis, cholangitis, choledocholithiasis)
  HF, hepatic flexure (obstruction)
Right lower quadrant
  A, appendix (appendicitis,* abscess)
  O, ovary (torsion, ruptured cyst, carcinoma)
Left upper quadrant
  Sp, spleen (rupture, infarct, abscess)
  SF, splenic flexure (obstruction)
Left lower quadrant
  LC, left colon (diverticulitis, ischemic colitis)
  O, ovary (torsion, ruptured cyst, carcinoma)
Epigastrium
  H, heart (myocardial infarction, pericarditis, aortic dissection)
  AAA, abdominal aortic aneurysm
  Lu, lung (pneumonia, pleurisy)
  SA, subphrenic abscess
  E, esophagus (gastroesophageal reflux disease)
  S, stomach and duodenum (peptic ulcer)
  P, pancreas (pancreatitis);
  K, kidney (pyelonephritis, renal colic)
Hypogastrium
  K, kidney (renal colic)
  PA, psoas abscess
  I, intestine (infection,* obstruction,* inflammatory bowel disease*)
  O, ovary (torsion, ruptured cyst, carcinoma)
  OT, ovarian tube (ectopic pregnancy, salpingitis, endometriosis)
  B, bladder (cystitis, distended bladder)
Generalized abdominal pain
  1. See conditions marked with an asterisk
  2. Peritonitis (any cause)
  3. Diabetic ketoacidosis
  4. Sickle cell crisis
  5. Acute intermittent porphyria
  6. Acute adrenocortical insufficiency due to steroid withdrawal

The causes of *generalized abdominal pain* are fewer. Disorders producing either localized or generalized pain are indicated by an asterisk, and additional causes of generalized abdominal pain alone are listed in the legend to Figure 5–1.

MAJOR THREAT TO LIFE

- Perforated or ruptured viscus
- Ascending cholangitis
- Necrosis of viscus
- Exsanguinating hemorrhage

A *perforated* or *ruptured viscus* may result in hypovolemic shock (from third space losses), septic shock (from bacterial peritonitis), or both. Progression of infection from an initial localized site (e.g., *ascending cholangitis*) to septic shock may occur rapidly (i.e., within hours of the patient's first presenting symptom). *Necrosis of a viscus*, as in severe pancreatitis, intussusception, volvulus, strangulated hernia, or ischemic colitis, may cause hypovolemic or septic shock and electrolyte and acid-base disturbances. *Exsanguinating hemorrhage* with hypovolemic shock may result from a leaking abdominal aortic aneurysm, a ruptured ectopic pregnancy, or a splenic rupture; occasionally it may have an iatrogenic cause, such as a liver or renal biopsy or a misdirected thoracentesis.

Patients with myocardial infarction and aortic dissection occasionally present with abdominal pain. These diagnoses should be considered, especially if no local abdominal signs can be identified.

BEDSIDE

Quick-Look Test

Does the patient look well (comfortable), sick (uncomfortable or distressed), or critical (about to die)?

Appearances are often deceptive in acute abdominal disease. If the patient has recently received narcotic analgesics or high-dose steroids, he or she may appear well despite a serious underlying problem.

Patients with severe colic are often restless, in contrast to those with peritonitis, who lie immobile, avoiding movement that exacerbates the pain. With peritonitis, patients may have their knees drawn up to reduce abdominal tension.

Airway and Vital Signs

What is the blood pressure (BP)?

Hypotension associated with abdominal pain is an ominous sign suggestive of impending hypovolemic, hemorrhagic, or septic shock.

Are there postural changes (lying and standing) in the BP and heart rate (HR)?

If the supine BP is normal, recheck the BP and HR with the patient standing.

> A drop in BP that is associated with an increased heart rate (>15 beats/min) suggests volume depletion.

What is the temperature?

Fever associated with abdominal pain is suggestive of intra-abdominal infection or inflammation. However, lack of fever in an elderly patient or in a patient receiving an antipyretic or immunosuppressive drug does not rule out infection.

Selective History and Chart Review

Diagnosis is often dependent on a careful history addressing (1) the pain at onset and its subsequent progression, (2) any associated symptoms, and (3) the past history.

Pain

Is the pain localized?

The location of the pain's maximum intensity can provide a clue to the site of origin (see Fig. 5–1). Remember that a patient may complain of diffuse abdominal pain, but on careful examination, the pain will be found to be localized.

How is the pain characterized (e.g., severe or mild, burning or knife-like, constant or waxing and waning, as in colic)?

There are characteristic descriptions of pain associated with certain diseases. The pain of a peptic ulcer tends to be burning, whereas that of a perforated ulcer is sudden, constant, and severe. The pain of biliary colic is sharp and constricting ("taking one's breath away"); that of acute pancreatitis is deep and agonizing; and that of obstructed bowel is gripping, with intermittent worsening.

Did the pain develop gradually or suddenly?

The severe pain of colic (renal, biliary, or intestinal) develops within hours. An acute onset with fainting suggests perforation of a viscus, ruptured ectopic pregnancy, torsion of an ovarian cyst, or a leaking abdominal aortic aneurysm.

Has the pain changed since its onset?

A ruptured viscus initially may be associated with localized pain that subsequently shifts or becomes generalized, with the development of chemical or bacterial peritonitis.

Does the pain radiate?

Pain radiates to the dermatome or cutaneous areas supplied by the same sensory cortical cells as the deep-seated structure (Fig. 5–2). For example, the diaphragm is supplied by cervical roots C3, C4, and C5. Many upper abdominal or lower thoracic conditions that cause irritation of the diaphragm refer pain to the cutaneous supply of C3, C4, and C5 (i.e., the shoulder and neck). The liver and gallbladder are derived from the right seventh and eighth thoracic segments. Thus, biliary colic-frequently refers pain to the inferior angle of the right scapula. The pain of pancreatitis may radiate to the midback or scapula.

Are there any aggravating or alleviating factors?

Pain that increases with meals, decreases with passage of bowel movements, or both suggests a hollow gut origin. An exception is pain from duodenal ulcer, which is often relieved by

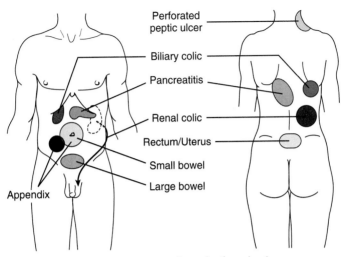

Figure 5–2 Common sites of referred pain.

the ingestion of food. The pain of pancreatitis is often worsened after eating and may be relieved by sitting up or leaning forward. Pain that increases with inspiration suggests pleuritis or peritonitis, and pain that is aggravated by micturition suggests a urogenital cause.

Associated Symptoms

Is there nausea or vomiting?

Vomiting that occurs with the onset of pain frequently accompanies acute peritoneal irritation or perforation of a viscus. It is also commonly associated with acute pancreatitis or obstruction of any muscular hollow viscus. Pain relieved by vomiting suggests a hollow gut origin (e.g., bowel obstruction). Vomiting many hours after the onset of abdominal pain may be a clue to intestinal obstruction or ileus.

What is the nature of emesis?

Brown, feculent emesis is pathognomonic of bowel obstruction, either paralytic or mechanical. Frank blood is suggestive of an upper gastrointestinal (GI) bleed. Vomiting food after fasting is consistent with gastric stasis or gastric outlet obstruction.

Is there diarrhea?

Diarrhea and abdominal pain are seen in infectious gastroenteritis, ischemic colitis, appendicitis, and partial small bowel obstruction. Diarrhea alternating with constipation is a common symptom of diverticular disease.

Is there fever or chills?

Fever and chills suggest an intra-abdominal infection. Check the temperature record since admission. Also check the medication sheet for antipyretic or steroid use—remember that fever may be masked by the administration of these medications.

Past History and Chart Review

Is there a history of peptic ulcer disease or antacid ingestion?

Peptic ulcer disease is a chronic, recurring disease. History repeats itself!

Is there a history of blunt or penetrating trauma to the abdomen? Has there been a liver or kidney biopsy or thoracentesis since admission?

A subcapsular hemorrhage of the spleen, liver, or kidney may result in hemorrhagic shock 1 to 3 days later.

Is there a history of alcohol abuse and ascites?

Spontaneous bacterial peritonitis must always be considered in an alcoholic patient with ascites and fever.

Is there a history of coronary or peripheral vascular disease?

Atherosclerosis is a diffuse process and may affect the vascular supply to several body systems. In addition to the possibility of a myocardial infarction presenting with abdominal pain, a leaking abdominal aortic aneurysm, aortic dissection, and ischemic colitis due to atherosclerosis of the mesenteric arteries should be considered.

If the patient is a premenopausal woman, what was the date of her last normal menstrual period?

Abdominal pain associated with a missed period raises the possibility of an ectopic pregnancy. Hypotension in this situation suggests a ruptured ectopic pregnancy, a life-threatening situation.

Is there a history of previous abdominal surgery?

Adhesions are responsible for 70% of bowel obstructions.

Has the patient received drugs that affect blood clotting?

Intra-abdominal hemorrhage may occur in the anticoagulated patient, especially if there is a history of peptic ulcer disease.

Is there a history of use of aspirin or nonsteroidal anti-inflammatory drugs (NSAIDs), alcohol, or other ulcerogenic drug?

Peptic ulcer should be a consideration in a patient receiving one or more of these agents.

Selective Physical Examination

Vitals	Repeat now
HEENT	Icterus (cholangitis, choledocholithiasis)
	Spider nevi (risk of spontaneous bacterial peritonitis if ascites is present)

Resp   Generalized or localized restriction of abdominal wall movement in respiration (localized or generalized peritoneal inflammation)

              Stony dullness to percussion, decreased breath sounds, decreased tactile fremitus (pleural effusion)

              Dullness to percussion, diminished or bronchial breath sounds, crackles (consolidation and pneumonia)

CVS   Decreased JVP (volume depletion)

              New onset of dysrhythmia or mitral insufficiency murmur (myocardial infarction)

ABD   Before examining the abdomen, make sure that your hands are warm and the head of the bed is flat. It may be helpful to flex the patient's hips to relax the abdominal wall. When examining for tenderness, begin in a nonpainful region. Watch the patient's face as you examine for the following:

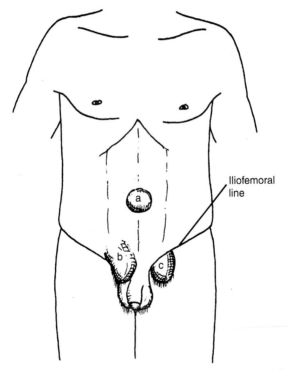

Iliofemoral line

Figure 5–3 Hernial orifices. a, Umbilical hernia; b, inguinal hernia; c, femoral hernia. Note that the "bulge" of the inguinal hernia begins superiorly to the inguinal ligament, whereas the "bulge" of the femoral hernia originates inferiorly to the inguinal ligament.

Visible peristalsis (bowel obstruction)
Bulging flanks (ascites)
Loss of liver dullness (perforated viscus)
Localized tenderness, masses (see Fig. 5–1)
Rigid abdomen, guarding, rebound tenderness (peritonitis)
Shifting dullness, fluid wave (ascites)
Absent bowel sounds (paralytic ileus or late bowel obstruction)
Check all hernia orifices (strangulated hernia) (Fig. 5–3)
Murphy's sign (cholecystitis) (Fig. 5–4)
Psoas sign (appendicitis) (Fig. 5–5)
Obturator sign (appendicitis) (Fig. 5–6)

Rectal   Tenderness (retrocecal appendicitis, prostatitis)
Mass (rectal carcinoma)
Rectal fissure (Crohn's disease)

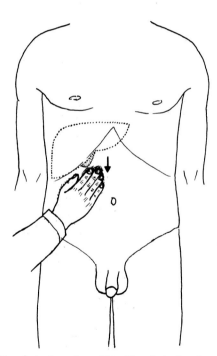

Figure 5–4 Murphy's sign. A positive Murphy's sign is manifested by pain and inspiratory arrest when the patient takes a deep breath while the examiner applies pressure against the abdominal wall in the region of the gallbladder. A positive Murphy's sign is often seen in the presence of cholecystitis.

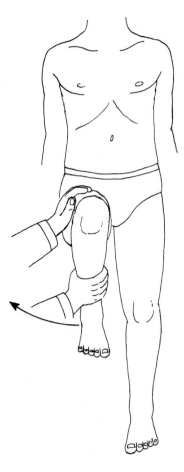

Figure 5–5 Psoas sign. A positive psoas sign is manifested by abdominal pain in response to passive hip extension. (This test also may be performed with the patient lying on his or her side.) This sign is often present in patients with appendicitis or a psoas abscess.

Figure 5–6 A positive obturator sign is manifested by abdominal pain in response to passive internal rotation of the right hip from the 90-degree hip-knee flexion position when the patient is supine. This sign is often present in patients with appendicitis.

Stool   positive for occult blood (ischemic colitis, peptic ulcer)

Pelvic   Tenderness (ectopic pregnancy, ovarian cyst, pelvic inflammatory disease)

Mass (ovarian cyst or tumor)

Management

Your assessment and investigation thus far may not have led you to a specific diagnosis of the cause of the patient's abdominal pain. You will, however, have determined from the physical examination whether the patient has developed shock, the most serious complication from disorders that cause abdominal pain.

Shock. The initial treatment of either *hypovolemic* or *septic shock* is the same and is aimed at immediate expansion of the intravascular volume.

1. Rapid volume repletion can be achieved using normal saline (NS) or Ringer's lactate 500 to 1000 mL IV as rapidly as possible, followed by an IV rate titrated to the jugular venous pressure (JVP) and vital signs. In this situation, IV fluids should be given through a large-bore peripheral IV or central line.

2. Blood should be drawn for a stat crossmatch for 4 to 6 units of packed red blood cells (RBCs), hemoglobin (Hb), prothrombin time (PT), activated partial thromboplastin time (aPTT), and platelet count. Baseline values of electrolytes, urea, creatinine, blood glucose, amylase, and white blood cell (WBC) count and manual differential are also useful. Two sets of blood cultures should be drawn if septic shock is suspected.

3. If hemorrhagic shock is suspected, packed RBCs should be given in place of, or in addition to, the crystalloid, NS, or Ringer's lactate as soon as the crossmatch has been completed. In extreme circumstances, O-negative blood may be used while waiting for the crossmatched supply.

4. When shock occurs in the setting of a disorder causing abdominal pain, urgent surgical consultation is almost always required. Ensure that the patient is NPO (nothing by mouth). Consider inserting a nasogastric (NG) tube if the patient is vomiting.

5. As resuscitation measures are being initiated, additional investigations can be arranged, as follows:

   a. Order three radiographic views of the abdomen (anteroposterior [AP] abdomen supine and erect or lateral decubitus, and posteroanterior [PA] chest erect). If the patient looks unwell or critical, these x-rays will need to be done on a stat portable basis.

      (1) *Toxic megacolon* is manifested by an increase in diameter of the midtransverse colon (>7 cm) and a

mucosal pattern of thumbprinting or thickening. This condition is a medical or surgical emergency.

(2) Look for air under the diaphragm in the chest film or between the viscera and subcutaneous tissue in the lateral decubitus film. This sign is indicative of a perforated viscus.

(3) Look for air-fluid levels that suggest bowel obstruction or ileus.

(4) Look for calcified gallstones, which could be a cause of cholecystitis or pancreatitis.

(5) Pancreatic calcifications, if present, may be a clue that the patient is having a recurrent attack of chronic pancreatitis.

b. If septic shock is suspected, specimens for Gram stain, culture, and sensitivity testing should be obtained immediately from sputum, if available; urine, which may require catheterization; and wounds. If there is ascites, an immediate diagnostic paracentesis should be performed.

6. In a case of suspected septic shock, once culture specimens have been obtained, empirical broad-spectrum antibiotics (e.g., a third-generation cephalosporin plus metronidazole) should be started immediately to treat infection due to coliforms and gut anaerobes.

Acute "Surgical" Abdomen. If the patient is not in shock or has been successfully resuscitated from shock, you must consider the possible underlying conditions responsible for the complaint of abdominal pain. Of utmost importance at this point is to determine whether the patient has an acute "surgical" abdomen (i.e., requiring surgery).

PERFORATED OR RUPTURED VISCUS. Finding air under the diaphragm on the upright chest x-ray (CXR) or between the viscera and subcutaneous tissue on the lateral decubitus film indicates a perforated or ruptured viscus. Immediate surgical consultation is required. Ensure that the patient is NPO.

INTRA-ABDOMINAL HEMORRHAGE. Abdominal pain due to an intra-abdominal hemorrhage almost always requires immediate surgical consultation. Ensure that the patient is kept NPO and that blood has been sent for a stat crossmatch for 4 to 6 units of packed RBCs.

RUPTURED INTRA-ABDOMINAL ABSCESS. An intra-abdominal abscess that has ruptured often results in acute peritonitis and, if left untreated, may progress to septic shock. Urgent surgical consultation for proper drainage is required. Ensure that the patient is kept NPO.

NECROSIS OF A VISCUS. Necrosis of an intra-abdominal viscus due to intussusception, volvulus, strangulated hernia, or ischemic colitis requires urgent surgical consultation. Ensure that the patient is kept NPO.

Other Conditions. Other conditions that may not cause an acute surgical abdomen are common and should be considered if none of

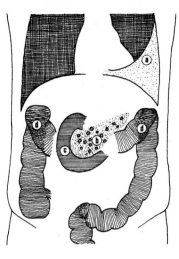

Figure 5–7 Radiographic features of pancreatitis. a, Left pleural effusion; b, calcification within the pancreas; c, sentinel loop; d, colonic distention.

the previously mentioned conditions is present. Each has features requiring specific attention from the physician on call.

PANCREATITIS. Pancreatitis should be suspected in any patient with abdominal pain but no evidence of an upper GI bleed or ascites. The abdominal x-ray films may reveal a sentinel loop, colonic distention, left pleural effusion, or calcification within the pancreas (Fig. 5–7). An elevated serum amylase or lipase level supports the diagnosis, but normal levels do not exclude the possibility of pancreatitis. The patient should be NPO. IV fluids with NS should be ordered to replace any losses. Narcotic analgesic agents are usually required. *Meperidine* (Demerol) 50 to 150 mg IM or SC every 3 to 4 hours PRN (as needed) is the drug of choice, because morphine can cause spasm of the sphincter of Oddi. If the patient develops a fever, an abdominal ultrasound or computed tomography (CT) scan should be ordered to search for a possible pancreatic abscess. In cases of severe pancreatitis with sepsis, abscess formation, or generalized peritonitis, broad-spectrum antibiotics directed against bowel flora (see page 42, point 6) are appropriate.

INTRA-ABDOMINAL ABSCESS. A contained intra-abdominal abscess requires delineation by either ultrasound or CT scan. This can be arranged in the morning, provided the patient is otherwise stable. Abscesses may be treated with ultrasound-guided percutaneous drainage, surgical drainage, or antibiotics alone, depending on the circumstance.

PEPTIC ULCER DISEASE OR GASTROESOPHAGEAL REFLUX DISEASE. Cases of suspected peptic ulcer disease or gastroesophageal reflux disease (GERD) should be considered for endoscopy, particularly if the patient has so-called alarm symptoms such as bleeding, anemia, dysphagia, or weight loss. Antisecretory agents may be initiated on call, even before the patient has had endoscopy. H_2 blockers are common initial therapy for both conditions, and once-daily dosing may be as effective as more frequent dosing. Commonly used agents include *cimetidine* (Tagamet) 800 mg PO at bedtime, *ranitidine* (Zantac) 300 mg PO at bedtime, *famotidine* (Pepcid) 40 mg PO at bedtime, and *nizatidine* (Axid) 300 mg PO at bedtime. Proton pump inhibitors *omeprazole* 20 mg PO daily, *lansoprazole* 15 mg PO daily, *pantoprazole* 40 mg PO daily, and *esomeprazole* 20 mg PO daily are very effective antisecretory agents but more expensive than the H_2 antagonists. Antacids may be given (e.g., *Gelusil* 30 to 60 mL PO every 1 to 2 hours) during the acute phase but are contraindicated if endoscopy is to be performed, because they may obscure the endoscopist's view of mucosal lesions.

Helicobacter pylori infection is a remediable risk factor in many patients with peptic ulcer disease. Eradication of this organism increases the rate of healing and decreases the likelihood of recurrence. Many effective regimens exist for the treatment of *H. pylori* and are commonly referred to as "triple therapy." Such regimens usually include an antisecretory agent (an H_2 antagonist or proton pump inhibitor) and two antimicrobial drugs (e.g., *metronidazole* 500 mg PO twice a day and *amoxicillin* 1 g PO twice a day). Unfortunately, it is not possible to distinguish which patients with peptic ulcer disease are infected on the basis of symptoms alone. When you are presented at night with a patient in whom peptic ulcer disease is suspected, empirical triple therapy for *H. pylori* is not recommended; this should be reserved for patients with peptic ulcer disease confirmed by endoscopy.

PYELONEPHRITIS. Pyelonephritis associated with severe systemic symptoms such as high fever, chills, and impending shock requires an immediate blood and urine culture and empirical IV antibiotics (ampicillin and an aminoglycoside) until the specific organism has been identified.

RENAL STONES. Patients with severe pain from renal stones may be managed acutely with *morphine* 3mg IV repeated (usually once or twice), as needed. *Diclofenac* 75 mg IM or 100 mg PR may be a useful adjunctive measure. Surgical removal, basket extraction, or lithotripsy may be required if the stone has not passed within a few days or if an associated persistent infection is present.

INFECTIOUS GASTROENTERITIS. Infectious gastroenteritis may require specific antibiotics if the stool culture results reveal a bacterial cause. Viral gastroenteritis is treated supportively with IV fluids and antiemetics. *Clostridium difficile* infection should be suspected in any patient who develops diarrhea during or after a course of antibiotics. Sigmoidoscopy may reveal a characteristic pseudomembrane, in which case *metronidazole* 500 mg PO every 6 hours or *vancomycin* 125 to 500 mg every 6 hours may be instituted before confirmation by *C. difficile* culture or toxin assay.

OVARIAN CYST, TUMOR, OR SALPINGITIS. These are best managed by referral to a gynecologist.

ABDOMINAL PAIN IN THE AIDS OR IMMUNOSUPPRESSED PATIENT

Symptoms such as chronic abdominal pain, nausea, and vomiting are common in the critically ill acquired immunodeficiency syndrome (AIDS) or immunosuppressed patient. Many AIDS patients already appear chronically ill, and this must be factored into one's assessment of the cause of abdominal pain. In addition, many of these patients already have abnormalities in baseline laboratory values, making *changes* in laboratory parameters more important than absolute values.

The following special features are pertinent in the evaluation of abdominal pain in an AIDS or immunosuppressed patient:

1. Fever is a sensitive sign of infection in an AIDS patient with abdominal pain. Unfortunately, it is a nonspecific finding and may be due to nonabdominal occult infections or to human immunodeficiency virus (HIV) itself. AIDS patients with temperatures ≥38.5°C should have blood cultures drawn twice, although frequently no causative agent is isolated.

2. Enteric infections are common causes of abdominal pain (usually cramping in quality and associated with diarrhea), including *Cryptosporidium, Shigella, Salmonella, Cytomegalovirus,* and *Campylobacter* enteritis.

3. AIDS and immunocompromised patients commonly have leukopenia due to the effect of HIV suppression of the bone marrow and to drugs. Thus, even a normal WBC level, especially if accompanied by a left shift, should be interpreted as a sign of possible infection in an AIDS patient with fever and abdominal pain. Neutropenic enterocolitis (typhlitis), consisting of transmural inflammation and submucosal hemorrhage in the cecum or ascending colon, is associated with severe abdominal pain in immunocompromised patients.

4. Drug-induced pancreatitis can result from the use of a variety of nucleoside reverse transcriptase inhibitors and may complicate the lipodystrophy syndrome associated with HIV disease and antiretroviral treatments.

5. Hepatic steatosis with lactic acidosis is a rapidly fatal condition that has about a 50% mortality. Fortunately, it is a rare syndrome associated with nucleoside reverse transcriptase therapy.

6. HIV-infected patients are at high risk for non-Hodgkin's lymphoma, which can present predominantly in the GI tract.

7. Acalculous cholecystitis is relatively common. However, gallbladder disease may also be caused by *Cryptosporidium, Cytomegalovirus,* or *Mycobacterium avium-intracellulare* infections.

ABDOMINAL PAIN IN THE ELDERLY

The investigation and management of abdominal pain in an elderly patient should proceed along the same lines as for other patient groups. Of note in the elderly is that abdominal pain may be very mild despite the presence of an acute abdomen. One should not underestimate the seriousness of mild abdominal pain in the elderly, especially if associated with acute confusion, fever, elevated WBC level, or metabolic acidosis.

Two conditions causing abdominal pain that are usually unique to the elderly are *colonic perforation* due to diverticular disease and *mesenteric ischemia* due to atherosclerosis.

Chest Pain

In developed countries, where coronary artery disease is the leading cause of death, it is logical that when a patient complains of "chest pain," you wonder whether he or she is having angina or, worse, a heart attack. There are, however, several other equally serious causes of chest pain that may go undiagnosed if they are not specifically looked for. In the assessment of chest pain, history taking is your most powerful tool.

PHONE CALL

Questions

1. How severe is the pain?
2. What are the vital signs?
3. What was the reason for admission?
4. Does the patient have a past history of angina or myocardial infarction (MI)? If yes, is the pain similar to his or her usual angina or previous MI?

Orders

If MI is suspected:
1. Electrocardiogram (ECG) stat
2. Oxygen by facemask or nasal prongs at 4 L/min
   If the patient is a carbon dioxide (CO_2) retainer, you must be cautious when giving oxygen (maximum FIO_2 0.28 by mask or 2 L/min by nasal prongs).
3. Nitroglycerin 0.3 to 0.6 mg sublingually (SL) every 5 minutes, provided the systolic blood pressure (BP) is >90 mm Hg
4. Ask the RN to take the patient's chart to the bedside

Inform RN

"I will arrive at the bedside in . . . minutes."

Most causes of chest pain are diagnosed by history. It is impossible to obtain an accurate and relevant history by speaking to the RN over the telephone; the history must be taken firsthand from the patient. Because some causes of chest pain represent medical emergencies, the patient should be assessed immediately.

ELEVATOR THOUGHTS

What causes chest pain?

Cardiac	Angina
	MI
	Aortic dissection
	Pericarditis
Resp	Pulmonary embolism or infarction
	Pneumothorax
	Pleuritis (± pneumonia)
GI	Esophageal spasm, reflux, dysmotility; esophagitis
	Peptic ulcer disease
MSS	Costochondritis
	Arthropathies
	Xiphodynia
	Rib fracture
Skin	Herpes zoster
Psych	Panic disorder
	Anxiety disorder

MAJOR THREAT TO LIFE

- Myocardial ischemia or MI
- Aortic dissection
- Pneumothorax
- Pulmonary embolus

Cardiogenic shock or fatal dysrhythmias may occur as a result of *myocardial ischemia* or *infarction*. *Aortic dissection* may result in death from cardiac tamponade, aortic rupture, acute aortic insufficiency, or MI and may damage other organ systems by compromising vascular supply. A *pneumothorax* may cause hypoxia by compressing the ipsilateral lung. A tension pneumothorax may also result in hypotension as a result of positive intrathoracic pressure decreasing venous return to the heart. *Pulmonary embolism* may cause hypoxia and, in more severe cases, may result in acute right ventricular failure.

BEDSIDE

Quick-Look Test

Does the patient look well (comfortable), sick (uncomfortable or distressed), or critical (about to die)?

Most patients with chest pain from MI or myocardial ischemia look pale and anxious. Patients with pericarditis, pneumothorax, or pulmonary embolism involving the pleural surface look apprehensive and breathe with shallow, painful respirations. If the patient looks well, suspect esophagitis or a musculoskeletal problem such as costochondritis.

Airway and Vital Signs

What is the BP?

Most patients with chest pain have a normal BP. Hypotension may be seen with MI, massive pulmonary embolism, aortic dissection resulting in cardiac tamponade, or tension pneumothorax. Hypertension, occurring in association with myocardial ischemia or aortic dissection, should be treated urgently (see Chapter 16, pages 162 to 163).

A wide pulse pressure should raise the suspicion of aortic insufficiency, which may be seen as a complication of a proximal aortic dissection.

A pulsus paradoxus (see page 266) may be a clue to the presence of a pericardial effusion, which may be seen with an aortic dissection or pericarditis.

What is the heart rate (HR)?

Does the patient have tachycardia?

Severe chest pain of any cause may result in sinus tachycardia. HRs of >100 beats/min should also alert you to the possibility of a tachydysrhythmia such as atrial fibrillation, other supraventricular tachycardias, or ventricular tachycardia, which may require immediate cardioversion.

Does the patient have bradycardia?

Bradycardia in a patient with chest pain may represent sinus or atrioventricular (AV) nodal ischemia (as may be seen with MI) or beta blockade or calcium channel blockade due to drugs. Immediate treatment of bradycardia is not required unless the rate is extremely slow (<40 beats/min) or the patient is hypotensive (see Chapter 18, pages 177 to 178).

What is the breathing pattern?

Tachypnea may accompany any type of chest pain. Shallow, painful breathing suggests a pleural (pleuritis, pneumothorax, pericarditis, pulmonary embolism) or musculoskeletal cause.

What does the ECG show?

The ECG should be reviewed immediately after taking of the vital signs to avoid delays in administering thrombolytic therapy if the patient is having an acute MI. Because thrombolysis is most effective when given within the first 4 hours of chest pain, if an MI is suspected based on the ECG, call your resident *immediately* to assess the patient for possible thrombolytic therapy. Remember, a normal ECG does not rule out the possibility of angina or MI.

The ECG in a case of aortic dissection may look perfectly normal. The presence of left ventricular hypertrophy (LVH) may provide a clue to long-standing hypertension, which is a risk factor for a dissection.

The most common ECG finding in a patient with pulmonary embolism is sinus tachycardia, but a rightward axis should also be looked for.

The ECG in a patient with pericarditis may show diffuse, usually mild, ST elevations and sometimes PR depression.

Management I

Is the patient receiving oxygen?

Ensure that the patient is receiving oxygen at an appropriate concentration. If you have access to a pulse oximeter, attach the patient, and keep the oxygen saturation level ≥93%.

Does the patient have chest pain now?

If yes, and myocardial ischemia is suspected, proceed as follows.

Chest Pain and Systolic BP >90 mm Hg

- If the last dose of SL nitroglycerin was given >5 minutes ago, give another dose immediately. If, after an additional 5 minutes, the pain is still present, give a third nitroglycerin dose.
- If the pain continues despite three doses of nitroglycerin, ask the RN to draw 10 mg (1 mL) of morphine into a syringe diluted with 9 mL of normal saline (NS). Give the *morphine* in 2- to 4-mg aliquots IV until the pain is relieved, provided the systolic BP is >90 mm Hg.

  Morphine sulfate may cause hypotension or respiratory depression. Take the patient's BP and respiratory rate (RR) before each dose is given. If necessary, *naloxone hydrochloride* (Narcan) 0.2 to 2 mg IV, IM, or SC may be given every 5 minutes to a total of 10 mg to reverse these side effects. Nausea or vomiting may also occur and can usually be controlled with *dimenhydrinate* 25 mg IV or IM or 50 mg PO every 4 to 6 hours as needed.

- If the chest pain requires the administration of morphine, arrange for assessment by the intensive care unit/cardiac care unit (ICU/CCU) team as soon as possible.

Chest Pain and Systolic BP <90 mm Hg

- What is the patient's normal BP? If the systolic BP is normally 90 mm Hg, you may proceed cautiously with nitroglycerin 0.3 mg SL, as described, provided there is no further drop in the BP.
- If the hypotension is an acute change, establish IV access immediately with a large-bore IV catheter (size 16 if possible). (Refer to Chapter 18, page 180, for management of hypotension.)

If the Patient Looks Sick or Critical

- Establish IV access using D5W if not already done.
- Draw an arterial blood gas (ABG) sample.
- Attach the patient to a pulse oximeter.

Selective History and Chart Review

How does the patient describe the pain?

Crushing, squeezing, viselike pain or pressure is characteristic of MI. Severe tearing or ripping pain is characteristic of an aortic dissection.

Is the pain the same as the patient's usual angina?

If the patient recognizes the current discomfort as his or her usual angina, the patient is probably right.

Is the chest pain worse with deep breathing or coughing?

Pleuritic chest pain suggests pleuritis, pneumothorax, rib fracture, pericarditis, pulmonary embolism, pneumonia, or costochondritis.

Does the pain radiate?

Radiation of the pain to the jaw, shoulders, or arms is suggestive of myocardial ischemia or infarction. Radiation of pain to the back suggests myocardial ischemia, MI, or aortic dissection distal to the left subclavian artery. Dissection proximal to the left subclavian artery characteristically causes nonradiating anterior chest pain. A burning sensation that radiates to the neck and is accompanied by an acid taste in the mouth is suggestive of esophageal reflux.

Is there any associated nausea, vomiting, diaphoresis, or lightheadedness?

Cardiogenic nausea and vomiting are associated with larger MIs but do not suggest a particular location, as was previously thought.

Is the chest pain worse with swallowing?

Chest pain that is made worse by swallowing suggests an esophageal disorder or pericarditis.

Selective Physical Examination

Vitals	Repeat now
Body habitus	Does the patient look marfanoid?
	A tall, thin patient with long limbs and arachnodactyly may have a connective tissue disorder predisposing him or her to aortic dissection.
HEENT	White exudate in oral cavity or pharynx (thrush with possible concomitant esophageal candidiasis)

Resp	Asymmetrical expansion of the chest (pneumothorax)
	Deviation of the trachea to one side (large pneumothorax on the side opposite the deviation)
	Hyperresonance to percussion (on the side of a pneumothorax)
	Diminished breath sounds (on the side of a pneumothorax)
	Crackles (CHF secondary to acute MI, pneumonia)
	Consolidation (pulmonary infarction, pneumonia)
	Pleural rub (pulmonary embolism, pneumonia)
	Pleural effusion (pulmonary embolism, pneumonia, ruptured aortic dissection)
Chest wall	Tender costal cartilage (costochondritis)
	Erythema, swelling of costal cartilage (costochondritis, arthritis)
	Tender xiphoid process (xiphodynia)
	Localized rib pain (rib fracture)
CVS	Unequal carotid pulses (aortic dissection)
	Unequal upper limb BP or diminished femoral pulses (aortic dissection)
	Elevated JVP (right ventricular failure secondary to MI or pulmonary embolism; tension pneumothorax)
	Right ventricular heave (acute RV failure secondary to pulmonary embolism)
	Left ventricular heave (CHF)
	Displaced apical impulse (away from the side of a pneumothorax)
	Loud P_2 (acute cor pulmonale), S_3 (CHF)
	Mitral insufficiency murmur (papillary muscle dysfunction due to ischemia or infarction)
	Aortic stenosis murmur (angina)
	Aortic insufficiency murmur (proximal aortic dissection)
	Pericardial rub (pericarditis)
	Pericardial rubs are biphasic or triphasic scratching sounds that vary with position.
ABD	Guarding, rebound tenderness (perforated ulcer)
	Epigastric tenderness (peptic ulcer disease)
	Generalized abdominal pain (mesenteric infarction from aortic dissection)

| CNS | Hemiplegia (aortic dissection involving a carotid artery) |
| Skin | Unilateral maculopapular rash or vesicles in a dermatomal pattern (herpes zoster) |

Look at the Chest X-ray

Review the chest x-ray (CXR) as soon as possible.

If a pneumothorax is suspected, upright inspiratory and expiratory films should be ordered. A pneumothorax is identified by a peripheral hyperlucent area, indicating free air in the pleural space and partial or complete collapse of the affected lung (Fig. 6–1). A tension pneumothorax is a medical emergency and should be treated urgently, as outlined in Chapter 20, page 207.

The CXR may be normal in a patient with angina or an MI. Sometimes pulmonary venous congestion is seen if there is significant associated left ventricular dysfunction.

If an aortic dissection is suspected, look specifically for a widened mediastinum or prominent aortic knuckle (Fig. 6–2). Suspected aortic dissection requires you to proceed urgently with the appropriate investigation and management (see page 55).

The CXR may be normal in a patient with pericarditis unless significant pericardial fluid has accumulated, in which case the cardiac silhouette may be enlarged.

The CXR of a patient with suspected pulmonary embolism may be entirely normal or may show any of the features illustrated in Figure 24–3.

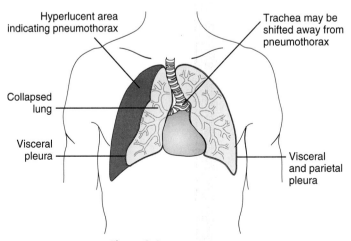

Hyperlucent area indicating pneumothorax

Trachea may be shifted away from pneumothorax

Collapsed lung

Visceral pleura

Visceral and parietal pleura

Figure 6–1 Pneumothorax.

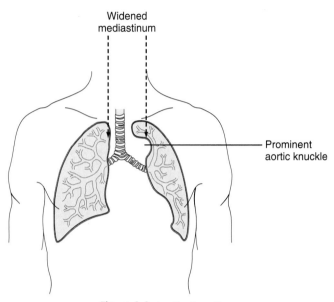

Widened mediastinum

Prominent aortic knuckle

Figure 6–2 Aortic dissection.

Management II

Angina. If *angina* has been relieved with one to three nitroglycerin tablets, review the precipitating cause. An adjustment in the antianginal medication may be required and should be made in consultation with your resident and the attending physician. However, if the angina occurred at rest or this is the first episode of angina, the patient should be assessed by the ICU/CCU staff regardless of whether the pain was relieved with three or fewer nitroglycerin tablets.

If the angina required more than three doses of nitroglycerin or IV morphine, serial cardiac enzymes and ECGs should be ordered. If the clinical impression is of possible MI, the patient should be transferred to the ICU/CCU for continuous ECG monitoring.

Myocardial Infarction. If an MI is suspected based on history or ECG changes (see Appendix D, page 422), the patient should be transferred to the ICU/CCU as soon as possible. The patient also should be evaluated immediately for possible thrombolytic therapy. Ongoing myocardial ischemia may also require treatment with aspirin, IV nitroglycerin, heparin, or beta blockers.

Aortic Dissection. Suspicion of aortic dissection requires urgent investigation and management as follows.

1. Arrange for an urgent computed tomography (CT) scan of the thorax or a transesophageal echocardiogram. If neither of these can be performed within the next hour, a transthoracic echocardiogram may detect a dilated aortic root, aortic valvular insufficiency, or a pericardial effusion, any of which may be a clue to the presence of a dissection. Occasionally, an aortic dissection flap is directly visualized with this test.

2. Draw blood for a stat crossmatch for 6 to 8 units of packed red blood cells (RBCs) and for analysis of electrolytes, urea, creatinine, glucose, complete blood cell count (CBC) and differential, prothrombin time (PT), and activated partial thromboplastin time (aPTT).

3. Review the ECG for evidence of an acute MI. This finding suggests that the aortic dissection involves the coronary ostia.

4. The patient should be transferred to the ICU/CCU as soon as possible for careful control of BP (see Chapter 16, page 162).

5. Surgical consultation should be obtained early if the diagnosis of dissection is apparent. The diagnosis can be confirmed by nuclear magnetic resonance imaging (MRI) or aortography.

Pericarditis. Patients with suspected pericarditis should have nonurgent echocardiograms performed to look for pericardial effusions or signs of hemodynamic compromise. *Indomethacin* (Indocin) 25 to 50 mg PO three times a day or aspirin 650 mg PO every 4 hours is helpful.

> Nonsteroidal anti-inflammatory drugs (NSAIDs) are contraindicated in a patient who has the syndrome of aspirin sensitivity, nasal polyps, and bronchospasm; in a patient who is anticoagulated; and in a patient who has active peptic ulcer disease. Because of their sodium-retaining properties, caution should be used in giving NSAIDs to patients in congestive heart failure (CHF). NSAIDs should also be used with caution in patients with renal insufficiency, because these drugs may inhibit renal prostaglandins, which are responsible for maintaining renal perfusion in those with prerenal conditions; sulindac (Clinoril) may not have this effect.

Pulmonary Embolus. The management of pulmonary embolus is discussed in Chapter 24, page 275.

Pneumothorax. A pneumothorax may require chest tube drainage, depending on its size. If the patient develops a tension pneumothorax, immediate treatment is necessary to relieve the pressure using a 16-gauge IV catheter, as described on page 207.

Pneumonia. Suggested antibiotics for pneumonia are discussed in Chapter 24, pages 278 to 280, and should be chosen according to the Gram stain results and patient's characteristics.

Esophagitis. The pain of esophagitis may be temporarily treated with antacids. Choose carefully. Magnesium-containing antacids (Gelusil, Maalox) may cause diarrhea, whereas antacids containing solely aluminum (Amphojel, Basaljel) may cause constipation. Do not substitute one GI complaint for another. *Gelusil* 30 to 60 mL every 1 to 2 hours during the acute phase and 30 to 60 mL PO every 1 to 4 hours after meals and at bedtime is a standard antacid order. More frequent doses may be required if the pain is severe. An alginate such as *Gaviscon* 10 to 20 mL PO or 2 to 4 tablets (chewed) after meals and at bedtime followed by a glass of water may also be used. Elevation of the head of the bed and avoidance of nighttime snacks may also be helpful.

An H_2 blocker such as *cimetidine* (Tagamet) 400 mg PO twice a day, *ranitidine* (Zantac) 150 mg PO twice a day, *famotidine* (Pepcid) 20 mg PO twice a day, or *nizatidine* (Axid) 150 mg PO twice a day should also be started to aid in the long-term treatment of this disease.[1] *Omeprazole* (Losec) 20 mg PO daily, *esomeprazole* 20 mg PO daily, *lansoprazole* 15 mg PO daily, pantoprazole 40 mg PO daily, and *rabeprazole* 20 mg PO daily are proton pump inhibitors; these drugs may be more expensive than H_2 blockers but are usually effective in treating erosive esophagitis resistant to the usual agents.

Esophageal candidiasis does not respond to antacids. Immunocompromised patients may experience severe chest pain from this condition. Diagnosis should be confirmed by endoscopy. Although useful in thrush, nystatin (Mycostatin) is not effective in esophageal candidiasis. In AIDS or immunocompromised patients, fluconazole (Diflucan) has been shown to be more effective than ketoconazole (Nizoral) in eradicating *Candida* from the esophagus; it also has a more rapid onset of action and resolution of symptoms. It may be given parenterally when necessary.[2] The dose is *fluconazole* 100 mg PO daily. An alternative is *itraconazole* (Sporanox) oral solution 200 mg PO daily on an empty stomach.

Peptic Ulcer. The pain of peptic ulcer disease may be temporarily treated with antacids. Gelusil 30 to 60 mL every 1 to 2 hours during the acute phase and 30 to 60 mL PO every 1 to 4 hours after meals and at bedtime is a standard antacid order. More frequent doses may be required if the pain is severe. An H_2 blocker such as *cimetidine* (Tagamet) 300 mg PO every 6 hours, *ranitidine* (Zantac) 150 mg PO twice a day, *famotidine* (Pepcid) 20 mg PO twice a day, or *nizatidine* (Axid) 150 mg PO twice a day may help in the long-term treatment of this disease. *Omeprazole* (Losec) 20 mg PO daily is more expensive but may be useful in ulcers resistant to H_2 blockade. A patient with suspected peptic ulcer disease should be referred for a possible endoscopic evaluation in the morning.

Costochondritis. Costochondritis may be treated with an NSAID, such as *naproxen* (Naprosyn) 250 mg PO every 6 to 8 hours (see precautions, page 55).

Herpes Zoster. Unilateral chest pain in a dermatomal distribution may precede the typical skin lesions of herpes zoster ("shingles") by 2 or 3 days. The rash begins as a reddened, maculopapular area that rapidly evolves into vesicular lesions. Treatment of acute herpes zoster neuritis may be difficult and often requires narcotic analgesics, amitriptyline hydrochloride, and, in some cases, steroids. Topical preparations of capsaicin (Zostrix) may also provide temporary relief of neuralgic pain but should not be applied directly to open skin lesions. Antiviral agents such as *acyclovir* 800 mg PO every 6 hours may reduce the severity and duration of localized herpes zoster. Immunocompromised patients may require larger doses such as 800 mg PO five times a day or 10 mg/kg IV every 8 hours.

Panic and Anxiety Disorders. *Panic attacks* are defined as "discrete periods of discomfort or fear" and are often associated with chest pain, dyspnea, diaphoresis, and dizziness. These symptoms may also be accompanied by feelings of depersonalization and a fear of dying, of "going crazy," or of "losing control." Chest pain may also be a feature of an *anxiety disorder*. Because of the possibility of a life-threatening cause of chest pain, panic and anxiety disorders should be diagnoses of exclusion. Short-acting benzodiazepines such as alprazolam 0.5 mg PO daily or lorazepam 1 to 2 mg PO daily as needed may be helpful in the short-term treatment of these disorders.

References

1. Pope CE: Acid-reflux disorders. N Engl J Med 1994;331:656-660.
2. Vasquez JA: Therapeutic options for the management of oropharyngeal and esophageal candidiasis in HIV/AIDS patients. HIV Clin Trials 2000;1:47-59.

Combativeness— The Out-of-Control Patient

Every once in a while, you will be paged by an exasperated nurse who has been trying to reason with an out-of-control patient. We are not referring here to moody or uncooperative patients; we are referring to hostile individuals whose temporary behavior poses a real physical threat to themselves, other patients, or hospital staff. Your job is not to act as the strong arm of the hospital law. Your role is to deem which medical reasons, if any, are responsible for the patient's behavior and to administer appropriate treatment.

PHONE CALL

Questions

1. What was the reason for admission?
2. What medications is the patient taking now?
3. Is there an obvious reason for the patient's combative behavior?
4. What measures have been used thus far to calm or reason with the patient?
5. What additional hospital personnel are there to help you now?
6. What is the patient's estimated height and weight?

Orders

1. Ask the RN to call the hospital's security personnel now, if this has not already been done. Your job is not to hurry to the ward to help hold down the patient. Your role is to determine the cause of the patient's behavior and to institute appropriate treatment.
2. *Lorazepam* (Ativan) 0.5 to 2 mg PO, SL, or IM. By the time the RN has called you, he or she has usually wrestled with the patient for 10 to 20 minutes, enlisted the aid of orderlies, and tried everything at his or her immediate disposal.

The initial dose depends on the patient's height and body weight: 0.5 mg may suffice for an elderly patient of slight build, whereas 2 mg may be necessary for a young, large football player.

Inform RN

"I will arrive at the bedside in . . . minutes."

The out-of-control patient requires your immediate attention.

ELEVATOR THOUGHTS

What causes dangerously combative behavior?

Any confusional state due to an acute or chronic medical or psychiatric condition can result in temporary hostile or combative behavior. How an individual reacts in a given situation is often a reflection of his or her premorbid personality. The most common out-of-control patient is a young individual who feels frustrated, confined, and overwhelmed by the illness and the hospital environment. A second common type of out-of-control patient is an elderly person who becomes disoriented and combative, particularly at night (the sundown phenomenon).

Numerous other medical conditions may set off this behavior in a hospitalized patient, including intracranial disease, systemic disorders (drugs, organ failure, metabolic and endocrine disorders, infection, inflammation), and psychiatric disorders. Once the patient is safely approachable, these conditions should be carefully sought (see Chapter 8, pages 63 to 64).

MAJOR THREAT TO LIFE

- Physical injury

    Patients who are acutely agitated and hostile are not reasoning properly and appear to be "looking for a fight." The typical out-of-control patient has pulled out the intravenous (IV) line, nasogastric (NG) tube, or Foley catheter and is cursing, threatening, and pummeling any hospital personnel within striking distance. The patient loses regard for his or her own safety and risks both new injury and worsening of the underlying medical condition that necessitated the hospitalization.

BEDSIDE

Quick-Look Test

Does the patient look well (comfortable), sick (uncomfortable or distressed), or critical (about to die)?

    The combative patient looks very much alive, agitated, and (often) ready for a fight.

Stand back from the situation for a moment and observe the patient. You must judge from a distance how dangerous the patient is and what immediate measures are required to calm him or her and regain control. Look for any obvious signs or conditions that may require specific treatment.

- Is the patient cyanotic or having difficulty breathing (hypoxia)?
- Does the patient appear to be hallucinating (drug intoxication or withdrawal)?
- Is the patient in pain?

Management

The first priority is to calm the patient and regain control of the situation. In performing this task, the first rule is to remain calm yourself. It is not necessary to jump into the brawl, and you will be far more effective if you use your head in this situation.

1. Some patients become calm simply because "the doctor" has arrived, and they feel less helpless and more in control of themselves with a physician there to address their immediate concerns. You will be able to judge within the first 30 seconds whether you are lucky and this is the case.

2. Some patients are so completely out of control that calm reasoning is futile. These patients may require temporary physical restraint while medication is given. You may try to explain that you are going to give the patient "a shot" to calm him or her down and make him or her feel better. If the patient does not allow you to approach because of aggressive behavior, the patient must be held down while medication is administered. Continued restraint may be required until the medication takes effect. Should you need to physically restrain a violent individual, the general rule is to have at least one person per limb plus one.

   - If the patient has already been given the lorazepam you ordered over the telephone and is still out of control, physical restraints may be necessary. Allow adequate time for the medication to take effect. If the patient remains agitated 30 minutes after the initial dose, you may give an additional dose of *lorazepam* 0.5 to 2 mg. The effective dose range is 0.5 to 2 mg every 1 to 6 hours. Always use the lowest effective dosage.

     > The two main side effects of lorazepam are respiratory depression and a clouding of consciousness that may attend the sedative effect, which may actually compound the behavioral problem.

   - An alternative is *haloperidol* (Haldol) 1 to 10 mg IM.

     > The two main acute side effects of haloperidol are hypotension and the occasional acute dystonic reaction (spasm of the face, tongue, back, or neck). The hypotension is

usually postural, and once the patient is cooperative, he or she should be assisted when initially going from the supine to the upright position. Acute dystonic reactions usually respond to *diphenhydramine* 25 to 50 mg PO, IM, or IV or *benztropine mesylate* 1 to 2 mg PO, IM, or IV.

3. Barbiturates should be avoided, because although they have valuable sedative properties, they tend to cloud consciousness and may actually compound the behavioral problem.

4. Call the patient's family, explain what has happened, and see whether the family can shed any light on the patient's behavior. If physical restraints (wrist and ankle restraints or a posey) were required, inform the family immediately and reassure them that the restraints will likely be needed only temporarily. Emphasize that these measures are intended to protect the patient from injuring himself or herself. Nothing is more upsetting than for uninformed and unsuspecting family members to walk into their loved one's room the next day and find the patient "tied down" to the bed.

5. Once the acute crisis is over, a thorough evaluation for underlying causes of confusion (any of which may lead to combative behavior) should be undertaken (see Chapter 8). Once the patient is safely approachable, a directed physical examination looking for life-threatening (see pages 65 to 67) or correctable (see pages 67 to 68) causes of confusion should be performed. You will have to use your judgment, because sometimes these patients are best left alone to sleep for a while. Just as often, however, a recently out-of-control patient will be grateful for the additional attention received from a concerned medical student or physician.

Bibliography

Citrome L, Volavka J: Violent patients in the emergency room setting. Emergency Psychiatry 1999;22:789-798.

Confusion/ Decreased Level of Consciousness

Confusion is a common problem in hospitalized patients, especially among the elderly. Unfortunately, the terms *delirium, toxic psychosis, acute brain syndrome,* and *acute confusional state* are often used interchangeably to refer to any cause of confusion. When the term *metabolic encephalopathy* is used, it implies that the confusion is not due to psychiatric disorders or structural intracranial lesions.

The two recommended terms are *delirium* and *dementia. Delirium* is characterized by restlessness, agitation, clouding of consciousness, and, in some patients, bizarre behavior, hallucinations, delusions, and illusions. *Dementia* refers to a state of irreversible loss of memory and a global cognitive deficit. The level of consciousness is an important distinguishing feature between delirium and dementia. Delirium is characterized by a clouding of consciousness (a decreased clarity of awareness of the environment), whereas dementia is associated with a normal level of consciousness. Also, the signs of delirium fluctuate, whereas the confusion seen with dementia is more constant.

Drowsiness, stupor, and *coma* refer to various degrees of unresponsiveness or diminished levels of consciousness.

PHONE CALL

Questions

1. Clarify the situation. In what way is the patient confused?
2. What are the vital signs?
3. Has there been a change in the level of consciousness?
4. Have there been previous episodes of confusion?
5. What was the reason for admission?
6. Is the patient diabetic?

Confusion can be caused by either too much or too little sugar in the blood. Hypoglycemia (due to excess insulin or oral hypoglycemic agents) and marked hyperglycemia (due to inadequate insulin or oral hypoglycemic agents) are prime considerations when confusion occurs in a diabetic patient.

7. **How old is the patient?**

A 30-year-old patient is much more likely to have a serious yet reversible cause of confusion than is an 80-year-old patient receiving multiple medications.

Orders

1. Blood glucose, Chemstrip, or glucose meter reading—hypoglycemia is a rapidly reversible cause of confusion.
2. O$_2$ saturation, if pneumonia or a respiratory disorder was the reason for admission—this can be measured by attaching a pulse oximeter to the patient.

Inform RN

"I will arrive at the bedside in . . . minutes."

Confusion in association with fever, decreased level of consciousness, or acute agitation (see Chapter 7) requires that you see the patient immediately.

ELEVATOR THOUGHTS

What causes confusion or a decreased level of consciousness?

Many disorders that begin with confusion may lead to a diminished level of consciousness and, ultimately, coma (note the items marked with an asterisk in the following list). To cause a diminished level of consciousness, both cerebral hemispheres must be affected (e.g., by drugs or toxins), or there must be suppression of the brain stem reticular activating system.

Central Nervous System (Intracranial)

1. Dementia
   a. Alzheimer's disease
   b. Multi-infarct dementia
   c. Parkinson's disease
   d. Normal-pressure hydrocephalus*
2. Malignancy (primary central nervous system [CNS] tumor, CNS metastasis, paraneoplastic syndrome)
3. Head trauma (subdural and epidural hematoma, concussion, cerebral contusion)*
4. Postictal state*
5. Transient ischemic attack (TIA)/stroke*

---

*Disorders that may begin with confusion but can lead to a diminished level of consciousness or coma.

6. Hypertensive encephalopathy*
7. Wernicke's encephalopathy (thiamine deficiency)
8. Vitamin B_{12} deficiency

Systemic

DRUGS

1. Alcohol withdrawal—in an alcoholic patient, confusion may occur when the patient is intoxicated, during early withdrawal, or later as part of delirium tremens
2. Narcotic and sedative drug excess* or withdrawal—even "normal" doses of these drugs frequently cause confusion in the elderly
3. Nonsteroidal anti-inflammatory drugs (NSAIDs), including aspirin
4. Antihypertensives (methyldopa, beta blockers)
5. Psychotropic medications (tricyclic antidepressants, lithium, phenothiazines, monoamine oxidase [MAO] inhibitors, benzodiazepines, selective serotonin reuptake inhibitors [SSRIs])*
6. Miscellaneous (steroids, cimetidine, antihistamines, anticholinergics)

ORGAN FAILURE*

1. Respiratory failure (hypoxia, hypercapnia)
2. Renal failure (uremic encephalopathy)
3. Liver failure (hepatic encephalopathy)
4. Congestive heart failure (CHF) (hypoxia), hypertensive encephalopathy

METABOLIC*

1. Hyperglycemia, hypoglycemia
2. Hypernatremia, hyponatremia
3. Hypercalcemia

ENDOCRINE

1. Hyperthyroidism or hypothyroidism*
2. Hyperadrenocorticism or hypoadrenocorticism

INFECTION OR INFLAMMATION

1. Meningitis,* encephalitis,* brain abscess*
2. Lyme disease
3. Cerebral vasculitis (systemic lupus erythematosus [SLE], polyarteritis nodosa)*

PSYCHIATRIC DISORDERS

1. Mania, depression
2. Schizophrenia

---

*Disorders that may begin with confusion but can lead to a diminished level of consciousness or coma.

MAJOR THREAT TO LIFE

- Intracranial mass
- Delirium tremens
- Meningitis

Patients with an *intracranial mass* (e.g., subdural or epidural hematoma, brain abscess, tumor) may initially present with confusion. Patients with untreated *delirium tremens* can have a mortality rate of up to 15%. *Meningitis* must be recognized early if antibiotic medication is to be effective.

BEDSIDE

Quick-Look Test

Does the patient look well (comfortable), sick (uncomfortable or distressed), or critical (about to die)?

Most patients with delirium look sick, whereas most patients with dementia look well.

Airway, Vital Signs, and Chemstrip Results

Is the patient receiving oxygen?

An FIO_2 of >0.28 given to a patient with chronic obstructive pulmonary disease (COPD) may depress the respiratory center, resulting in confusion from hypercapnia.

What is the blood pressure (BP)?

Hypertensive encephalopathy is rare; diastolic BP is usually >120 mm Hg. Confusion in association with a systolic BP of <90 mm Hg may be due to impaired cerebral perfusion secondary to shock. Drug overdose, adrenal insufficiency, and hyponatremia are metabolic causes that should be considered in a hypotensive, confused patient.

What is the heart rate?

A tachycardia suggests sepsis, delirium tremens, hyperthyroidism, or hypoglycemia, but it may also occur in any agitated, anxious patient.

What is the temperature?

Fever suggests infection, delirium tremens, or cerebral vasculitis.

What is the respiratory rate?

Confusion in association with tachypnea should alert you to the possibility of hypoxia. Tachypnea with confusion and petechiae in a young patient with a femoral fracture is a classic presentation of fat embolism syndrome.

What is the blood glucose result?

Hypoglycemia is most commonly seen in a patient with diabetes mellitus who has received the usual insulin dose but has not eaten. Rarely, an incorrect dose of insulin, surreptitious insulin use, or an insulinoma is the cause (see Chapter 32, page 354, for the management of hypoglycemia and pages 349 to 353 for the management of hyperglycemia).

Selective Physical Examination I

Is there evidence on physical examination of one of the major threats to life?

HEENT	Nuchal rigidity (meningitis)
	Papilledema (hypertensive encephalopathy, intracranial mass)
	Pupil size and symmetry
	> Dilated pupils suggest increased sympathetic outflow, such as may be seen in delirium tremens or cocaine ingestion, whereas pinpoint pupils suggest narcotic excess or recent application of constricting eyedrops
	Palpate the skull for fractures, hematomas, and lacerations (subdural or epidural hematoma, concussion)
	Hemotympanum or blood in the ear canal (basal skull fracture)
Neuro	General appearance—behavior and attitude
	Level of consciousness—alert, drowsy
	Mood, affect—depressed, agitated, restless
	Form of thought—flight of ideas, circumstantiality, loosening of associations, perseveration
	Thought content—delusions, concrete thinking
	Perceptions—illusions, hallucinations (auditory, visual)
	Mental status: a detailed mental status examination is required in the assessment of a confused patient; however, if the patient has a decreased level of consciousness or is agitated or uncooperative, not all the categories listed will be appropriate
	Orientation—time, place, and person
	Registration—name three objects (e.g., apple, pencil, car) and have the patient repeat them
	Attention and calculation—serial 7s
	Recall—ask for the three aforementioned objects (apple, pencil, car)
	Language—point to and identify objects; follow a three-stage command; write a sentence
	Long-term memory—birth date, name of hometown
	Judgment—test hypothetical situations

A full neurologic examination is required (within the limits posed by the mental status examination)

Is there any tremor (delirium tremens, Parkinson's disease, hyperthyroidism)?

Is there any asymmetry of pupils, visual fields, eye movement, limbs, tone, reflexes, or plantars?

| Asymmetry suggests structural brain disease

Management I

Bacterial Meningitis. If there is a suspicion of bacterial meningitis, refer immediately to Chapter 12, pages 97 to 98, for further investigation and management.

Intracranial Lesion. A structural intracranial lesion (e.g., stroke, tumor, subdural hematoma, epidural hematoma) should be suspected in a patient with new findings of asymmetry on neurologic examination. An urgent computed tomography (CT) head scan will help define the intracranial lesion. Prompt referral to a neurosurgeon is required for a subdural or epidural hematoma and for a cerebellar hemorrhage.

Delirium Tremens. Delirium tremens (confusion, fever, tachycardia, dilated pupils, diaphoresis) and alcohol withdrawal must be treated urgently with sedation. Benzodiazepines are of proven benefit. The loading dose of *diazepam* (Valium) is 5 to 10 mg IV as a bolus every 5 to 15 minutes until the patient is sedated (i.e., drowsy but rouses when stimulated). The maintenance dose is 10 to 20 mg PO four times a day, with subsequent tapering. Alternatively, give chlordiazepoxide 50 to 100 mg IV as a bolus until sedated. The maintenance dose is 100 mg PO four times a day for several days, with subsequent gradual tapering of the dose. Thiamine 100 mg IV (given slowly over 5 minutes), IM, or PO daily for up to 3 days, if not already administered during this hospitalization, should be given to prevent the development of Wernicke's encephalopathy in an alcoholic or malnourished patient. If necessary, IV 5% dextrose in normal saline (D5NS) may be given to correct volume depletion after the initial dose of thiamine. Barbiturates may be useful in refractory patients. However, respiratory depression is common with the higher doses that are required. Call your resident or attending physician for help before instituting them.

Selective Physical Examination II

Are there other correctable causes of confusion?

Vitals   Hypertension and bradycardia may signify rising intracranial pressure

Hypothermia suggests myxedema or alcohol, barbiturate, or phenothiazine intoxication

HEENT	Subhyaloid hemorrhage (subarachnoid hemorrhage)
	Conjunctival and fundal petechiae (fat embolism syndrome) (Fig. 8–1)
	Lacerated tongue or cheek (postictal)
	Goiter (hyperthyroidism or hypothyroidism)
Resp	Cyanosis (hypoxia)
	Barrel chest (COPD with hypoxia or hypercapnia)
	Bibasilar crackles (CHF with hypoxia)
CVS	Elevated JVP ⎤
	S₃ ⎬ CHF
	Pitting edema ⎦
ABD	Costovertebral angle tenderness (pyelonephritis)
	Liver, spleen, or kidney tenderness (infection)
	Guarding, rebound tenderness (intra-abdominal infection)
	Shifting dullness, dilated superficial veins, caput medusae (liver failure)
Neuro	Argyll Robertson pupils—accommodate but do not react to light (syphilis) (Fig. 8–2)
	Cranial nerve palsies (Lyme disease)
	Asterixis, constructional apraxia (liver failure) (Fig. 8–3)
Skin	Axillary fold, neck, upper chest petechiae (fat embolism syndrome)

Selective History and Chart Review

What drugs is the patient receiving?

Even the "usual" doses of some drugs can cause confusion in the elderly because of alterations in intestinal, renal, or hepatic blood flow; drug protein binding; or changes in body fluid compartments.

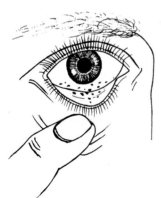
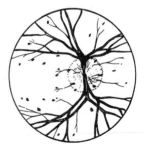

Figure 8–1 Conjunctival and fundal petechiae seen in fat embolism syndrome.

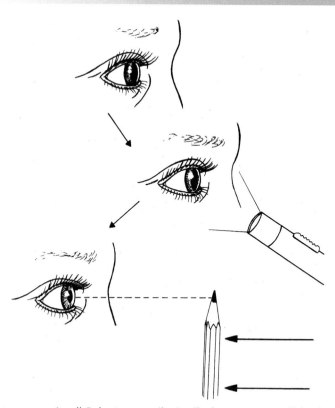

Figure 8–2 Argyll Robertson pupils. Pupils do not react to light, but they accommodate.

Is there a history of alcohol abuse?

It is important to establish when alcohol was last ingested, because withdrawal symptoms are unlikely after 1 week of abstinence.

Is the patient postoperative?

Postoperative patients are predisposed to confusion because of central nervous system (CNS) effects of anesthetic and analgesic medications, nutritional deficiencies (e.g., thiamine), and fluid and electrolyte disturbances. These physiologic abnormalities may be exacerbated in an elderly patient because of sensory impairment (reduced visual or auditory acuity), psychological factors, and cultural expectations.

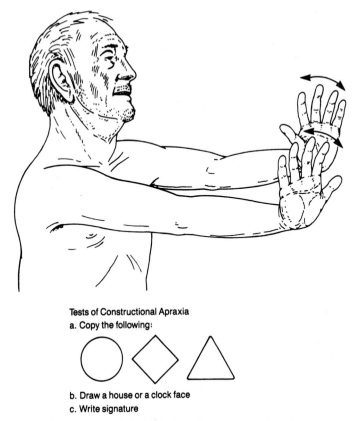

Tests of Constructional Apraxia
a. Copy the following:

b. Draw a house or a clock face
c. Write signature

Figure 8–3 *Top,* Asterixis. Wrist flapping is seen when the arms are outstretched. *Bottom,* Tests of constructional apraxia.

If there is a decreased level of consciousness, was the change gradual or sudden?

A sudden decrease in the level of consciousness is usually due to drug ingestion or an acute intracranial catastrophe (hemorrhage, trauma). Gradually developing unresponsiveness (over days or weeks) is usually due to a preceding systemic medical disorder (e.g., metabolic or endocrine disorders, hepatic or renal failure).

Does the patient have acquired immunodeficiency syndrome (AIDS)?

Human immunodeficiency virus (HIV) infection may result in cognitive impairment in an otherwise asymptomatic patient with AIDS. Patients in the more advanced stages of AIDS may suffer a wide variety of neurologic problems associated with confusion, including HIV-1–associated cognitive-motor complex (impaired concentration, slowness of hand movements, and difficulty walking), CNS opportunistic infections (e.g., toxoplasmosis, cryptococcal meningitis), and neoplasms (e.g., primary lymphoma of the brain).

Examine the most recent laboratory test results for those that may indicate the reason for confusion in the patient. Not all the tests listed will be available or pertinent.

- Blood glucose (hypoglycemia, hyperglycemia)
- Urea, creatinine (renal failure)
- Liver function (liver failure)
- Sodium (hyponatremia, hypernatremia)
- Calcium (hypercalcemia)
- Hemoglobin (Hb), mean corpuscular volume (MCV), red blood cell (RBC) morphology (anemia with oval macrocytes suggests vitamin B_{12} or folate deficiency)
- White blood cell count (WBC) and differential (infection)
- Arterial blood gases (ABG) (hypoxia or CO_2 retention)
- Thyroxine (T_4), triiodothyronine (T_3), thyroid-stimulating hormone (TSH) (hyperthyroidism, hypothyroidism)
- Antinuclear antibody (ANA), rheumatoid factor, erythrocyte sedimentation rate (ESR), C3, C4 (vasculitis)
- Drug levels (digoxin, lithium, aspirin, antiepileptic drugs)

Management II

Drugs. If the confusion is secondary to drugs, stop the medication.

If reversal of postoperative narcotic depression is indicated, give *naloxone* (Narcan) 0.2 to 2 mg IV, IM, or SC every 5 minutes (maximum total dose, 10 mg) until the desired improved level of consciousness is achieved. Maintenance doses every 1 to 2 hours may be required to maintain reversal of the CNS depression. Naloxone should be used with caution in patients known to be physically dependent on opiates.

Reversal of the benzodiazepine effect can be achieved by administering *flumazenil* (Romazicon) 0.2 mg IV over 15 seconds. Wait 1 minute. If ineffective, this may be followed by additional doses of 0.2 mg IV every 60 seconds to a maximum dose of 1 mg. If the patient becomes resedated, this regimen may be repeated again in 20 minutes. No more than 3 mg total dose should be given in 1 hour. The effect of flumazenil on respiratory depression caused by benzodiazepines is inconsistent. Also, reversal of benzodiazepine effect may be associated with seizures. Flumazenil is contraindicated in cyclic antidepressant overdose because of an increased risk of seizures. Its duration of action is relatively short, so overdose cases must be monitored for resedation.

Dementia. Dementia is a diagnosis of exclusion. The following investigations are required to rule out a treatable cause of dementia:

- Complete blood cell count (CBC), electrolytes, urea, creatinine
- Calcium, phosphorus

- Serum bilirubin (liver disease)
- Serum vitamin B_{12}, folate
- T_4, T_3, TSH
- Serologic test for syphilis (STS)
- CT or magnetic resonance imaging (MRI) head scan

Renal and Hepatic Failure. In *end-stage* kidney and liver failure, ensure that the problem has not been compounded by hepatotoxic or nephrotoxic medications. Aggressive treatment of the kidney failure (dialysis, if necessary) or liver failure (lactulose, neomycin) should be undertaken when indicated.

Hyponatremia or Hypernatremia. For the management of hyponatremia or hypernatremia, refer to Chapter 34.

Hypercalcemia. For the management of hypercalcemia, see Chapter 30.

Vitamin B_{12} Deficiency. Suspected vitamin B_{12} deficiency needs to be confirmed with a serum vitamin B_{12} level.

Mania, Depression, or Schizophrenia. Suspected mania, depression, or schizophrenia requires psychiatric consultation for confirmation of diagnosis. Agitation in a confused patient may require *haloperidol* 1 to 5 mg PO or IM every 4 to 6 hours.

Cerebral Vasculitis. Cerebral vasculitis is rare. High-dose steroid therapy is the accepted initial treatment.

Fat Embolism. Fat embolism syndrome can have a mortality rate of up to 8%. The mainstay of treatment is oxygen therapy. If the patient requires an FIO_2 of >0.5, transfer to the intensive care or cardiac care unit for probable intubation and mechanical ventilation with postive end-expiratory pressure (PEEP) is recommended.

Decreased Urine Output

Decreased urine output is a problem frequently seen on both medical and surgical services. Proper management of these patients calls on your skills in assessing volume status.

PHONE CALL

Questions

1. **How much urine has been passed in the last 24 hours?**
   Urine output of <400 mL/day (<20 mL/hr) is *oliguria*. *Anuria* suggests a mechanical obstruction of the bladder outlet or a blocked Foley catheter.
2. **What are the vital signs?**
3. **What was the reason for admission?**
4. **Is the patient complaining of abdominal pain?**
   Abdominal pain is a clue to the possible presence of a distended bladder, as may be seen with bladder outlet obstruction.
5. **Does the patient have a Foley catheter?**
   If the patient has a Foley catheter in place, the assessment of urine output can usually be assumed to be accurate. If not, you will have to ensure that the total volume of voided urine has been collected and measured.
6. **What is the most recent serum potassium level?**

Orders

1. If a Foley catheter is in place and the patient is anuric, ask the nurse to flush the catheter with 20 to 30 mL normal saline (NS) to ensure patency.
   A Foley catheter clogged with sediment is a common problem and a satisfying one to treat before beginning a more detailed investigation for decreased urine output.
2. Obtain serum electrolytes, urea, creatinine.
   A serum potassium level of >5.5 mmol/L indicates that hyperkalemia is present. This is the most serious complication of renal insufficiency. A serum HCO_3 measurement of <20 mmol/L

suggests metabolic acidosis due to renal insufficiency. A serum HCO_3 of <15 mmol/L should prompt you to determine the arterial pH. Elevations in serum urea and creatinine levels can be used as guidelines to assess the degree of renal insufficiency present.

Inform RN

"I will arrive at the bedside in . . . minutes."

Provided that the patient is not in pain and that a recent serum potassium level is not elevated, an assessment of decreased urine output can wait 1 or 2 hours if other problems of higher priority exist.

ELEVATOR THOUGHTS

What causes decreased urine output?

Prerenal Causes (Underperfusion of Kidney)

1. Volume depletion
2. Reduced cardiac output (congestive heart failure [CHF], constrictive pericarditis, cardiac tamponade)
3. Drugs that reduce effective glomerular perfusion (diuretics, angiotensin-converting enzyme inhibitors, nonsteroidal anti-inflammatory drugs [NSAIDs], cyclosporine)
4. Hepatorenal syndrome

Renal Causes

1. Glomerulonephritic syndromes (acute glomerulonephritis, subacute bacterial endocarditis [SBE], systemic lupus erythematosus [SLE], other vasculitides)
2. Tubulointerstitial problems
   a. Acute tubular necrosis due to
      (1) Hypotension
      (2) Nephrotoxins
         (a) Exogenous (aminoglycosides, amphotericin B, IV contrast materials, chemotherapy)
         (b) Endogenous (myoglobin, uric acid, oxalate, amyloid, Bence Jones protein)
   b. Acute interstitial nephritis due to drugs (penicillin, other beta-lactam antibiotics, NSAIDs, diuretics), autoimmune disease (e.g., SLE), infiltrative disease, infection
3. Vascular problems
   a. Emboli (from aortic atheroma, SBE, left heart thrombi)
   b. Renal artery thrombosis

Postrenal Causes

1. Bilateral ureteric obstruction (e.g., stones, clots, sloughed papillae, retroperitoneal fibrosis, retroperitoneal tumor)

2. Bladder outlet obstruction (e.g., prostatic hypertrophy, carcinoma of the cervix, stones, clots, urethral strictures)
3. Blocked Foley catheter

MAJOR THREAT TO LIFE

- Renal failure
- Hyperkalemia

Decreased urine output from any cause may result in or be a manifestation of progressive renal insufficiency, leading to renal failure. Of the complications of renal failure, hyperkalemia is the most immediately life threatening because it can lead to potentially fatal cardiac dysrhythmias.

BEDSIDE

Quick-Look Test

Does the patient look well (comfortable), sick (uncomfortable or distressed), or critical (about to die)?

A sick- or critical-looking patient suggests advanced renal insufficiency. A restless patient suggests pain from a distended bladder. However, both of these conditions can be present in a patient who appears to be deceptively well.

Airway and Vital Signs

Check for postural changes.

A postural rise in heart rate of >15 beats/min, a fall in systolic blood pressure (BP) of >15 mm Hg, or any fall in diastolic BP suggests significant hypovolemia. *Caution:* A resting tachycardia alone may indicate decreased intravascular volume. Fever suggests concomitant urinary tract infection.

Selective Physical Examination I

Examine for *prerenal* (volume status), *renal*, or *postrenal* (obstructive) causes of decreased urine output. *Caution:* More than one cause may be present.

HEENT	Jaundice (hepatorenal syndrome)
	Facial purpura ⎫ Amyloidosis
	Enlarged tongue ⎭
Resp	Crackles, pleural effusions (CHF)
CVS	Pulse volume, JVP
	Skin temperature and color
ABD	Enlarged kidneys (hydronephrosis secondary to obstruction, polycystic kidney disease)
	Enlarged bladder (bladder outlet obstruction, neurogenic bladder, blocked Foley catheter)

Rectal	Enlarged prostate gland (bladder outlet obstruction)
Pelvic	Cervical or adnexal masses (ureteric obstruction secondary to cervical or ovarian cancer)
Skin	Morbilliform rash (acute interstitial nephritis)
	Livedo reticularis on lower extremities (atheromatous embolic renal failure)

Selective Chart Review

- Review the patient's history and hospital course, looking specifically for factors that may predispose to prerenal, renal, or postrenal causes of decreased urine output (see Elevator Thoughts).
- Look for recent blood urea and creatinine values.

  A creatinine-to-urea ratio of <12 suggests a prerenal cause. A urine specific gravity of >1.020 or urine sodium concentration of <20 mmol/L also suggests a prerenal cause.

- Look for specific combinations of factors that may predispose to renal failure, such as a patient receiving both angiotensin-converting enzyme inhibitors and diuretics, aminoglycosides in a septic patient, IV contrast material in a patient receiving an angiotensin-converting enzyme inhibitor, or a patient with CHF who was given an NSAID.[1]

Management I

Your job becomes simpler when you can find a *prerenal* or *postrenal* cause for decreased urine output.

Prerenal. First ensure that the intravascular volume is normal. If the patient is in CHF, initiate diuresis, as discussed in Chapter 24, pages 270 to 272. If the patient is volume depleted, replenish the intravascular volume with NS. Do not add a potassium supplement to the IV solution until the patient passes urine. Do not give Ringer's lactate because it contains potassium.

Postrenal. Lower urinary tract obstruction can be adequately excluded by passage of a Foley catheter into the bladder.

1. If there has been bladder outlet obstruction, the initial urine volume on catheterization is usually >400 mL, and the patient experiences immediate relief.

   Remember to listen carefully for heart murmurs before catheterizing the patient. If there is documented evidence of a cardiac valvular abnormality requiring bacterial endocarditis prophylaxis, refer to Chapter 21, pages 244 to 245.

   After catheterization, watch for the development of postobstructive diuresis by monitoring urine volume status carefully for the next few days.

2. If a Foley catheter is already in place, ensure that flushing the catheter with 20 to 30 mL of NS allows free flow of fluid from the bladder. This maneuver excludes an intraluminal blockage of the Foley catheter as a cause of postrenal obstruction.

3. The presence of a Foley catheter in the bladder rules out only lower urinary tract obstruction. If the preceding two steps fail to restore urine output, a *renal ultrasound* examination should be ordered first thing in the morning to exclude upper urinary tract obstruction. Although bilateral ureteric obstruction is rare, additional useful information, such as documentation of the presence of both kidneys and an estimate of renal size, may be obtained.

Renal. If prerenal and postrenal factors are not causing the patient's decreased urine output, you are left in the murky waters of renal causes. A search for the renal causes of decreased urine output can wait until some additional important questions are answered (see Management II).

Management II

Regardless of the cause of decreased urine output (prerenal, renal, or postrenal), you must now answer the following four questions.
1. Are any of the following five life-threatening complications of decreased urine output present?
   a. Hyperkalemia (the most immediately serious problem)
      (1) Order a stat serum potassium level, if not already done.
      (2) Review the chart for a recent serum potassium level.
      (3) Order a stat electrocardiogram (ECG) if suspicion of hyperkalemia exists.
         > Peaked T waves are early signs of hyperkalemia (Fig. 9–1). More advanced ECG manifestations include depressed ST segments, prolonged PR intervals, loss of P waves, and wide QRS complexes.
      (4) Discontinue any potassium supplements.
      (5) Treat as outlined in Chapter 33, pages 358 to 359.
   b. CHF—suggested by tachypnea, elevated jugular venous pressure (JVP), crackles on pulmonary auscultation, an S_3, and sacral or pedal edema. Refer to Chapter 24, pages 270 to 272, for management of CHF.
   c. Severe metabolic acidemia (pH <7.2)—suggested by the presence of (compensatory) hyperventilation and confirmed by arterial blood gas (ABG) measurement. Investigation should take place as outlined in Chapter 28, page 315.
   d. Uremic encephalopathy—manifests as confusion, stupor, or seizures and is managed by dialysis. If seizures occur, they should be managed as outlined in Chapter 23 until dialysis can be initiated.
   e. Uremic pericarditis—suggested by the presence of pleuritic chest pain, pericardial friction rub, or diffuse ST segment elevation on the ECG. It is managed best with dialysis.

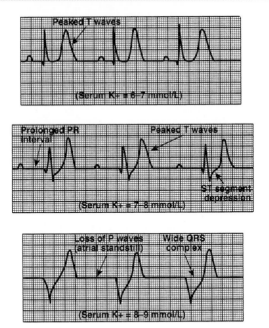

Figure 9–1 Progressive electrocardiographic features of hyperkalemia.

2. Is the patient receiving any drugs that may worsen the situation?
   a. Potassium supplements
   b. Potassium-sparing diuretics (spironolactone, triamterene, amiloride)
   c. Nephrotoxic drugs (NSAIDs, aminoglycosides)
   Review the need for these agents and discontinue immediately if possible. If aminoglycosides are required, doses will need to be adjusted based on serum levels.
3. Is the patient in oliguric renal failure?
   If the patient's urine production is <480 mL/day (<20 mL/hr), he or she has oliguric renal failure. Although this has a higher mortality rate than nonoliguric renal failure, there is little evidence to support efforts to convert oliguric to nonoliguric renal failure through the aggressive use of diuretics. In fact, diuretics may worsen the situation if the renal failure has been caused by IV contrast agents.[2] In general, loop diuretics should be used in this situation only if there is coexisting CHF.

4. Does the patient need dialysis?
  a. If the patient does not pass urine despite high doses of diuretics, the indications for urgent dialysis are as follows:
    (1) Hyperkalemia
    (2) CHF
    (3) Metabolic acidemia (pH <7.2)
    (4) Severe uremia (urea level >35 mmol/L; creatinine level >800 mmol/L) ± uremic seizures
    (5) Uremic pericarditis
  b. If the patient is in renal failure and if one or more of these conditions are present, request an urgent nephrology consultation to dialyze the patient. While awaiting the nephrologist's arrival, all of the following problems can be treated temporarily with nondialysis measures:
    (1) Hyperkalemia—glucose with insulin infusion, $NaHCO_3$, calcium, sodium polystyrene sulfonate (refer to Chapter 33).
    (2) CHF—preload measures (sit the patient up, morphine, nitroglycerin ointment); give O_2 (refer to Chapter 24, pages 270 to 272).
    (3) Metabolic acidemia—$NaHCO_3$ (refer to Chapter 28, page 315, for assessment of metabolic acidosis).
    (4) Uremic encephalopathy—keep the patient calm and at bed rest until dialysis can be initiated.
    (5) Uremic pericarditis—treat symptomatically for pain with an NSAID until dialysis can be initiated.

Once these questions have been addressed, you can sit down and think about possible *renal causes* of decreased urine output. The majority of renal causes are diagnosed by history, physical examination, and laboratory findings. Occasionally, a renal biopsy is required. A simple urinalysis can often provide valuable clues to the diagnosis.

- Urine dipstick
  Hematuria and proteinuria together suggest *glomerulonephritis*. A positive orthotoluidine test for blood may represent red blood cells (RBCs), free hemoglobin, or myoglobin. Suspect *rhabdomyolysis* if there is a positive orthotoluidine test result on dipstick but few or no RBCs on urine microscopy. (In this case, order tests for serum levels of creatine phosphokinase [CPK], calcium, and PO_4 and urine levels of myoglobin.)
  A positive test result for urinary protein alone should prompt you to do a serum albumin and 24-hour urine collection for protein and creatinine clearance to identify the *nephrotic syndrome*, if present.
- Urine microscopy
  RBC casts are diagnostic of *glomerulonephritis*. White blood cell casts, particularly eosinophil casts, may be seen in cases of *acute interstitial nephritis*. Pigmented granular casts may be seen

with *acute tubular necrosis*. Oval fat bodies are suggestive of *nephrotic syndrome*.

- Urine for eosinophils
  Ask for this test if there is a suspicion of *acute interstitial nephritis*.

In most cases, beyond these simple tests, no further investigation is required at night. For any suspected *renal* cause of decreased urine output, however, ensure that prerenal and postrenal factors are not additional contributors to the poor urine output.

REMEMBER

All medications that the oliguric or anuric patient is receiving should be reviewed, and any potential nephrotoxins should be discontinued. Many drugs depend on renal excretion and may require dosage adjustment. If you are uncertain about the route of excretion of a drug that has been ordered for a patient, it may be safest to discontinue the drug until you find out.

References

1. Thadhani R, Pascual M, Bonventre JV: Acute renal failure. N Engl J Med 1996;334:1448-1460.
2. Solomon R, Werner C, Mann D, et al: Effects of saline, mannitol, and furosemide on acute decreases in renal function induced by radiocontrast agents. N Engl J Med 1994;331:1416-1420.

Diarrhea

Avoid treating diarrhea as a diagnosis. Diarrhea is always a symptom of another underlying disorder and seldom warrants nonspecific "antimotility therapy." Your job at night is to determine the likely cause of the diarrhea, whether additional investigations should be performed, and whether complications have arisen that require treatment.

PHONE CALL

Questions

1. What are the vital signs?
2. What was the reason for admission?
3. Is this a new problem? If not, has the cause of the diarrhea been diagnosed?
4. Has the patient had recent surgery?
5. Is the patient HIV positive?
6. Is there blood, pus, or mucus in the stool?

    Bloody stools with pus or mucus suggest inflammation, as may be seen with infection, inflammatory bowel disease, or ischemic colitis.

7. Does the patient have abdominal pain?

    Moderate or severe abdominal pain suggests ischemic colitis, diverticulitis, or inflammatory bowel disease.

Orders

None.

Inform RN

"I will arrive at the bedside in . . . minutes."

A single episode of diarrhea in an otherwise well patient does not usually require bedside assessment. If the diarrhea is frequent, severe, or associated with the passage of blood, the patient should be evaluated at the bedside as soon as possible. If the patient is hypotensive, tachycardic, or febrile, he or she should be assessed immediately.

ELEVATOR THOUGHTS

What causes diarrhea?

Acute Diarrhea (<2 Weeks' Duration)

"THE FOUR I'S"

Infection	Inflammation and toxins (Table 10–1)
Iatrogenic	Drugs (laxatives, stool softeners, magnesium-containing antacids, sorbitol-containing liquid dosage forms, digoxin, quinidine, colchicine, and xanthines) and surgery (gastrectomy, vagotomy, cholecystectomy, intestinal resection)
Ischemia	Mesenteric thrombosis, vascular embolus to the mesenteric artery, volvulus
Impaction	Fecal impaction

Chronic Diarrhea (>2 Weeks' Duration)

"THE FIVE I'S AND TWO M'S"

Infection	Amebiasis, giardiasis, *Clostridium difficile*
Inflammatory bowel disease	Ulcerative colitis, Crohn's disease, collagenous colitis, lymphocytic colitis, radiation enteritis or colitis
Infiltrative disorders	Amyloid, lymphoma
Irritable bowel syndrome	
Intake	Laxative abuse, caffeine, sweeteners (sorbitol, fructose, xylitol)
Malabsorption	Celiac disease, short bowel syndrome, bacterial overgrowth
Metabolic/hormonal	Enzyme deficiencies (lactase deficiency, pancreatic insufficiency)
	Hormone production (gastrinoma, carcinoid, VIPoma, villous adenoma, medullary carcinoma of the thyroid)
	Endocrinopathies (diabetic diarrhea, hyperthyroidism, Addison's disease)

Any of the causes of acute diarrhea, if left untreated, may cause chronic diarrhea.

MAJOR THREAT TO LIFE

- Intravascular volume depletion; electrolyte imbalance
- Systemic infection

Volume depletion and *electrolyte disturbances* are the reasons that many children in underdeveloped countries die from diarrhea.

TABLE 10–1 Etiologic Agents in Infectious Diarrhea

Inflammatory

Bacteria

Salmonella spp.
Shigella spp.
Campylobacter spp.
Yersinia enterocolitica
Vibrio parahaemolyticus (uncooked shellfish)
Plesiomonas shigelloides (uncooked shellfish)
Aeromonas hydrophila (untreated well water, brackish water)
*Mycobacterium avium-intracellulare**
*Mycobacterium tuberculosis**
*Chlamydia**
Escherichia coli[†]

Viruses

Norwalk virus
Rotavirus
Cytomegalovirus*
Herpes simplex*
Epstein-Barr virus*
HIV enteropathy*

Nematode

*Strongyloides stercoralis**

Protozoa

*Entamoeba histolytica**
*Giardia lamblia**
Cryptosporidium spp.*
*Isospora belli**
Enterocytozoon bieneusi (Microsporida)*
Cyclospora spp.*

Toxins

Toxins Produced in Vivo

Clostridium difficile (after antibiotic administration)
Clostridium perfringens (beef, poultry)
Vibrio cholerae
Bacillus cereus (fried rice)
Enterotoxigenic *E. coli* (hamburger)[†]

Preformed Toxins

Staphylococcus aureus (potato salad, mayonnaise, pudding)
Bacillus cereus (fried rice)

---

*Prevalent in HIV-positive patients.
[†]Enteroinvasive, enterohemorrhagic, and enteroaggregative *E. coli* strains produce an inflammatory diarrheal illness. Enteropathogenic *E. coli* produces a noninflammatory diarrheal illness by attachment to the intestinal brush border, resulting in a disaccharidase deficiency and loss of absorptive surface. Enterotoxigenic *E. coli* attaches to the small intestinal mucosa and produces toxins that result in a secretory diarrhea.[1]

HIV, human immunodeficiency virus.

This is seldom seen in hospitalized adult patients, but if left untreated, diarrhea can certainly progress to serious volume depletion and electrolyte imbalance. Some bacterial causes of diarrhea, if left untreated, may become *systemic* life-threatening disorders.

BEDSIDE

Quick-Look Test

Does the patient look well (comfortable), sick (uncomfortable or distressed), or critical (about to die)?

Most patients with acute diarrhea do not look unwell. However, if the diarrhea is due to an invasive organism (e.g., *Salmonella, Shigella*), the patient may look sick and complain of headache, diffuse myalgia, chills, and fever.

Airway and Vital Signs

What is the blood pressure (BP)?

Resting hypotension suggests significant volume depletion. If the resting BP is normal, examine for postural changes. A postural rise in heart rate (HR) of >15 beats/min, a fall in systolic BP of >15 mm Hg, or any fall in diastolic BP indicates significant hypovolemia.

What is the HR?

Intravascular volume depletion usually results in tachycardia unless the patient has a coexisting disorder (e.g., autonomic dysfunction due to beta blockade, sick sinus syndrome [SSS], or autonomic neuropathy) that prevents the generation of a tachycardia. However, in diarrheal diseases, tachycardia may also be due to anxiety, pain, or fever. A relative bradycardia despite fever raises the suspicion of *Salmonella* infection.

What is the temperature?

Fever in a patient with diarrhea is nonspecific but suggests the presence of inflammation, as may be seen with infectious diarrhea, diverticulitis, inflammatory bowel disease, intestinal lymphoma, tuberculosis, and amebiasis. Some organisms (*Shigella* and *Salmonella* spp.) may cause systemic sepsis. However, remember that sepsis may occur in the absence of fever, especially in the elderly.

Selective Physical Examination I

Is the patient volume depleted? Is there evidence of systemic sepsis?

Vitals	(See above)
CVS	Pulse volume, JVP (flat neck veins)
	Skin temperature, color

Management I

What immediate measures need to be taken to correct intravascular volume depletion?

1. Normalize the intravascular volume. This can be achieved quickly by administering an IV fluid that remains in the intravascular space at least temporarily, such as normal saline (NS) or Ringer's lactate. Give NS 250 to 500 mL IV over 1 to 2 hours, titrating the IV fluid to the patient's vital signs and jugular venous pressure (JVP). Reassess the volume status after each bolus of IV fluid, aiming for a JVP of 2 to 3 cm H_2O above the sternal angle and concomitant normalization of HR and BP.
2. Check the chart for a recent electrolyte determination. If the patient has not had electrolytes checked within the last 24 hours, order serum electrolytes, urea, and creatinine levels now.
3. In a patient with fever >38.5°C, two sets of blood cultures should be drawn. If the patient is also hypotensive, volume replacement should be instituted with NS, and consideration should be given to empirical antibiotic coverage (see Chapter 12, page 97).
4. A rectal examination should be performed and stool samples sent for occult blood, culture, ova and parasite determination, *Clostridium difficile* toxin, and white blood cell (WBC) stain. If unusual organisms are suspected (e.g., in an acquired immunodeficiency syndrome [AIDS] patient), the laboratory should be alerted so that appropriate culture techniques and media can be used.

Selective Chart Review

Are potential causes of diarrhea apparent from the chart?

Is the patient on any medications that may cause diarrhea?

Medications are the most common cause of diarrhea in the hospital. Frequent offenders include laxatives, stool softeners, magnesium-containing antacids, sorbitol-containing liquid dosage forms, digoxin, quinidine, colchicine, and xanthines. Laxatives and stool softeners should be discontinued. Magnesium-containing antacids may be withheld or switched to aluminum-containing preparations. Do not discontinue other medications without first asking your resident or attending physician. Remember, also, that some medications (e.g., Anacin, Dristan, Dyazide) contain gluten, which is relevant in a patient with celiac disease.

Has the patient received antibiotics recently?

Many antibiotics cause transient diarrhea through alteration of the intestinal flora. In addition, *pseudomembranous colitis* due to

C. difficile enterotoxin may result in persistent diarrhea during or after antibiotic use. Diagnosis is usually made using an enzyme-linked immunoassay (ELISA), which has a sensitivity of 85% and a specificity of 100%.[2] Treatment includes discontinuing the offending antibiotic and administering *metronidazole* 500 mg PO every 6 hours for 10 to 14 days. *Vancomycin* 125 to 500 mg PO every 6 hours for 10 to 14 days is an alternative therapy, but it is more expensive and no more effective than metronidazole.

Does the patient have AIDS?

Immunocompromised patients and patients with AIDS may develop diarrhea for many reasons, including infections due to a variety of pathogens, medications (especially protease inhibitors), and AIDS enteropathy. The most common infectious causes include *Cryptosporidium, Microsporidium, Mycobacterium avium-intracellulare, Salmonella, Shigella,* and *Cytomegalovirus.* If this is the first documented episode of diarrhea, stool samples should be sent for acid-fast stain, WBC stain, bacterial and mycobacterial culture, and ova and parasite determination. The test with the highest yield is microscopic examination with a search for ova and parasites. The correct transport medium must be used for specific pathogen cultures, and laboratories often require identification of the possible pathogens, such as *Cryptosporidum, Yersinia, Aeromonas,* and *Escherichia coli* 0157, in order to select the most appropriate laboratory techniques. Diagnosis of anorectal infections may require proctoscopy or sigmoidoscopy, with specimens taken for gonorrhea, herpes simplex viral culture, and dark-field examination for syphilis; this can be arranged in the morning.

Has the patient had recent surgery?

Postgastrectomy dumping of hypertonic boluses of stomach contents into the jejunum is associated with vasomotor symptoms of flushing, anxiety, palpitations, sweating, and dizziness, and there may be associated diarrhea. Resections of the ileum and right colon may result in diarrhea due to bile acid malabsorption.

Does the patient have known inflammatory bowel disease, celiac disease, lactase deficiency, or other conditions known to cause chronic diarrhea?

Has there been recent travel abroad?

E. coli enterotoxin is the most common cause of "traveler's diarrhea," although *Salmonella* spp., *Shigella* spp., and *Campylobacter jejuni* may be responsible for some cases of acute, self-limited traveler's diarrhea. Giardiasis, amebiasis, and tropical sprue may cause a more chronic picture.

Has the patient been admitted for the investigation of diarrhea?

If so, a plan of investigation has probably already been outlined. If the patient is not volume depleted and is otherwise comfortable, no additional measures are required at night.

Is the patient receiving tube feedings?

Diarrhea often complicates enteral tube feedings, but in many cases it is due to factors other than the feeding formula itself, such as medications or underlying illnesses. Occasionally, diarrhea may develop because of the formula's composition (e.g., high fat, high osmolarity, presence of lactose), the manner in which it is delivered (bolus versus continuous infusion), or contamination of the formula.[3] In most cases, decisions regarding a change in formula or in the manner or rate of delivery can wait until morning.

Selective Physical Examination II

Look for clues to specific causes of diarrhea.

Vitals	Repeat now
HEENT	Lymphadenopathy (lymphoma, Whipple's disease, AIDS)
ABD	Surgical scars (gastrectomy, cholecystectomy, intestinal resection)
	Hepatosplenomegaly (*Salmonella* infection)
	Epigastric tenderness (Zollinger-Ellison syndrome)
	RLQ mass or tenderness (Crohn's disease, ischemic colitis)
	LLQ mass or tenderness (diverticulitis, tumor, inflammatory bowel disease, ischemic colitis, fecal impaction)
Rectal	Rectal fissure (Crohn's disease)
	Hard mass (fecal impaction, tumor)
	Fresh blood or stool positive for occult blood (inflammatory bowel disease, infection, tumor)
MSS	Arthritis (inflammatory bowel disease, Whipple's disease)
Skin	Rose spots (*Salmonella* infection)
	Dermatitis herpetiformis (celiac disease)
	Pyoderma gangrenosum (Crohn's disease)
	Hyperpigmentation (Whipple's, Addison's, or celiac disease)
	Flushing (carcinoid)

Management II

It is unusual to be able to pinpoint the specific cause of diarrhea when seeing a patient for the first time at night. Occasionally a patient will say, "I'm sure it's my Crohn's disease acting up," or "I have lactose intolerance and the kitchen gave me yogurt for dinner." In these cases, the patient usually turns out to be right. When the diagnosis is not obvious at night, your goals are to ensure that the patient is adequately hydrated, does not have a serious electrolyte imbalance, and does not have a systemic infection. Additional specialized investigations for diarrhea can, in most cases, wait until the morning to be arranged.

Remember, in many cases of infectious diarrhea, frequent loose stools are the body's way of expelling the offending organism or toxin. Do not compound the problem by inhibiting the body's ability to do this. Diarrhea is always best treated by addressing the underlying cause, which may take a few days (and sometimes weeks) to identify. Unless the diarrhea is profuse or disabling, nonspecific antidiarrheal agents are best avoided. Explain this to the patient and to the nurses caring for him or her so that everyone is clear about the treatment approach.

If the patient's diarrhea is severe and disabling, use of *one* of the nonspecific antidiarrheal agents listed below is occasionally warranted. However, none of these agents should be prescribed before you examine the patient (including a rectal examination and possibly sigmoidoscopy) and decide on an appropriate plan of investigation.

Loperamide (Imodium) 4 mg PO every 4 hours until diarrhea is controlled, to a maximum dose of 16 mg in 24 hours. The drug is less effective if given on an as-needed basis (PRN). Side effects include dry mouth, abdominal distention and cramping, occasionally nausea and vomiting, and rarely toxic megacolon. Other side effects include rash, drowsiness, dizziness, and tiredness.

Diphenoxylate hydrochloride (Lomotil) 5 mg PO three or four times a day until diarrhea is controlled, to a maximum dose of 20 mg in 24 hours. It is as effective as loperamide for treating acute nonspecific diarrhea but has a slower onset of antidiarrheal action. Diphenoxylate is contraindicated in patients with hepatic failure or cirrhosis. Respiratory depression may occur when it is used in combination with phenothiazines, tricyclic antidepressants, or barbiturates. Toxic megacolon may result if ulcerative colitis is present.

Bismuth subsalicylate (Pepto-Bismol) 30 mL or 2 tablets (262 mg/tablet) PO every 30 minutes, to a maximum of eight doses per day. Blackening of the tongue and stools is known to occur. It may inhibit the absorption of tetracycline. Salicylate overdose may occur, especially if the patient is also receiving aspirin.

Agents such as anticholinergics, kaolin, and pectin do not reduce fecal water loss in diarrheal illnesses and are best avoided.

References

1. Hart CA, Batt RM, Saunders JR: Diarrhea caused by *Escherichia coli*. Ann Trop Paediatr 1993;13:121-131.
2. Hurley BW, Nguyen CC: The spectrum of pseudomembranous enterocolitis and antibiotic-associated diarrhea. Ann Intern Med 2002;162:2177-2184.
3. Eisenberg PG: Causes of diarrhea in tube-fed patients: A comprehensive approach to diagnosis and management. Nutr Clin Pract 1993;8:3.

Fall Out of Bed

Patients always seem to be falling out of bed, but they can fall while in other places, too. This chapter applies to any fall occurring in the patient's room or elsewhere in the hospital.

PHONE CALL

Questions

1. Was the fall witnessed?
2. Is there an obvious injury?
3. What are the vital signs?
4. Has there been a change in the level of consciousness?
5. Is the patient receiving anticoagulant, antineoplastic, or other drugs affecting coagulation, or antiseizure medications?
6. What was the reason for admission?

Orders

Ask the RN to call immediately if the level of consciousness changes before you are able to assess the patient.

Inform RN

"I will arrive at the bedside in . . . minutes."

A change in the level of consciousness, a suspected fracture, or a coagulation disorder requires that you see the patient immediately. However, when other sick patients are in need of assessment, they take priority over a patient who has had an uncomplicated fall.

ELEVATOR THOUGHTS

Why does a patient fall?

Cardiac	Postural hypotension (volume depletion, drugs, autonomic failure)
	Vasovagal attack
	Dysrhythmia
	MI

Neuro	Confusion and cognitive impairment (particularly in the elderly)
	Drugs (narcotics, sedatives, antidepressants, tranquilizers, antihypertensive agents)
	Metabolic disorders (electrolyte abnormalities, renal failure, hepatic failure)
	Dementia (Parkinson's disease, Alzheimer's disease, multi-infarction, normal-pressure hydrocephalus) resulting in poor safety awareness
	Gait and balance disorders
	Visual impairment
	TIA, stroke
	Seizure
Environmental/ accidental	Disorientation at night
	Call bell inaccessible
	Restraints
	Improper bed height
	Wet floors
	Unsafe clothing (e.g., long hospital gowns or pajamas, tractionless slippers)
	Obstacles (e.g., bed rails, IV poles, clutter around bed)

There are many potential environmental hazards in the hospital setting. Elderly persons are particularly prone to accidental falls due to a combination of environmental hazards, poor vision, diminished muscular strength, and impaired righting reflexes.

MAJOR THREAT TO LIFE

- Head injury

  The most remediable critical situation is an acute epidural or subdural bleed. Any patient who may have hit his or her head during a fall requires a complete neurologic examination immediately. Even seemingly minor trauma can result in a serious intracranial bleed in an anticoagulated patient. If a new neurologic problem is identified, an immediate computed tomography (CT) scan of the head may be helpful. Immediate reversal of anticoagulation should be considered and discussed with the resident and a hematologist (see Chapter 31, pages 341 to 342, for reversal of anticoagulation). If no neurologic deficit is identified at this time, observation with frequent assessment of the neurovital signs is required.

BEDSIDE

Quick-Look Test

Does the patient look well (comfortable), sick (uncomfortable or distressed), or critical (about to die)?

Most patients do not have life-threatening problems as a result of falling. Usually, they look well, and the vital signs are normal.

Airway and Vital Signs

What are the heart rate (HR) and rhythm?

Tachycardia, bradycardia, or irregular rhythm may indicate a dysrhythmia as the cause of the fall.

Are there postural (lying and standing) changes in blood pressure (BP) and HR?

A postural fall in BP together with a postural rise in HR (>15 beats/min) suggests volume depletion. A drop in BP without a change in HR suggests autonomic dysfunction. An initial drop in BP that corrects on standing also suggests autonomic dysfunction. Drugs are common causes of postural hypotension in elderly patients, particularly antihypertensive agents, sedatives, and antidepressants.

Selective History

Does the patient know why he or she fell out of bed?

What was the patient doing just before the fall?

Coughing, micturating, or straining are examples of maneuvers that may result in vasovagal syncope. Question any witnesses who observed the fall. Did the patient trip or slip?

Were there any warning symptoms before the fall?

Lightheadedness and visual disturbances on standing may indicate postural hypotension. Palpitations suggest a dysrhythmia. A preceding aura would be rare in this situation but, if present, is highly suggestive of a seizure disorder.

Is there a history of previous falls?

Recurrent falls suggest an underlying disorder that has gone unrecognized. Although your main duty at night is to detect, document, and treat any injuries that have been sustained, a pattern of falling behavior may be an important clue to an unrecognized but treatable disorder.

Is the patient diabetic?

Hyperglycemia or hypoglycemia may cause confusion, contributing to a fall. Order a finger-prick blood glucose (FPBG) reading. Check the diabetic record for the past 3 days.

Is the patient aware of any injury sustained during the fall?

Patients may fracture a wrist or hip as a result of falling. Elderly women are at particular risk because of osteoporosis.

Selective Physical Examination

Look for both the cause and the consequences of the fall.

Vitals	Repeat now—only supine BP and HR are necessary, provided that both supine and standing measurements were already taken
HEENT	Tongue or cheek lacerations (seizure) Hemotympanum (basal skull fracture)
CVS	Pulse rate and rhythm (dysrhythmia) Decreased JVP (volume depletion)
MSS	Palpate skull and face ⎫ Palpate spine and ribs ⎪ Fractures, hematomas, and Palpate long bones ⎬ lacerations Check passive ROM ⎪ of all four limbs ⎭
Neuro	Complete neurologic examination—pay particular attention to level of consciousness and any asymmetrical neurologic findings ⎸New findings of asymmetry suggest structural ⎸brain disease

Selective Chart Review

Search for the cause of the fall.
1. **What was the reason for admission?**
2. **Is there a past history of cardiac dysrhythmia, seizure disorder, autonomic neuropathy, disorientation at night, or diabetes mellitus?**
3. **What drugs is the patient receiving?**
   - Antihypertensive agents
   - Diuretics (volume depletion)
   - Antidysrhythmic agents
   - Antiseizure medications
   - Narcotics
   - Sedatives, tranquilizers
   - Antidepressants
   - Insulin, oral hypoglycemic agents
4. **Check the most recent laboratory results.**
   - Glucose: ↑ or ↓ may cause confusion
   - Na: ↑ or ↓ may cause confusion
   - K: ↑ can cause atrioventricular (AV) block; ↓ can cause weakness or tachydysrhythmias
   - Ca: ↑ causes confusion; ↓ may cause seizures
   - Urea, creatinine (uremia can result in confusion and seizures)

- Antiseizure drug levels (subtherapeutic levels may result in seizure breakthrough; toxic levels may be associated with ataxia)

Management

Treat the Cause. Investigate and treat the suspected cause. A fall is a symptom, not a diagnosis! Establish the reason for the fall (provisional diagnosis). The cause is often multifactorial. For example, diuretic-induced nocturia forces an elderly patient, under the influence of nighttime sedation, to struggle to the bathroom in an unfamiliar, dimly lit hospital room.

Reversible Factors. Reversible factors must be corrected, especially volume depletion and inappropriate drug therapy in the elderly.

Nocturia. The majority of elderly patients who fall out of bed at night are on their way to the bathroom because of nocturia. Make sure that the nocturia is not iatrogenic (e.g., an evening diuretic order or an unnecessary IV infusion).

Elderly Patient. If the patient is disoriented at night, ensure that the call bell is easily accessible, a nightlight is left on, and the evening's fluid intake is limited. The use of physical restraints (poseys and bed rails) may actually contribute to falls and should be discouraged.[1] It is best to leave the side rails down or lower the bed height.

Complications. Are there any complications resulting from the fall, giving rise to a second diagnosis? For example, a stroke patient may have unknowingly dislocated or subluxated his or her shoulder on the paralyzed side during the fall. An anticoagulated patient may develop a serious, delayed hemorrhage at any site of trauma. Reexamine these patients frequently.

Reference

1. Tinetti ME, Liu WL, Ginter SF: Mechanical restraint use and fall-related injuries among residents of skilled nursing facilities. Ann Intern Med 1992;116:369-374.

Fever

It is unusual to spend an entire night on call without being called about a febrile patient. The majority of fevers seen in hospitalized patients are due to infections. Locating the source of a fever usually requires some detective work. Whether the cause of a fever requires specific immediate treatment depends on both the clinical status of the patient and the suspected diagnosis.

PHONE CALL

Questions

1. **How high is the temperature, and by what route was it taken?**

   37°C oral = 37.5°C rectal or 36.5°C axillary.

2. **What are the other vital signs?**

3. **Are there any associated symptoms?**

   Pain may help localize a site of infection or inflammation. A headache, neck ache, seizure, or change in sensorium, together with fever, suggests meningitis or encephalitis.

4. **Is this a "new" fever?**

5. **What was the reason for admission?**

6. **Is this a postoperative patient?**

   Postoperative fever is very common and may be due to atelectasis, pneumonia, pulmonary embolism, wound infection, infected intravenous (IV) sites, or urinary tract infection from a Foley catheter.

Orders

1. If febrile and hypotensive, give 500 mL of normal saline (NS) IV as rapidly as possible.

2. If febrile with meningitis symptoms (headache, neck ache, seizure, or change in sensorium), order a lumbar puncture (LP) tray to the bedside now.

Inform RN

"I will arrive at the bedside in . . . minutes."

An elevated temperature alone is seldom life threatening. However, fever in association with hypotension or meningitis symptoms requires that you see the patient immediately.

ELEVATOR THOUGHTS

What causes fever?

- Infection—by far the most common cause of fever in a hospitalized patient
    Common sites of infection are the lung, urinary tract, wounds, and IV sites. Less common are central nervous system (CNS), abdominal, and pelvic infections. An *immunocompromised patient* is not only predisposed to infection but also more susceptible to serious complications of infection.
- Pulmonary embolism and deep vein thrombosis (DVT)
- Drugs
- Neoplasm
- Connective tissue diseases
- Postoperative atelectasis

MAJOR THREAT TO LIFE

- Septic shock
- Meningitis

Fever is most commonly a manifestation of infection in the hospitalized patient. Most infections can be brought under control by a combination of the body's natural defense mechanisms and judicious antibiotic use. Infection at any site, if progressive, may lead to septicemia with attendant *septic shock*. *Meningitis*, by virtue of its location, can result in permanent neurologic deficit or death if allowed to go untreated.

BEDSIDE

Quick-Look Test

Does the patient look well (comfortable), sick (uncomfortable or distressed), or critical (about to die)?
    Toxic signs, such as apprehension, agitation, or lethargy, suggest serious infection.

Airway and Vital Signs

What is the heart rate (HR)?
    Tachycardia, proportionate to the temperature elevation, is an expected finding in a febrile patient. Normally, the HR rises by 16 beats/min for each degree Celsius of temperature rise.

A relative bradycardia in a febrile patient has been observed in *Legionella* pneumonia, *Mycoplasma pneumoniae* pneumonia, ascending cholangitis, typhoid fever, and *Plasmodium falciparum* malaria with profound hemolysis.

What is the blood pressure (BP)?

Fever in association with supine or postural hypotension indicates relative hypovolemia and can be the forerunner of septic shock. Ensure that an IV line is in place. Infuse NS or Ringer's lactate to correct the intravascular volume deficit.

Selective Physical Examination I

What is the volume status? Is the patient in septic shock? Are there signs of meningitis?

Vitals	Repeat now
HEENT	Photophobia, neck stiffness
CVS	Pulse volume, JVP
	Skin temperature, color
Neuro	Change in sensorium
	Special maneuvers

> *Brudzinski's sign:* With the patient supine, passively flex the neck forward; flexion of the patient's hips and knees in response to this maneuver constitutes a positive test result (see Fig. 14–3*A*)
>
> *Kernig's sign:* With the patient supine, flex one hip and knee to 90 degrees, then straighten the knee; pain or resistance in the ipsilateral hamstrings constitutes a positive test result (see Fig. 14–3*B*)

Septic shock is a clinical diagnosis consisting of two states. Early in the development of septic shock, the patient may be warm, dry, and flushed because of peripheral vasodilatation and increased cardiac output (*warm shock*). As septic shock progresses, the patient becomes hypotensive, and the skin becomes cool and clammy (*cold shock*) as a result of peripheral vasoconstriction. Serious delays in treatment may result from failure to recognize the first state.

Fever in an elderly patient, regardless of cause, can produce changes in sensorium ranging from lethargy to agitation. If a specific site of infection is not obvious, an LP should be performed to rule out meningitis (see pages 97 to 98).

Management I

What immediate measures need to be taken to prevent septic shock or to recognize meningitis?

Septic Shock

If the patient is febrile and hypotensive, determine the volume status and give IV fluids (NS or Ringer's lactate) promptly until the volume status returns to normal.

> *Caution:* Aggressive volume repletion in a patient with a history of congestive heart failure (CHF) may compromise cardiac function. Do not overshoot the mark!

While IV fluid resuscitation is taking place, obtain samples for necessary cultures, usually including blood from two different sites, urine (for Gram stain and culture), sputum, and any other potentially infected body fluid.

Septic shock is a major threat to life, and once culture samples are taken, antibiotics must be given to cover both gram-positive and gram-negative organisms. The choice of antibiotic also depends on a knowledge of local antibiotic susceptibility patterns. Many institutions have protocols to guide empirical antibacterial therapy, particularly in neutropenic patients. A common empirical broad-spectrum regimen includes a third- or fourth-generation cephalosporin (cefotaxime or ceftriaxone) together with an amino-glycoside (gentamicin, tobramycin, or amikacin). Alternatives to cephalosporins include piperacillin/tazobactam or imipenem. If methicillin-resistant staphylococci or bacterial endocarditis is suspected and therapy must be started, a combination of van-comycin and gentamicin can be used.

> Some patients are allergic to penicillin. Ensure that the patient is *not* allergic before ordering penicillin or cephalosporin. Aminoglycosides are common causes of nephrotoxicity and ototoxicity. Select maintenance dosing intervals according to the patient's calculated creatinine clearance (see Appendix E, page 425). Follow the serum aminoglycoside concentrations, usually after the third or fourth dose, and the serum creatinine concentration.

If the volume status is normal and the patient is still hypotensive, transfer him or her to the intensive care unit/cardiac care unit (ICU/CCU) for inotropic or vasopressor support. (Refer to Chapter 18 for further discussion of septic shock.)

A Foley catheter should be placed in a patient with septic shock to monitor urine output.

Meningitis

Fever plus headache, seizure, stiff neck, or change in sensorium is considered to be meningitis until proved otherwise.

An LP should be performed without delay to confirm the diagnosis and guide antimicrobial therapy. This procedure should not be undertaken if there are focal neurologic findings or signs of increased intracranial pressure such as papilledema (see Fig. 14–2), coma, irregular respirations, bradycardia, or decerebrate posture. Other contraindications include a coagulopathy, owing to the risk of intrathecal hematoma formation, which may result in cord compression.

In bacterial meningitis, the cerebrospinal fluid (CSF) usually shows a pleocytosis ($>10^9$/L), protein >0.4 g/L, and glucose <2 mmol/L. However, these findings may not be present early in the course.

Gram stain is positive in 80% of patients not previously treated with antibacterial agents. In patients who have been partially treated, detection of bacterial antigens with latex agglutination is helpful but unreliable in detecting group B meningococcal antigen.

If you are unable to visualize the fundi or if there is papilledema or focal neurologic signs (suggesting a mass lesion), give the first dose of antibiotics and arrange for an urgent computed tomography (CT) scan of the head to exclude a space-occupying lesion before performing the LP. An LP done in the presence of an intracranial space-occupying lesion can result in uncal herniation and brain stem compression (coning).

Selective Chart Review

If the patient is not in septic shock and does not have symptoms or signs of meningitis, perform a selective chart review, looking for *localizing clues* (Table 12–1). Also check the chart for the following:

- Temperature pattern during hospital stay
- Recent white blood cell (WBC) count and differential
- Evidence of immunodeficiency (e.g., cancer chemotherapy, hematologic malignancy, human immunodeficiency virus [HIV] infection, CD4 lymphocyte count)
- Allergies to antibiotics
- Other possible reasons for fever (e.g., connective tissue disease, neoplasm)
- Antipyretics, antibiotics, or steroids that may modify the fever pattern

Selective Physical Examination II

Confirm localizing symptoms or signs already documented in the chart review.

Vitals	Repeat now
HEENT	Fundi—papilledema (intracranial abscess), Roth's spots (infective endocarditis) (Fig. 12–1)
	Conjunctival or scleral petechiae (infective endocarditis)
	Ears—red tympanic membranes (otitis media, a complication of intubation)
	Sinuses—tenderness, inability to transilluminate (sinusitis)
	Oral cavity—dental caries, tender tooth on tongue blade percussion (periodontal abscess)
	Pharynx—erythema, pharyngeal exudate (pharyngitis, thrush)
	Neck—stiff (meningitis)
Resp	Crackles, friction rub, signs of consolidation (pneumonia, pulmonary embolism)

TABLE 12–1 **Selective Chart Review—Looking for Localizing Clues**

Localizing Clue	Diagnostic Considerations	Comments
Recent surgery	Atelectasis	Postoperative fever due to atelectasis is a diagnosis made only after excluding infection
	Pneumonia	
	Pulmonary embolism	
	Infected surgical wound, biopsy site, or deeper infection of biopsy organ	Despite modern surgical techniques, any incision or puncture site may serve as a portal for bacteremia
Blood transfusion	Transfusion reaction	See Chapter 27
Headache, seizure, stiff neck, changes in sensorium	Meningitis	Delirium tremens can mimic meningitis in some patients; is the patient withdrawing from alcohol?
	Intracranial abscess	
	Encephalitis	
Sinus discomfort	Sinusitis	
Dental caries, toothache	Periodontal abscess	
Sore throat	Pharyngitis	
	Tonsillitis	
Dysphagia	Retropharyngeal abscess	Either of these diagnoses is a medical emergency; consult ENT or anesthesia immediately
	Epiglottitis	
SOB, cough, or chest pain	Pneumonia	
	Lung abscess	
	Pulmonary embolus	
Murmur, CHF, or peripheral embolic lesions	Infective endocarditis	
Pleuritic chest pain	Pneumonia	
	Empyema	
	Pulmonary embolus	
	Pericarditis	
Costovertebral angle tenderness	Pyelonephritis	
	Perinephric abscess	
Foley catheter, dysuria, hematuria, or pyuria	Cystitis	Condom catheters and Foley catheters predispose patients to urinary tract infections
	Pyelonephritis	

Continued

TABLE 12–1 **Selective Chart Review—Looking for Localizing Clues—cont'd**

Localizing Clue	Diagnostic Considerations	Comments
Abdominal pain		If there are peritoneal signs, consider surgical consultation
RUQ	Subphrenic abscess Hepatic abscess Hepatitis RLL pneumonia Cholecystitis	
	Ascending cholangitis	Does the patient have Charcot's triad (fever, RUQ pain, jaundice)? If so, consider surgical consultation
RLQ	Appendicitis Crohn's disease Salpingitis	
LUQ	Splenic abscess Subphrenic abscess Infected pancreatic pseudocyst LLL pneumonia	
LLQ	Diverticular abscess Salpingitis	
Ascites	Peritonitis	Perform abdominal paracentesis to exclude spontaneous bacterial peritonitis in any ascitic patient who becomes unwell
Diarrhea	Enteritis Colitis	
Swollen, red, tender joint	Septic arthritis	A monoarticular effusion or a disproportionately inflamed joint in polyarticular disease must be tapped to exclude infection
	Gout or pseudogout	
Prosthetic joint	Infected prosthesis	
Vaginal discharge	Endometritis Salpingitis	
Red or tender IV site	Septic phlebitis	
TPN line	Catheter sepsis	Fever may be the only symptom

CHF, congestive heart failure; ENT, ear, nose, and throat; IV, intravenous; LLL, left lower lobe; LLQ, left lower quadrant; LUQ, left upper quadrant; RLL, right lower lobe; RLQ, right lower quadrant; RUQ, right upper quadrant; SOB, shortness of breath; TPN, total parenteral nutrition.

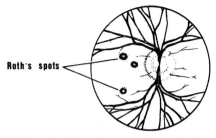

Roth's spots

Figure 12–1 Roth's spots. Round or oval hemorrhagic retinal lesions with central pallor.

CVS	New murmurs (infective endocarditis)
ABD	Localized tenderness (see page 32)
Rectal	Tenderness or mass (rectal abscess)
MSS	Joint erythema or effusion (septic arthritis)
Skin	Decubitus ulcers (cellulitis)
	Osler's nodes and Janeway's lesions, petechiae (infective endocarditis)
	IV sites (phlebitis, cellulitis)
	All surgical wounds must be examined (that means taking off the dressings)
Pelvis	A pelvic examination should be done if a pelvic source of fever is possible

Management II

Any patient with an unexplained fever >38.5°C (orally) that has developed in the hospital should have the following performed:

- Blood cultures immediately from two different sites
- Urinalysis (routine and microscopic) and urine culture immediately
- WBC count and differential

The performance of other, more *selective tests* depends on the *localizing clues* you elicited from your chart review, history, and physical examination. For example:

- Throat swab for Gram stain and culture
- Sputum for Gram stain and culture
- Chest x-ray (CXR)
- LP
- Blood culture for infective endocarditis (refer to your institution's protocol)
- Cervical culture (obtain the specific medium for gonococcal isolation before performing the pelvic examination)
- Joint aspiration
- Swab of decubitus ulcers or infected or draining wounds for Gram stain and culture

Fluid from any source should be examined microscopically immediately to guide your choice of antibiotics.

Remove *suspected IV lines* and replace if necessary at a new site. Central total parenteral nutrition (TPN) lines that may be infected should be replaced in consultation with your resident or TPN service. Catheter tips should be sent to the laboratory for culture.

Remove a Foley catheter in a patient suspected of having a *urinary tract infection*. A few days of incontinence is an annoyance for the nursing staff but will not harm the patient if there is no perineal skin breakdown. An exception to this is when a Foley catheter has been placed to treat urinary retention, because urinary stasis predisposes the patient to infection.

Broad-Spectrum Antibiotics

Three types of patients need broad-spectrum antibiotics now:

1. A patient with *fever and hypotension* (see page 97).
2. A patient with *fever and neutropenia* ($<500/mm^3$ or $<1000/mm^3$ and falling) in whom a localizing site of infection is not apparent. Anticipate this event in an immunocompromised patient (e.g., on chemotherapy) and agree on an appropriate broad-spectrum regimen with the hematologist or oncologist well ahead of time.
3. A patient who is febrile, appears toxic and acutely ill, and is suspected of having an infection despite no evidence of a clear-cut source.

A minimal workup includes the following:

* Blood cultures

  Although blood cultures have a low yield for diagnosing bacteremia, they are very valuable when true-positive. Optimally, two 20-mL aliquots of blood should be obtained from two venipuncture sites separate from any established venous access sites. This technique helps reduce contamination and false-positive results.[1]
* Urinalysis and urine culture
* Sputum for Gram stain and culture
* CXR

The selection of the initial antibiotics should be based on the most likely source or site of infection, the most likely causative organisms, and their likely antibiotic sensitivities. Your institution should have policies about the availability and appropriateness of specific antibiotics. Often more than one antibiotic is required. Common choices include a third-generation cephalosporin (e.g., ceftazidime, ceftriaxone, ceftizoxime, or cefotaxime) or extended-spectrum penicillin (e.g., imipenem/cilastatin, piperacillin/tazobactam, or ticarcillin/clavulanate) and an aminoglycoside (e.g., gentamicin, tobramycin, or amikacin). However, a gastrointestinal or female pelvic source may require additional coverage of anaerobic organisms (e.g., metronidazole), and intravascular device or prosthetic cardiac valve sources may require an antibiotic effective against methicillin-resistant staphylococci (e.g., vancomycin or other glycopeptide such as teicoplanin).

Specific Antibiotics

Two types of patients need specific antibiotics now:

1. A patient with *fever and meningitis symptoms* requires antibiotics immediately after the LP is done. However, do not delay initial antibiotic treatment if a CT scan of the head must be done before the LP (see pages 97 to 98).
2. A patient with *fever and clear localizing clues* should be given specific antibiotics after collection of culture specimens. Antibiotic therapy should be considered an urgent requirement in a diabetic patient.

No Antibiotics until a Specific Microbiologic Diagnosis Is Made

A patient who does not look sick or critical, who is immunologically competent, and in whom the source of fever is not readily apparent (e.g., a patient admitted for workup of fever of unknown origin [FUO]) should not have antibiotics until a specific microbiologic diagnosis is made.

Choice of Antibiotics

Unfortunately, infecting organisms can develop resistance to antibiotics, and the presence of these resistant strains is encouraged by widespread antibiotic use. Specific antibiotic choices depend on knowledge of your institution's local microbial flora and their antibiotic susceptibilities. Most parenteral antibiotics are expensive. Your institution should have guidelines for antibiotic use to diminish the development of resistant organisms and to control costs.

Fever in the HIV-Positive Patient

In patients with HIV disease, fever is usually caused by infection or lymphoma. In these patients, one should assume that fever is due to infection until proved otherwise. Occasionally, no specific cause of fever is found. In this case, the fever may be due to the HIV infection itself, but this should be considered a diagnosis of exclusion.

Although HIV-positive patients are susceptible to any of the common infections, a number of opportunistic pathogens should be considered. The organ system involved in such a patient may suggest the offending organism (Table 12–2). More than in any other patient population, multiple infections are often present in HIV-positive patients.

TABLE 12–2 **Common Infecting Organisms Responsible for Fever in Patients with HIV Disease, by System Involved**

Organ System	Organism	Diagnostic Test
Lungs (cough, SOB)	*Pneumocystis carinii*	Induced sputum or bronchoscopy specimens for toluidine blue or silver stain
	Bacteria (*Pneumococcus, Haemophilus influenzae, Staphylococcus aureus*)	Sputum culture and Gram stain, blood cultures
	Mycobacteria (*Mycobacterium tuberculosis, Mycobacterium avium-intracellulare*)	Sputum smears for AFB × 3; sputum and blood for mycobacterial culture
	Occasionally fungi (cryptococcosis, histoplasmosis, aspergillosis)	Sputum and blood for fungal culture
	Occasionally CMV	Definitive diagnosis requires lung biopsy, which is rarely indicated CMV is often recovered on bronchoscopy specimens but does not indicate CMV pneumonia
CNS (meningitis)	*Cryptococcus neoformans*	Serum cryptococcal antigen; CSF: cryptococcal antigen, India ink stain, fungal culture
	Bacteria (*Pneumococcus, Meningococcus, Listeria*)	CSF: Gram stain, culture, and bacterial antigens
	Mycobacterium (*M. tuberculosis*)	CSF: smears and culture for TB
	Treponema pallidum (syphilis)	Serum and CSF: VDRL, serum MHA-TP or FTA-ABS
	HIV	By exclusion
CNS (mass lesion)	*Toxoplasma gondii*	CT scan head (with contrast); serology (IgG ± IgM) usually positive but not diagnostic—if serology is negative, argues against diagnosis; brain biopsy may be required if no response to empirical treatment

TABLE 12–2 **Common Infecting Organisms Responsible for Fever in Patients with HIV Disease, by System Involved—cont'd**

Organ System	Organism	Diagnostic Test
	Occasionally tuberculoma, cryptococcoma, histoplasmoma	Brain biopsy
CNS (diffuse disease)	JC virus (progressive multifocal leuko-encephalopathy)	CT scan head ± brain biopsy
	Herpes simplex encephalitis	CT scan head ± brain biopsy
	CMV encephalitis	CT scan head ± brain biopsy
	HIV dementia complex	Clinical diagnosis plus exclusion of other causes
GI tract		
Esophagitis (dysphagia, odynophagia)	*Candida albicans*	Empirical antifungal treatment (ketoconazole, fluconazole, or itraconazole)—if no reponse, endoscopy brushings and biopsy; smears/cultures
	CMV	Endoscopy for biopsy and viral culture
	Herpes simplex	Endoscopy for biopsy and viral culture
Diarrhea	Bacteria (*Salmonella, Shigella, Campylobacter, Yersinia, Clostridium difficile*)	Stool culture for bacterial pathogens, stool toxin assay and culture for *C. difficile*
	Parasites (*Cryptosporidium, Microsporidium, Giardia, Entamoeba histolytica, Isospora belli, Enterocytozoon bieneusi*)	Stools for ova and parasites ×3; stools for cryptosporidia (modified AFB smear or fluorescent stain)
	CMV	Sigmoidoscopy ± colonoscopy and biopsy
	M. avium-intracellulare	Stool smear for AFB, culture, ± endoscopy and biopsy, blood cultures for mycobacteria
Disseminated infection	Mycobacteria (*M. avium-intracellulare, M. tuberculosis*)	Blood, sputum, urine, stool for smears and mycobacterial culture

Continued

TABLE 12–2 **Common Infecting Organisms Responsible for Fever in Patients with HIV Disease, by System Involved—cont'd**

Organ System	Organism	Diagnostic Test
	CMV	Blood (buffy coat) and urine viral cultures; + biopsies
	Cryptococcosis	Blood, CSF, and urine fungal cultures; serum and CSF for cryptococcal antigen
	Histoplasmosis	Blood, sputum, and bone marrow biopsy for fungal culture; buffy coat smear for yeast forms in WBCs
	Herpes zoster	Tzanck smear, viral culture of skin lesions
	Coccidioidomycosis	Sputum, blood, and CSF for fungal culture; serology
	Bacillary angiomatosis (*Bartonella* spp.)	Biopsy of skin lesion, blood culture

AFB, acid-fast bacillus; CMV, cytomegalovirus; CNS, central nervous system; CSF, cerebrospinal fluid; CT, computed tomography; FTA-ABS, fluorescent treponemal antibody absorption; GI, gastrointestinal; HIV, human immunodeficiency virus; IgG, immunoglobulin G; IgM, immunoglobulin M; MHA-TP, microhemagglutination assay—*Treponema pallidum*; SOB, shortness of breath; TB, tuberculosis; WBC, white blood cell.

REMEMBER

1. An immunocompromised patient is especially susceptible to infection and liable to develop complications. You should not hesitate to call for the help of the resident or attending physician.
2. The definition of FUO is a temperature >38.3°C for 3 weeks with no cause found despite thorough in-hospital investigation for 1 week.
3. Fever due to neoplasm, connective tissue disorder, or drug reaction is a diagnosis that should be made only *after* excluding fever due to infection.
4. Fever may result from the use of prescription or nonprescription drugs. Even such commonly used drugs as antibiotics can cause a "drug fever," which usually occurs within 7 days of beginning the offending drug.

   Antipsychotic medications may cause the *neuroleptic malignant syndrome*, characterized by fever, muscular rigidity, an altered sensorium, tachycardia, and elevations in creatine phosphokinase (CPK), WBC count, and liver enzymes. The symptoms respond to discontinuation of the offending drug.

Overdoses of some psychostimulants, such as amphetamines and cocaine, may acutely elevate the temperature, resulting in rhabdomyolysis and contributing to fatal cardiac dysrhythmias.[2] Prompt cooling, the use of antipyretics, and the judicious use of tranquilizers may be indicated in this setting.

5. Administering antipyretics for a fever due to infection treats only the symptom. In fact, there is evidence that the ability to mount a febrile response is an adaptive mechanism that inhibits bacterial replication and enhances the ability of macrophages to kill bacteria.[3] It is useful to observe the fever pattern, and if the fever is not very high (>40°C) and the patient is not uncomfortable, it is not necessary to treat with aspirin or acetaminophen.

6. If antipyretics are ordered, ask the RN to indicate with an arrow the time of administration on the bedside temperature chart. Assessment of the therapeutic response is also made easier by charting the antibiotics given (Fig. 12–2).

7. Steroids may elevate the WBC count and suppress the fever response, regardless of the cause. Defervescence with steroids should be interpreted cautiously.

8. Microorganisms love foreign bodies. Look for foreign bodies at sites of infection—IV lines, Foley catheters, ventriculoperitoneal

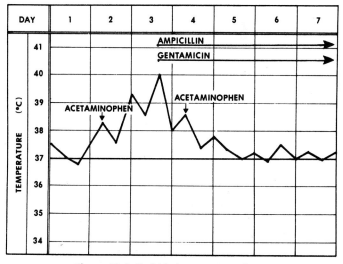

Figure 12–2 Bedside temperature chart.

(VP) shunts, prosthetic joints, peritoneal dialysis catheters, and porcine or mechanical heart valves.

9. Fever that occurs while the patient is already on antibiotics may mean the following:
   a. You are using an inappropriate antibiotic.
   b. You are giving an inadequate dose.
   c. You are not treating the right organism, or resistance or superinfection has developed.
   d. The antibiotic is not getting to the right place (e.g., thick-walled abscess requiring surgical drainage).
   e. The fever may not be due to an infection.

10. Delirium tremens is a serious cause of fever that is occasionally seen in patients withdrawing from alcohol. It is associated with confusion, including delusions and hallucinations; agitation; seizures; and signs of autonomic hyperactivity, such as fever, tachycardia, and sweating. This condition is sometimes fatal and requires high doses of benzodiazepines to stabilize the patient (see page 67).

References

1. Shafazand S, Weinacker AB: Blood cultures in the critical care unit. Chest 2002;122:1727-1736.
2. Callaway CW, Clark RF: Hyperthermia in psychostimulant overdose. Ann Emerg Med 1994;24:68-76.
3. Saper CB, Breder CD: The neurologic basis of fever. N Engl J Med 1994;330:1880-1886.

Gastrointestinal Bleeding

Gastrointestinal (GI) bleeding is common in hospitalized patients. Whether the bleeding is from minor gastric stress ulceration or from life-threatening exsanguination of an aortoduodenal fistula, the initial principles of assessment and management are the same.

PHONE CALL

Questions

1. **Clarify the situation. Is the blood old or new, and from where is it coming?**

   Vomiting of bright red blood or "coffee grounds" and most cases of melena indicate an upper GI bleed. Bright red blood passed rectally (i.e., hematochezia) usually indicates a lower GI bleed but may be seen in upper GI bleeds when blood loss is sudden and massive.

2. **How much blood has been lost?**

3. **What are the vital signs?**

   This information helps determine the urgency of the situation.

4. **What was the admitting diagnosis?**

   Recurrent bleeding from duodenal ulcer or esophageal varices carries a high mortality rate.

5. **Is the patient receiving anticoagulants (heparin, warfarin), thrombolytic therapy (streptokinase, tissue plasminogen activator [tPA]), or agents that affect platelet number (chemotherapy) or function (aspirin, clopidogrel, ticlopidine, glycoprotein IIb/IIIa inhibitors)?**

   Anticoagulants or thrombolytic agents may require immediate discontinuation or reversal in an actively bleeding patient.

Orders

1. Large-bore intravenous (IV) line (size 16 if possible) immediately, if not already in place.

IV access is a priority in a bleeding patient. Two IV sites may be required if the patient is hemodynamically unstable.

2. Hemoglobin (Hb) stat.

   Caution: The Hb level may be normal during an acute bleed and drops only with correction of the intravascular volume by a shift of fluid from the extravascular space.

3. Crossmatch: Is there blood on hold? If not, order stat crossmatch of 2, 4, or 6 units of packed red blood cells (RBCs), depending on your estimation of blood loss.

4. If the admitting diagnosis is bleeding esophageal varices and the patient is hypotensive, order a Minnesota (or Sengstaken-Blakemore) tube to be at the bedside immediately. If you are not familiar with the use of this tube, call your resident for assistance now. Also, commence *octreotide* 50-µg bolus followed by 25 µg/hr IV infusion.

5. Ask the RN to take the patient's chart to the bedside.

Inform RN

"I will arrive at the bedside in . . . minutes."

Hypotension or tachycardia requires you to see the patient immediately.

ELEVATOR THOUGHTS

What causes GI bleeding?

1. Upper GI bleed
   a. Esophagitis
   b. Esophageal varices
   c. Mallory-Weiss syndrome (tear)
   d. Gastric ulcer, gastritis
   e. Duodenal ulcer, duodenitis
   f. Neoplasm (esophageal cancer, gastric cancer)
2. Lower GI bleed
   a. Angiodysplasia
   b. Diverticulosis
   c. Neoplasm
   d. Colitis (ulcerative, ischemic, infectious)
   e. Mesenteric thrombosis
   f. Meckel's diverticulum
   g. Hemorrhoids
3. GI bleeding may also occur in the absence of structural pathology in a patient who has recently received a thrombolytic agent, is anticoagulated, or is receiving medications that cause thrombocytopenia or affect platelet function.

GI bleeding in a patient with human immunodeficiency virus (HIV) may be caused by any of the conditions listed, which are unrelated to the HIV-positive state. However, additional causes should be considered. Upper GI bleeding may result from Kaposi's sarcoma, gastric lymphoma, cytomegalovirus (CMV) infection of the esophagus or duodenum, or herpes simplex infection of the esophagus. Lower GI bleeding may result from Kaposi's sarcoma or from colitis caused by CMV, bacterial pathogens (including atypical mycobacteria), or herpes simplex.

MAJOR THREAT TO LIFE

- Hypovolemic shock

The major concern with GI bleeding is the progressive loss of intravascular volume in a patient whose bleeding lesion is not identified and managed correctly. If allowed to progress, even minor intermittent or continuous bleeding may eventually result in hypovolemic shock, with hypoperfusion of vital organs.

Initially, lost blood volume can be corrected by infusion of normal saline (NS) or Ringer's lactate, but if bleeding continues, the replacement of lost RBCs will also be required in the form of packed RBC transfusion. Hence, your initial assessment should be directed at the patient's volume status to determine whether a significant amount of intravascular volume has been lost.

BEDSIDE

Quick-Look Test

Does the patient look well (comfortable), sick (uncomfortable or distressed), or critical (about to die?)

A patient in hypovolemic shock due to blood loss appears pale and apprehensive and may have other symptoms and signs, including cold and clammy skin, due to stimulation of the sympathetic nervous system.

Airway and Vital Signs

Are there any postural changes in blood pressure (BP) or heart rate (HR)?

First, check for changes with the patient in the lying and sitting (with legs dangling) positions. If there are no changes, the BP and HR should then be checked with the patient standing.

A rise in HR >15 beats/min, a fall in systolic BP >15 mm Hg, or any fall in diastolic BP indicates significant hypovolemia.

Caution: A resting tachycardia alone may indicate decreased intravascular volume. If the resting systolic BP is <90 mm Hg, order a second large-bore IV line immediately.

Selective Physical Examination I

What is the patient's volume status? Is the patient in shock?

Vitals	Repeat now
CVS	Pulse volume, JVP
	Skin temperature and color
Neuro	Mental status

> Shock is a clinical diagnosis, as follows: systolic BP <90 mm Hg with evidence of inadequate tissue perfusion, such as cold and clammy skin and central nervous system (CNS) changes (agitation or confusion). In fact, the kidney is a sensitive indicator of shock (i.e., urine output <20 mL/hr). The urine output of a patient who is hypovolemic ordinarily correlates with the renal blood flow, which in turn is dependent on cardiac output and is an extremely important measurement. However, placement of a Foley catheter should not take priority over resuscitation measures.

Management I

What immediate measures need to be taken to correct shock or prevent it from occurring?

Replenish the intravascular volume by giving IV fluids. The best immediate choice is a crystalloid (NS or Ringer's lactate), which stays in the intravascular space at least temporarily. Albumin or banked plasma can be given, but it is expensive, carries a risk of hepatitis, and is not readily available.

Blood has been lost from the intravascular space, and ideally, blood should be replaced (see Box 13–1 for steps to take if the patient refuses a blood transfusion). If there is no blood on hold for the patient, a stat crossmatch usually takes 50 minutes. If blood is on hold, it should be available at the bedside in 30 minutes. In an emergency, O-negative blood can be given, although this practice is usually reserved for acute trauma victims.

> The incidence of transfusion-associated hepatitis can be minimized by transfusing only when necessary. *Rule of thumb:* Maintain an Hb level of 90 to 100 g/L.

Order the appropriate IV rate, which depends on the patient's volume status. *Shock* requires running IV fluid wide open through at least two large-bore IV sites. Elevating the IV bag, squeezing the IV bag, or using IV pressure cuffs may help increase the rate of delivery of the solution. *Moderate volume depletion* can be treated with 500 to 1000 mL of NS given as rapidly as possible, with serial measurements of volume status and assessment of cardiac status. If blood is not at the bedside within 30 minutes, delegate someone to find out why there is a delay.

> Aggressive volume repletion in a patient with a history of congestive heart failure (CHF) may compromise cardiac function. Do not overshoot the mark!

BOX 13–1 Patients Who Refuse Blood Transfusion

There are some patients who, for religious or other reasons, may refuse blood transfusions.[1] This should be respected, and local laws should be followed as appropriate. In this case, call your resident or attending physician for help. In general, the following principles apply:

- Immediate endoscopy, with a view toward therapeutic intervention (e.g., sclerotherapy, heater coagulation, laser therapy), is recommended, as is early surgical consultation.
- Avoid resuscitation with synthetic colloids, which may interfere with coagulation.
- Normal saline may be used, but avoid overaggressive fluid replacement in this patient group, because attempts to achieve normotension before bleeding is controlled may inhibit spontaneous hemostasis and cause further bleeding. A rule of thumb in this situation is to aim for a systolic blood pressure of 90 to 100 mm Hg in a previously normotensive patient, or 20 to 30 mm Hg below a hypertensive patient's usual systolic readings.
- Agents such as IV desmopressin acetate (to raise factor VIII and von Willebrand factor and reduce bleeding time) and antifibrinolytics (e.g., tranexamic acid) may help prevent ongoing blood loss, but they should be used only after consultation with a hematologist or the patient's attending physician.
- If the hemorrhage is severe, these patients may benefit from hyperbaric oxygen therapy, if available.

What can you do at this time to stop the source of bleeding?

Treat the underlying cause. Treating hypovolemia is treating a symptom.

1. Upper GI bleed (hematemesis and most cases of melena)

   Many clinicians begin a parenteral acid-suppressing agent, even though studies have not confirmed any influence on complications such as rebleeding, need for surgery, or death within the first 48 to 72 hours.[2,3] Parenteral H_2-blocking drugs used include *cimetidine* (Tagamet) 300 mg IV every 6 hours, *ranitidine* (Zantac) 50 mg IV every 8 hours, and *famotidine* (Pepcid) 20 mg IV every 8 hours. These agents may be just as effective orally. *Nizatidine* (Axid) is another H_2 blocker available only in the oral form at a dose of 150 mg PO every 12 hours. *Omeprazole* 20 mg PO daily, *lansoprazole* 15 mg PO daily, *pantoprazole* 40 mg PO daily (also available IV), and *rabeprazole* 20 mg PO daily are potent antisecretory agents but are more expensive than the H_2 blockers. Antacids are contraindicated if endoscopy or surgery is anticipated. They obscure the field in endoscopy and increase the risk of aspiration in surgery.

2. Lower GI bleed (usually bright red blood per rectum and, occasionally, melena)

No other treatment is required until the specific site of bleeding is identified, but continue to monitor the volume status.

3. Abnormal coagulation

If the international normalized ratio (INR) or activated partial thromboplastin time (aPTT) is prolonged, or if the patient is thrombocytopenic, fresh frozen plasma (2 units) or platelet infusion (6 to 8 units), respectively, may be required. If the patient has recently received thrombolytic therapy, additional agents, such as aprotinin (Trasylol), may be required, but these should be initiated only after consultation with your resident or attending physician. If the patient is receiving an antiplatelet medication, it should be stopped, although the effect of the agent may persist for days. Bleeding disorders resulting from drug-induced platelet dysfunction may require platelet transfusion or other specialized measures (see page 343).

Selective Chart Review

What was the reason for admission?

Has the cause of this GI bleed already been identified during this admission?

Is the patient on any medication that may worsen the situation?

NSAIDs	Counteract the protective effect of prostaglandins on gastric mucosa and may result in gastric erosions or peptic ulcers
Steroids	Increased frequency of ulcer disease in patients on steroids; most disease processes for which a patient is receiving steroids do not allow their immediate discontinuation
Heparin	Prevents clot formation by enhancing the action of antithrombin III
Warfarin	Prevents activation of vitamin K–dependent clotting factors
Streptokinase	Converts free plasminogen to plasmin, which then causes lysis of fibrin
tPA	Binds specifically to fibrin, becoming active, and then converts plasminogen to plasmin on the tissue surface
Antiplatelet agents	Aspirin, clopidogrel, ticlopidine, and the glycoprotein IIb/IIIa inhibitors (e.g., tirofiban) interfere with platelet activation, adhesion, or aggregation and may result in bleeding

What laboratory data should be obtained?
- Most recent Hb value

- INR, aPTT, platelets. Are there any platelet or coagulation abnormalities that may predispose the patient to bleeding?
- Bleeding time (if a platelet disorder is suspected)
- Urea, creatinine levels (uremia prolongs bleeding time)

> Remember, in prerenal failure, the urea level may be more markedly elevated than the creatinine level. This difference may be accentuated in the presence of GI bleeding by absorption of urea from the breakdown of blood in the GI tract.

Selective Physical Examination II

Where is the site of bleeding?

Vitals	Repeat now
HEENT	Nosebleed
ABD	Epigastric tenderness (peptic ulcer disease)
	RLQ tenderness or mass (cecal cancer)
	LLQ tenderness (sigmoid cancer, diverticulitis, ischemic colitis)
Rectal	Bright red blood, melena, hemorrhoids, or mass (rectal cancer)

Also, look for signs of chronic liver disease (hepatosplenomegaly, ascites, parotid gland hypertrophy, spider angiomata, gynecomastia, palmar erythema, testicular atrophy, dilated abdominal veins), which may suggest the presence of esophageal varices.

Management II

Once hypovolemia is corrected, ongoing management includes maintaining adequate intravascular volume while trying to determine the specific site of bleeding.

What procedures are available to determine the site of bleeding?
- Esophagogastroduodenoscopy
- Tagged RBC scan
- Angiography
- Sigmoidoscopy
- Colonoscopy

In a patient with an *upper GI bleed* that has stopped and who is hemodynamically stable, elective endoscopy can be performed within the next 24 hours. Urgent endoscopy may be required if bleeding continues or the patient is hemodynamically unstable.

Some conditions can be temporarily stabilized at the time of endoscopy. *Esophageal varices* can be treated with sclerotherapy or banding, *octreotide* (50-μg bolus, then 25 μg/hr IV infusion), or a Minnesota (or Sengstaken-Blakemore) tube (Fig. 13–1). In most cases, the presence of bleeding varices should be documented endoscopically before initiating any treatment. Sclerotherapy or banding is the preferred emergency treatment. Sclerotherapy plus *octreotide* (25 μg/hr IV for 5 days) is more effective than sclerotherapy alone in controlling variceal bleeding in patients with cirrhosis.[4] A Minnesota

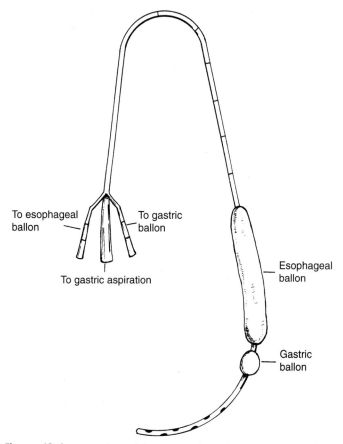

Figure 13–1 Sengstaken-Blakemore tube. The Minnesota tube is similar, with an additional port for esophageal aspiration.

tube is a temporizing measure reserved for a life-threatening bleed. *Gastric* or *duodenal ulcers* with a visible vessel at the base may be treated with electrocoagulation, heater probe therapy, or direct injection (epinephrine, ethanol, or polidocanol).

Patients with *lower GI bleeds* who are hemodynamically stable should be scheduled for colonoscopy. For unstable patients, an urgent tagged RBC scan should be arranged, followed by angiography, if possible. Tagged RBC scans and mesenteric angiography are most sensitive if performed while there is still active bleeding, but they should not take priority over resuscitation measures.

Angiographic diagnosis and management of upper GI bleeds are rarely necessary, owing to recent improvements in endoscopic therapy. Intra-arterial infusion of vasoconstrictors or selective arterial embolization may be helpful if severe or persistent bleeding occurs in a patient at high risk for surgery or in centers where endoscopic therapy is unavailable.

When is early surgical consultation appropriate?

- Exsanguinating hemorrhage
- Continued bleeding with transfusion requirements >5 units/day
- Second bleed from an ulcer, requiring transfusion during the same hospital stay
- Ulcer with a visible vessel at the base on endoscopy
- Patient who refuses blood transfusion (see Box 13–1)

Order an electrocardiogram and cardiac enzyme tests if there are any risk factors for coronary artery disease. A hypotensive episode in a patient with atherosclerosis may result in myocardial infarction.

REMEMBER

1. Keep the patient NPO (nothing by mouth) for endoscopy or possible surgery.
2. Insertion of a nasogastric (NG) tube to look for bright red blood may help identify an upper GI source of bleeding. However, negative NG returns do not rule out an upper GI bleed. Do not leave the NG tube in place to monitor bleeding. The patient's volume status is the best indicator of further blood loss, and an NG tube may cause mucosal artifacts, hampering interpretation of endoscopic findings.
3. Bismuth compounds (e.g., Pepto-Bismol) and iron supplements can turn stools black. True melena is pitch black, sticky, and tarlike, with an odor that is hard to forget.
4. An aortoduodenal fistula can appear as a sentinel (minor) bleed followed by rapid exsanguination. Consider this possibility in any patient who has undergone abdominal vascular surgery or in any patient with a midline abdominal scar who is unable to give a history.
5. Never attribute a GI bleed to hemorrhoids before thorough exclusion of other sources of bleeding.

References

1. Thomas JM, Wong CJ: Management of gastrointestinal hemorrhage in patients who refuse blood transfusion. Ann R Coll Physicians Surg Can 1999;32:76-77.
2. Zuckerman G, Welch R, Douglas A, et al: Controlled trial of medical therapy for active upper gastrointestinal bleeding and prevention of rebleeding. Am J Med 1984;76:361-366.

3. Daneshmend TK, Hawkey CJ, Langman MJS, et al: Omeprazole versus placebo for acute upper gastrointestinal bleeding: Randomized double blind controlled trial. BMJ 1992;304:143-147.
4. Besson I, Ingrand P, Person B, et al: Sclerotherapy with or without octreotide for acute variceal bleeding. N Engl J Med 1995;333:555-560.

Headache

Patients in the hospital often complain of headache. You must decide whether the headache is chronic and of no urgent concern or a symptom of a more serious problem.

PHONE CALL

Questions

1. **How severe is the headache?**
   Most headaches are mild and not of major concern unless associated with other symptoms.
2. **Was the onset sudden or gradual?**
   The sudden onset of a severe headache is suggestive of subarachnoid hemorrhage.
3. **What are the vital signs?**
4. **Has there been a change in the level of consciousness?**
5. **Is there a past history of chronic or recurrent headaches?**
6. **What was the reason for admission?**

Orders

1. Ask the RN to take the patient's temperature if it has not been recorded within the past hour.
   Bacterial meningitis may present with only fever and headache.
2. If you are confident that the headache represents a chronic or previously diagnosed, recurrent problem, the patient can be given medication that has relieved the headache in the past or a non-narcotic analgesic agent (e.g., acetaminophen). Ask the RN to call back in 2 hours if the headache has not been relieved by the medication.

Inform RN

"I will arrive at the bedside in . . . minutes."
   Headaches associated with fever, vomiting, or a decreased level of consciousness and severe headaches with an acute onset require you

to see the patient immediately. Chronic, recurrent headaches must be assessed at the bedside if the headache is more severe than usual or if the character of the pain is different.

ELEVATOR THOUGHTS

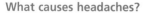

What causes headaches?

Chronic (Recurrent) Headaches

1. Muscle contraction
   a. Psychogenic—depression, anxiety, stress (tension headaches)
   b. Cervical osteoarthritis
   c. Temporomandibular joint disease
2. Vascular
   a. Migraine
   b. Cluster
3. Drugs
   a. Nitrates
   b. Calcium channel blockers
   c. Nonsteroidal anti-inflammatory drugs (NSAIDs)

Acute Headaches

1. Infectious
   a. Meningitis
   b. Encephalitis
2. Post trauma
   a. Concussion
   b. Cerebral contusion
   c. Subdural or epidural hematoma
3. Vascular
   a. Subarachnoid hemorrhage
   b. Intracerebral hemorrhage
4. Increased intracranial pressure
   a. Space-occupying lesions
   b. Malignant hypertension
   c. Benign intracranial hypertension
5. Local causes
   a. Temporal arteritis
   b. Acute angle-closure glaucoma

MAJOR THREAT TO LIFE

- Subarachnoid hemorrhage
- Bacterial meningitis
- Herniation (transtentorial, cerebellar, central)

Subarachnoid hemorrhage is associated with a very high mortality rate if it is not recognized and treated to prevent rebleeding. *Bacterial meningitis* must be recognized early if antibiotic treatment is to be successful. Any intracranial mass lesion (e.g., tumor, blood, pus) may result in *herniation* (Fig. 14–1).

BEDSIDE

Quick-Look Test

Does the patient look well (comfortable), sick (uncomfortable or distressed), or critical (about to die)?

Most patients with chronic headaches look well. Those with subarachnoid hemorrhage, meningitis, or severe migraines look sick.

Airway and Vital Signs

What is the temperature?

Fever associated with a headache requires that you make a prompt decision whether a lumbar puncture (LP) should be performed.

What is the blood pressure (BP)?

Malignant hypertension (hypertension with papilledema) is usually associated with a systolic BP >190 mm Hg and a diastolic BP >120 mm Hg. Headache is not usually a symptom of hypertension unless there has been a recent increase in pressure and the diastolic BP is >120 mm Hg.

What is the heart rate (HR)?

Hypertension in association with bradycardia may be a manifestation of increasing intracranial pressure.

Selective Physical Examination I

Does the patient have increased intracranial pressure or meningitis?

HEENT	Nuchal rigidity (meningitis or subarachnoid hemorrhage)
	Papilledema (increased intracranial pressure)—see Figure 14–2 for the funduscopic features of papilledema; an early sign of increased intracranial pressure is absence of venous pulsations
Neuro	Mental status
	Pupil symmetry
	A finding of asymmetrical pupils associated with a rapidly decreasing level of consciousness represents a life-threatening situation; ask for a neurosurgical consult immediately for assessment and treatment of probable uncal herniation
	Kernig's sign and Brudzinski's sign (meningitis or subarachnoid hemorrhage) (Fig. 14–3)

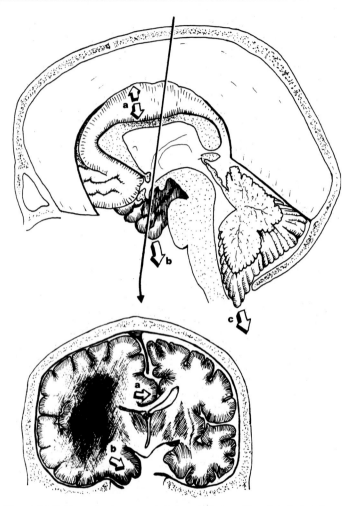

Figure 14–1 Central nervous system herniation. a, Cingulate herniation; b, uncal herniation; c, cerebellar herniation.

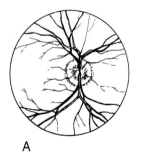
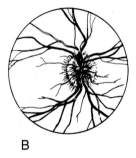

A

B

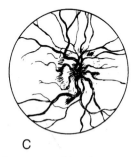
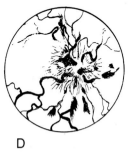

C

D

Figure 14–2 Disc changes seen in papilledema. *A*, Normal. *B*, Early papilledema. *C*, Moderate papilledema with early hemorrhage. *D*, Severe papilledema with extensive hemorrhage.

	A full neurologic examination is required if there is nuchal rigidity, pupillary asymmetry, or papilledema
Skin	Maculopapular rash, petechiae, or purpura may be seen in bacterial meningitis

Management I

If there is *papilledema*, there is likely increased intracranial pressure. In the context of "headache," this should suggest a mass lesion (tumor, pus, or blood), but it may also be seen with less localized processes such as subarachnoid hemorrhage or meningitis. An immediate computed tomography (CT) scan of the head helps differentiate among these possibilities. An LP is contraindicated because of the risk of brain herniation.

If *fever* is present in addition to papilledema, empirical antibiotic coverage should be implemented before the CT scan, as follows.

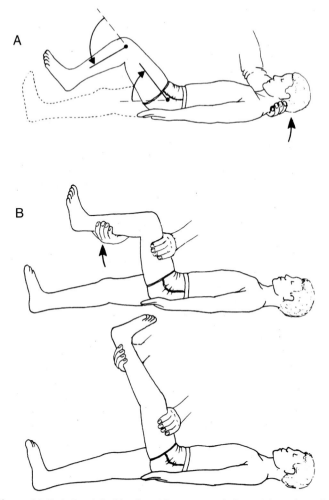

Figure 14–3 *A*, Brudzinski's sign. The test result is positive when the patient actively flexes his or her hips and knees in response to passive neck flexion by the examiner. *B*, Kernig's sign. The test result is positive when pain or resistance is elicited by passive knee extension from the 90-degree hip-knee flexion position.

Suspected Bacterial Meningitis

1. Adult, community-acquired infection (most often *Streptococcus pneumoniae*, *Neisseria meningitidis*, *Listeria monocytogenes*, streptococci)—pending culture results:
   - *Cefotaxime* 2 g IV every 6 hours or *ceftriaxone* 2 g IV every 12 hours, with
   - *Ampicillin* 2 g IV every 4 hours for older patients to cover the possibility of *Listeria* infection, and
   - *Vancomycin* 15 mg/kg IV every 12 hours with or without *rifampin* 20 mg/kg PO daily in one or two divided doses in cases of serious risk of infection due to penicillin-resistant pneumococci[1]
   - *Dexamethasone* 10 mg PO every 6 hours for 4 days, starting before or with the first dose of antibiotics[2]
2. Immunosuppressed, alcoholic, or older than 60 years (gram-negative bacilli, staphylococci)—either *cefotaxime* 2 g IV every 6 hours or *ceftriaxone* 2 g IV every 12 hours, both with *vancomycin* 15 mg/kg IV every 12 hours
3. Postcraniotomy, head trauma, or cerebrospinal fluid (CSF) shunt—either *cefotaxime* 2 g IV every 6 hours or *ceftriaxone* 2 g IV every 12 hours, both with *vancomycin* 15 mg/kg IV every 12 hours

   > Vancomycin in usual doses may not reach adequate concentrations at the site of infection. Higher doses, up to 4 g/day, may be required in some cases.

Suspected Subdural Empyema or Brain Abscess

1. Secondary to frontoethmoid sinusitis, otitis media, mastoiditis, or lung abscess—cloxacillin plus a third-generation cephalosporin plus metronidazole

   > Sixty percent to 90% of subdural empyemas are caused by extension of sinusitis or otitis media.

2. After trauma—cloxacillin or nafcillin plus a third-generation cephalosporin

In addition to beginning antibiotics, a patient with a subdural empyema or a brain abscess should be referred for neurosurgical assessment. Also, prophylactic antiepileptic therapy should be administered routinely, as follows: *phenytoin* (Dilantin) loading dose 18 mg/kg IV at a rate no faster than 25 to 50 mg/min IV, followed by a maintenance dosage of 100 mg IV every 8 hours or 300 mg PO daily. Steroid treatment, surgery, or both may be required to relieve increased intracranial pressure due to cerebral edema.

If there is *fever, nuchal rigidity, and no papilledema*, the likelihood of meningitis is high. In this case, perform an LP, followed immediately by IV antibiotics, as recommended earlier. If there is a delay of 1 hour or longer in performing the LP, antibiotic therapy should be initiated first—the initial dose will have little effect on the evaluation of the CSF obtained later.

If there is *nuchal rigidity, no fever, and no papilledema,* a subarachnoid hemorrhage should be considered. In this case, noncontrast CT of the brain should be performed before the LP. If a subarachnoid hemorrhage is present, the CT scan will show subarachnoid blood in most cases. If the CT brain scan is normal and a subarachnoid hemorrhage is still suspected, an LP should be performed, looking for xanthochromia. Confirmation of a subarachnoid hemorrhage requires immediate neurosurgical consultation.

If there is *no papilledema, no fever, and no nuchal rigidity,* a more detailed history and chart review can be performed.

Selective History and Chart Review

Was the onset of the headache sudden or insidious?

The abrupt onset of severe headache suggests a vascular cause, with the most serious being subarachnoid or intracerebral hemorrhage.

How severe is the headache?

Most muscle contraction headaches are mild and not incapacitating. However, when migraine headaches are associated with severe pain, the patient may look sick.

Is the headache improved or worsened in the supine position?

Most muscle contraction headaches are improved by lying down. Headaches made worse by lying down suggest increasing intracranial pressure, and an intracranial mass should be considered.

Were there any prodromal symptoms?

Nausea and vomiting are associated with increased intracranial pressure but may also occur with migraine or acute angle-closure glaucoma. Photophobia and neck stiffness are associated with meningitis. The classic visual aura (scintillations, migratory scotomata, and blurred vision) that precedes a migraine headache is helpful in making the diagnosis, but the absence of an aura does not rule out migraine.

Is there a past history of chronic, recurring headaches?

Migraine and muscle contraction headaches follow a pattern. Ask the patient whether this headache is the same as his or her "usual" headache. The patient will probably make the diagnosis for you.

Is there a history of recent head trauma?

An epidural hematoma may occur after even a relatively minor head injury, particularly in teenagers or young adults. Subdural hematomas can appear insidiously 6 to 8 weeks after seemingly minor trauma and are not uncommon in alcoholic patients.

Does the patient have joint disease in the neck or upper back?

Muscle contraction headaches in the elderly are often caused by cervical osteoarthritis. These headaches characteristically start in the neck region and radiate to the temple or forehead.

Does the patient have clicking or popping when opening or closing the jaw?

These symptoms are a clue to the presence of temporomandibular joint dysfunction. In addition, the pain may be located predominantly in the ear or face.

Has an ophthalmologist or another physician (MD) dilated the patient's pupils within the past 24 hours?

Acute angle-closure glaucoma can be precipitated by pupillary dilatation. The patient typically complains of a severe unilateral headache located over the brow and may experience nausea, vomiting, and abdominal pain.

Is there any decrease or loss in vision? Is there a history of jaw claudication?

Temporal arteritis is a systemic illness (fever, malaise, weight loss, anorexia, weakness, myalgia) seen in patients older than 50 years. If this condition is suspected, order a stat erythrocyte sedimentation rate (ESR). Visual loss in temporal arteritis is a medical emergency and should be managed in consultation with a neurologist or rheumatologist (for treatment, see page 129).

What drugs is the patient receiving?

Drugs such as nitrates, calcium channel blockers, and NSAIDs can cause headaches. Any head trauma or unusual headache occurring in a patient receiving anticoagulants or thrombolytic therapy should raise the suspicion of an intracranial hemorrhage. In this case, a CT scan of the head should be performed, and reversal of the anticoagulant or thrombolytic agent should be considered.

Selective Physical Examination II

Vitals	Repeat now
HEENT	Red eye (acute angle-closure glaucoma)
	Hemotympanum or blood in the ear canal (basal skull fracture)
	Tender, enlarged temporal arteries (temporal arteritis)
	Retinal hemorrhages (hypertension)
	Lid ptosis, dilated pupil, eye deviated down and out (posterior communicating cerebral artery aneurysm)
	Tenderness on palpation or failure of transillumination of the frontal and maxillary sinuses (sinusitis or subdural empyema)

Inability to fully open the jaw (temporomandibular joint dysfunction)

Cranial bruit (arteriovenous malformation)

Neuro — Complete neurologic examination

What is the level of consciousness?

> Drowsiness, yawning, and inattentiveness associated with headache are ominous signs. In a patient with a small subarachnoid hemorrhage, these may be the only signs.

Is there any asymmetry of pupils, visual fields, eye movements, limbs, tone, reflexes, or plantar responses?

> Asymmetry suggests structural brain disease; if this is a new finding, a CT scan of the head is required.

MSS — Palpate skull and face, looking for fractures, hematomas, and lacerations

> Evidence of recent head trauma suggests the possibility of a subdural or epidural hematoma.

Management II

Muscle Contraction Headache. Chronic muscle contraction headache can be treated temporarily with non-narcotic analgesics. This is the most common type of headache seen in the hospital. A long-term treatment plan, if not already established, can be discussed in the morning.

Mild Migraine Headache. A mild migraine headache can be treated adequately with analgesics such as *aspirin* 650 to 1300 mg PO every 4 hours for two doses, *ibuprofen* 400 to 800 mg PO every 6 hours for two doses, or *naproxen sodium* 275 to 550 mg PO every 2 to 6 hours.[3] Patients with allergies to these medications may be given *acetaminophen* 650 to 1300 mg PO every 4 hours for two doses or *codeine* 30 to 60 mg PO or IM every 3 to 4 hours PRN.

Severe Migraine Headache. A severe migraine headache is best treated immediately during the prodromal stage, but it is unlikely that you will be called until the headache is well established. Ask the patient what he or she usually takes for migraine headaches; this is probably the most effective agent to prescribe immediately.

Serotonin receptor agonists, such as dihydroergotamine or sumatriptan succinate (Imitrex), are first-line therapy for most severe migraines. *Dihydroergotamine* 0.5 to 1 mg IM, SC, or IV may be given and repeated in 1 hour if ineffective. Alternatively, *sumatriptan* 50 to 100 mg PO or 6 mg SC may be given. Sumatriptan should not be given within 24 hours of the administration of dihydroergotamine.[4]

> These agents are contraindicated in uncontrolled hypertension, unstable coronary artery disease, coronary spasm, or

pregnancy and in the presence of hemiplegic migraine. Side effects of sumatriptan include chest or throat tightness, tingling in the head or limbs, and nausea. Dihydroergotamine is less likely to induce chest pain but more likely to cause nausea.

In patients with severe migraines in whom vasoconstrictors are contraindicated, one of the following dopamine antagonists may be tried:

- *Metoclopramide* 10 mg IV
- *Chlorpromazine* 0.1 mg/kg IV over 20 minutes; repeat after 15 minutes to a maximum dose of 37.5 mg (pretreatment with 5 mL/kg normal saline IV may prevent the hypotensive effects of chlorpromazine)
- *Prochlorperazine* 5 to 10 mg IV or IM or 25 mg PR

Cluster Headache. Cluster headaches are difficult to treat. Most last less than 45 minutes, and oral treatment has minimal effect. If a cluster headache develops in the hospital and is severe, a parenteral narcotic, such as *codeine* 30 to 60 mg IM or *meperidine* (Demerol) 50 to 100 mg IM, may be tried. Alternatively, *dihydroergotamine* or *sumatriptan* in the same doses recommended for migraine headaches may be effective.

Postconcussion Headache. If intracranial hemorrhage has been ruled out by a CT scan of the head, postconcussion headache should be treated with an analgesic agent that is unlikely to cause sedation, such as acetaminophen or codeine. Aspirin is contraindicated in a post-trauma patient because the inhibition of platelet aggregation may predispose the patient to bleeding complications.

Hemorrhages and Space-Occupying Lesions. Patients with subdural, epidural, and subarachnoid hemorrhages and space-occupying lesions (brain abscess, tumor) causing raised intracranial pressure should be referred to a neurosurgeon as soon as possible. While awaiting neurosurgical consultation, *nimodipine* 60 mg PO every 4 hours may improve the outcome in patients with subarachnoid hemorrhage.[5]

Malignant Hypertension. Malignant hypertension (hypertension and papilledema) should be managed by careful reduction of BP (see Chapter 16, page 161).

Benign Intracranial Hypertension. Benign intracranial hypertension (pseudotumor cerebri) is a syndrome of unknown cause. There is increased intracranial pressure (headache and papilledema) but no evidence of a mass lesion or hydrocephalus. Refer the patient to a neurologist in the morning for further investigation and management.

Temporal Arteritis. Temporal arteritis should be treated immediately to prevent irreversible blindness. *Prednisone* 60 mg PO daily can be started immediately when this diagnosis is suspected and supported by an ESR of >60 mm/hr (Westergren method). Confirmation by temporal artery biopsy should be arranged within the next 3 days.

Glaucoma. A patient with acute angle-closure glaucoma should be referred to an ophthalmologist immediately.

References

1. British Infection Society (BIS): Early management of suspected bacterial meningitis and meningococcal septicemia in adults. London, BIS, 2003. Available at www.britishinfectionsociety.org/meningitis.html.
2. DeGans J, Van De Beek D: Dexamethasone in adults with bacterial meningitis. N Engl J Med 2002;347:1549-1556.
3. Pryse-Phillips W, Dodick D, Edmeads J, et al: Guidelines for the diagnosis and management of migraine in clinical practice. Can Med Assoc J 1997;156:1273-1287.
4. Kubacka RT: Practical approaches to the management of migraine. Am Pharm 1994;34:34-44.
5. Pickard JD, Murray GD, Illingworth R, et al: Effect of oral nimodipine on cerebral infarction and outcome after subarachnoid hemorrhage: British Aneurysm Nimodipine Trial. BMJ 1989;298:636-642.

ɹrt Rate and
thm Disorders

There are only three abnormalities in heart rate (HR) or rhythm that you will be called to assess at night—too fast, too slow, and irregular. Remember that the main purpose of the HR is to keep cardiac output high enough to perfuse three vital organs: heart, brain, and kidney. Your task is to find out why the heart is beating too quickly, too slowly, or irregularly before it results in hypoperfusion of the patient's vital organs. Begin by asking whether the HR is too fast or too slow. (Rapid HRs are discussed first; slow HRs are addressed on page 149 of this chapter.) Next, decide whether the rhythm is regular or irregular.

RAPID HEART RATES

PHONE CALL

Questions

1. **What is the HR?**
2. **Is the rhythm regular or irregular?**
3. **Is this a new problem since admission?**
4. **What is the blood pressure (BP)?**
    Remember that hypotension may be a *cause* of tachycardia (i.e., compensatory) or a *result* of tachycardia that does not allow adequate diastolic filling of the left ventricle to maintain cardiac output.
5. **Is the patient having chest pain or shortness of breath (SOB)?**
    Dysrhythmias are common in patients with underlying coronary artery disease. A rapid HR may be the result of myocardial ischemia or congestive heart failure (CHF), or it may precipitate ischemia or CHF in such a patient.
6. **What is the respiratory rate?**
    Any illness causing hypoxia may result in tachycardia.
7. **What is the temperature?**
    Tachycardia, proportional to the temperature elevation, is an expected finding in a febrile patient. However, you must

examine the patient to ensure that there is no other cause for the rapid HR.

Orders

1. If the patient is experiencing tachycardia and *hypotension*, order a large-bore (size 16 if possible) intravenous (IV) line immediately.
2. If the patient is having *chest pain,* ask the RN to put the cardiac arrest cart in the room and attach the patient to the electrocardiogram (ECG) monitor.
3. Order a stat 12-lead ECG and rhythm strip.

Inform RN

"I will arrive at the bedside in . . . minutes."

A rapid HR in association with chest pain (angina), SOB (CHF), or hypotension requires you to see the patient immediately.

ELEVATOR THOUGHTS

What causes rapid heart rates?

Rapid Irregular Heart Rates

1. Atrial fibrillation
2. Atrial flutter with variable block
3. Multifocal atrial tachycardia
4. Sinus tachycardia with premature atrial contractions (PACs) or premature ventricular contractions (PVCs)

Rapid Regular Heart Rates

1. Sinus tachycardia
2. Atrial flutter
3. Other supraventricular tachycardias (SVTs)
   a. Reentrant
      (1) Atrioventricular (AV) nodal reentry
      (2) Accessory pathways (e.g., Wolff-Parkinson-White [WPW] syndrome, concealed pathways)
   b. Nonreentrant
      (1) Unifocal atrial tachycardia
      (2) Junctional tachycardia
      (3) Ventricular tachycardia
          As electrophysiologic studies have enhanced our knowledge, the classification of SVTs has become more mechanistic but sometimes less practical. Although sinus tachycardia, atrial fibrillation, and atrial flutter are tachycardias with a supraventricular origin, their mechanisms are sufficiently distinct from those of the other SVTs that they are often classified separately. The term *supraventricular tachycardia* is

commonly reserved for (usually narrow-complex) tachycardia that is not clearly sinus, atrial fibrillation, or atrial flutter. Do not be distressed because you cannot differentiate an SVT due to AV nodal reentry from one resulting from orthodromic reentry using a concealed bypass tract. The precise mechanism of an SVT often is not apparent on the surface ECG, and in most cases, the initial management is the same.

MAJOR THREAT TO LIFE

- Hypotension, leading to shock
- Angina, progressing to myocardial infarction (MI)
- CHF, leading to hypoxia

It is useful to recall the determinants of BP, as expressed in the following two formulas:

$$BP = \text{cardiac output (CO)} \times \text{total peripheral resistance (TPR)}$$
$$CO = HR \times \text{stroke volume (SV)}$$

As demonstrated by the first equation, any decrease in CO will result in a decrease in BP, unless it is accompanied by a compensatory increase in TPR. Although in most instances a rapid HR increases CO, many of the rapid HRs do not allow adequate time for diastolic filling of the ventricles, resulting in a low SV and, hence, a decreased CO. The low CO may result in *hypotension*, in *angina* in a patient with underlying coronary artery disease, or in *CHF* in a patient with inadequate left ventricular reserve.

BEDSIDE

Quick-Look Test

Does the patient look well (comfortable), sick (uncomfortable or distressed), or critical (about to die)?

A patient with SVT or ventricular tachycardia may look deceptively well if adequate BP is maintained. Patients with tachycardia that is sufficiently severe to cause hypotension, angina, or pulmonary edema usually look sick or critical and are likely to be unstable.*

---

*The term *unstable tachycardia* is used in the American Heart Association's ECC Guidelines 2000 to refer to a situation in which the heart beats too fast for the patient's cardiovascular condition. In this situation, the patient displays serious symptoms (shortness of breath, chest pain, altered mental status) or is hypotensive or in pulmonary edema, *and* the symptoms can be attributed to the tachycardia. The term *unstable tachycardia* more accurately refers to an unstable *patient*, rather than an unstable rhythm disorder.

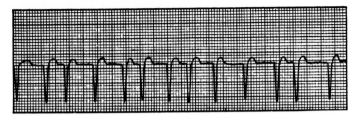

Figure 15–1 Atrial fibrillation with rapid ventricular response.

Airway and Vital Signs

What is the HR? Is it regular or irregular?

Read the ECG and rhythm strip.

What is the BP?

If the patient is hypotensive (systolic BP <90 mm Hg), you must decide the following quickly:

1. Whether the tachycardia is a result of the hypotension (i.e., compensatory tachycardia)

or

2. Whether the hypotension is a result of the tachycardia (i.e., inadequate diastolic filling leading to low CO with low BP).

> Three rapid heart rhythms occasionally can cause hypotension due to decreased diastolic filling, resulting in hypoperfusion of vital organs: atrial fibrillation with rapid ventricular response, SVT, and ventricular tachycardia (Figs. 15–1 to 15–3). If the patient is hypotensive, it is important to recognize these rhythms immediately, because prompt treatment is required to restore adequate CO.

What is the respiratory rate?

A patient with tachypnea may be in pulmonary edema—an important determination. If pulmonary edema is present, the patient qualifies as unstable and is probably in need of cardioversion.

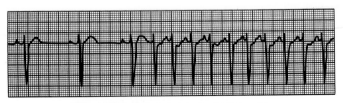

Figure 15–2 Supraventricular tachycardia.

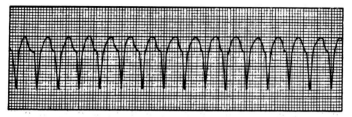

Figure 15–3 Ventricular tachycardia.

Management

If the patient is *hypotensive* and has atrial fibrillation with a rapid ventricular response, SVT, or ventricular tachycardia, emergency cardioversion may be required.

- Ask the RN to immediately call for your resident and an anesthetist.
- Ask the RN to bring the cardiac arrest cart into the room. Attach the patient to the ECG monitor.
- Give the patient 100% O_2 by mask (28% if the patient has chronic obstructive pulmonary disease [COPD]).
- Ensure that an IV line is in place.
- Ask the RN to have available *midazolam* 5 mg IV.

  > Premedication to alleviate the pain of electrical shocks is required whenever possible. Your anesthesia team may have its own protocols or preferences for conscious sedation. Unless you are faced with a life-threatening situation, it is best to await the arrival of your resident and the anesthetist before administering premedication or proceeding to electrical cardioversion.

- If the patient has an SVT, you may attempt carotid sinus massage (see page 145) or instruct the patient in a vagal maneuver (see page 145) while you await the arrival of more experienced help.

  > Occasionally, these maneuvers "break" an SVT, obviating the need for pharmacologic or electrical conversion of the arrhythmia. If these maneuvers are unsuccessful, you need to proceed to pharmacologic or electrical cardioversion.

- If the patient has an SVT, ask the RN to draw *adenosine* 6 mg IV into a syringe.

  > Adenosine has a very brief half-life, may be given to an unstable patient, and may terminate an SVT such as AV nodal reentry without the need for electrical cardioversion. This **should not be given**, however, without the guidance of your resident.

If the patient is *hypotensive* and none of these three rhythms is present, the tachycardia is most likely *secondary* to hypotension. You must perform a selective physical examination to decide which of the four major causes of hypotension is resulting in compensatory tachycardia: (1) cardiogenic causes, (2) hypovolemic causes, (3) sepsis, or (4) anaphylaxis. (Refer to Chapter 18 for the investigation and management of hypotension.)

Evaluation of Rapid Heart Rates in the Stable Patient

Fortunately, most of the patients you will see with rapid HRs are not unstable. In these cases, you can relax for a minute. Look at the ECG and rhythm strip and decide which rapid rhythm the patient is experiencing.

RAPID IRREGULAR RHYTHMS
- Atrial fibrillation (Fig. 15–4A)
- Atrial flutter with variable block (see Fig. 15–4B)
- Multifocal atrial tachycardia (Fig. 15–5)
- Sinus tachycardia with PACs (Fig. 15–6)
- Sinus tachycardia with PVCs (Fig. 15–7)

RAPID REGULAR RHYTHMS
- Sinus tachycardia (Fig. 15–8)
- Atrial flutter (Fig. 15–9)
- SVT—for example, unifocal atrial tachycardia (Fig. 15–10); AV nodal reentry or orthodromic WPW tachycardia (Fig. 15–11)
- Ventricular tachycardia (Fig. 15–12)

Note: A wide-complex regular tachycardia such as that shown in Figure 15–3 may in fact represent either ventricular tachycardia or

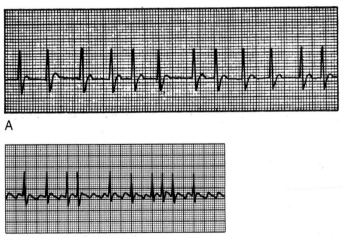

A

B

Figure 15–4 Rapid irregular rhythms. *A,* Atrial fibrillation. *B,* Atrial flutter with variable block.

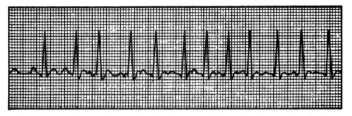

Figure 15–5 Rapid irregular rhythms—multifocal atrial tachycardia.

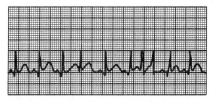

Figure 15–6 Rapid irregular rhythms—sinus tachycardia with premature atrial contractions.

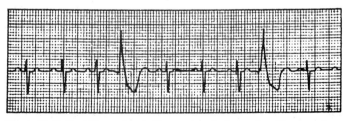

Figure 15–7 Rapid irregular rhythms—sinus tachycardia with premature ventricular contractions.

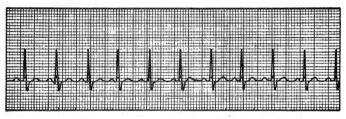

Figure 15–8 Rapid regular rhythms—sinus tachycardia.

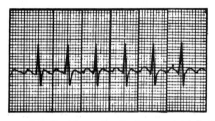

Figure 15–9 Rapid regular rhythms—atrial flutter.

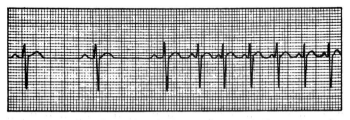

Figure 15–10 Rapid regular rhythms—supraventricular tachycardia: ectopic atrial tachycardia.

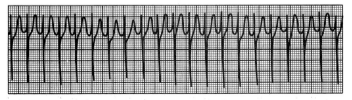

Figure 15–11 Rapid regular rhythms—supraventricular tachycardia: atrioventricular nodal reentry or Wolff-Parkinson-White orthodromic tachycardia.

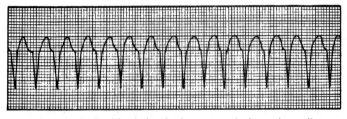

Figure 15–12 Rapid regular rhythms—ventricular tachycardia.

SVT with aberrancy. Most cases of wide-complex tachycardia in hospitalized patients are ventricular tachycardia, particularly if it occurs in a patient with known or suspected coronary artery disease or cardiomyopathy. Do not assume that a wide-complex tachycardia is SVT with aberrancy just because the rhythm is well tolerated by the patient or the patient is young. If you are uncertain, call your resident for help. A trial of *adenosine* 6 mg IV may help differentiate between these two dysrhythmias. Verapamil can be dangerous in this situation and may result in cardiovascular collapse in a patient with ventricular tachycardia. If uncertainty remains, IV procainamide may be effective in treating both dysrhythmias.

Management of Rapid Irregular Rhythms

Atrial Fibrillation. If the patient is *unstable*—is hypotensive, has chest pain (angina), or has SOB (CHF)—and if atrial fibrillation is of recent onset (<2 days), the treatment of choice is cardioversion, beginning with 100 J.

Atrial fibrillation with ventricular rates of >150/min and without evidence of hemodynamic compromise (no hypotension, angina, or CHF) can be treated with negative dromotropes. The decision whether to give the agents orally or intravenously depends on whether the patient looks unwell or is completely asymptomatic. A patient who looks unwell may be on the way to becoming unstable or may be having symptoms that do not technically qualify as "unstable" (e.g., anxiety, diaphoresis, palpitations); in this case, IV administration of one of these medications may be warranted. *Continuous ECG monitoring is required when any of these agents is given intravenously.* If the patient is completely asymptomatic, rate control can be undertaken at a more leisurely (and safer) pace with oral agents that slow conduction through the AV node. Although IV digoxin has been a traditional choice for rate control, beta blockers and calcium channel blockers are more effective. One of the following may be used to achieve rate control:

- *Metoprolol* 1 to 2 mg/min IV up to a total of 5 mg if necessary. The oral dose is 25 to 50 mg twice a day

or

- *Esmolol* 0.5 mg/kg per minute IV over 1 minute, followed by an infusion of 0.05 to 0.2 mg/kg per minute

or

- *Diltiazem* 0.25 mg/kg (usual dose, 15 to 25 mg) IV over 2 minutes. The oral dose of the short-acting preparation is 30 to 90 mg every 6 hours, and this can be switched to a longer-acting preparation once dosing requirements and tolerability are established

or

- *Verapamil* 2.5 to 15 mg (initial dose, usually 2.5 to 5 mg) IV over 1 to 2 minutes. The oral dose of the short-acting preparation is 80 to 120 mg every 8 hours, and this can be switched to a longer-acting preparation once dosing requirements and tolerability are established

or

- *Digoxin* 1 mg IV or PO in divided doses over 24 hours, followed by 0.125 to 0.25 mg PO daily thereafter.

  > Because digoxin is excreted predominantly by glomerular filtration, smaller maintenance doses are required in the presence of renal dysfunction.

  In a patient already receiving digoxin, additional doses should be given with caution and careful observation.

  > Digoxin overdose is a common cause of morbidity in both community and hospital settings. Common side effects include dysrhythmia, heart block, anorexia, nausea, vomiting, and neuropsychiatric symptoms, such as hallucinations. It is unusual for these side effects to develop acutely when digoxin is prescribed in the regimen previously outlined. The subsequent development of these side effects can be minimized by adjusting maintenance doses according to renal function. The risk of digoxin-induced ventricular dysrhythmias can be reduced by avoiding hypokalemia.

Atrial fibrillation with ventricular rates of <100/min in an untreated patient suggests underlying AV nodal dysfunction. These patients do not require immediate treatment unless they are hemodynamically compromised (e.g., hypotension, angina, CHF).

SELECTIVE HISTORY AND CHART REVIEW. Once the ventricular rate is controlled, perform a selective history and chart review, looking for the following causes of atrial fibrillation:

- Coronary artery disease
- Hypertension
- Hyperthyroidism (check T_4, TSH)
- Pulmonary embolism (check for risk factors, see page 273)
- Mitral or tricuspid valve disease (stenosis or regurgitation)
- Cardiomyopathy
- Congenital heart disease (e.g., atrial septal defect)
- Pericarditis, recent cardiac surgery
- Recent alcohol ingestion (holiday heart syndrome)
- Sick sinus syndrome (SSS)
- Hypoxia
- Idiopathic (lone fibrillator)

SELECTIVE PHYSICAL EXAMINATION. Look for specific causes of atrial fibrillation. Note that this process takes place after you have already begun to treat the patient.

Vitals	Repeat now
HEENT	Exophthalmos, lid lag, lid retraction (hyperthyroidism)
Resp	Tachypnea, cyanosis, wheezing, pleural effusion (pulmonary embolus)

CVS	Murmur of mitral regurgitation or mitral stenosis (mitral valve disease)
Ext	Swelling, erythema, calf tenderness (DVT)
	Tremor, hyperactive deep tendon reflexes (hyperthyroidism)

Multifocal Atrial Tachycardia. This rhythm does not always require specific management. The underlying cause should be treated; this is usually pulmonary disease, which is probably already being treated. Check for the following underlying causes:

- Pulmonary disease (especially COPD)
- Hypoxia, hypercapnia
- Hypokalemia
- CHF
- Drugs—theophylline toxicity
- Caffeine, tobacco, alcohol use

Multifocal atrial tachycardia can be a forerunner of atrial fibrillation. If no remediable causes can be found, *verapamil* 80 to 120 mg PO three times daily or *diltiazem* 30 to 90 mg PO four times daily may provide rate control and diminish the frequency of ectopics.

Sinus Tachycardia with PACs. Treatment is the same as for multifocal atrial tachycardia. Although PACs may be forerunners of multifocal atrial tachycardia or atrial fibrillation, they do not need to be treated unless atrial fibrillation develops.

Sinus Tachycardia with PVCs. Although certain features of PVCs that have been described as "malignant" (e.g., R on T phenomenon, multifocal PVCs, couplets or salvos [three or more PVCs in a row], frequent PVCs [more than five per minute]) have some relevance (Fig. 15–13), it is more important to look at the patient and determine the context in which the PVCs are occurring. If the patient has myocardial ischemia, is hemodynamically unstable, has a serious metabolic or electrolyte abnormality, or is taking pro-arrhythmic medications (see page 149), and the patient is having very frequent PVCs or runs of nonsustained ventricular tachycardia, he or she should be transferred to a telemetry ward or the intensive care unit/ cardiac care unit (ICU/CCU) for further investigation and continuous ECG monitoring.

Look for the following common causes of PVCs in the hospital:

- *Myocardial ischemia* (symptoms or signs of angina or MI).
  This is the most important cause of PVCs to identify, if present. PVCs are not generally associated with an increased risk of death unless they occur in the setting of myocardial ischemia or MI.
- *Hypokalemia.* Look for a recent serum potassium value in the chart, and order a repeat measurement if a recent one is not available. Check the 12-lead ECG for evidence of hypokalemia (Fig. 15–14). Determine whether the patient is

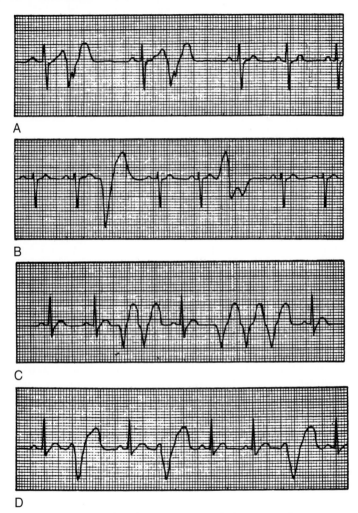

A

B

C

D

Figure 15–13 Examples of premature ventricular contractions. *A*, R on T phenomenon. *B*, Multifocal. *C*, Couplets or salvos. *D*, Frequent.

on diuretics that may cause hypokalemia (refer to Chapter 33 for treatment).

- *Hypoxia.* Obtain arterial blood gas (ABG) measurements if hypoxia is suspected clinically.
- *Acid-base imbalance.* Check the chart for a recent HCO_3^- determination. Obtain ABGs if acidosis or alkalosis is suspected.

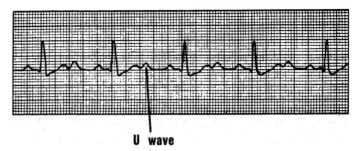

U wave

Figure 15–14 Electrocardiographic features of hypokalemia.

- *Cardiomyopathy.* Patients with cardiomyopathy that is sufficiently severe to cause PVCs almost always have a cardiologist and an established diagnosis of cardiomyopathy before you see them. Consult the patient's cardiologist for guidance in treating cardiomyopathy-related PVCs.
- *Drugs.* Drugs such as digoxin and other antiarrhythmic agents may actually *cause* PVCs.

Conditions such as *mitral valve prolapse* and *hyperthyroidism* can also cause PVCs, but these arrhythmias are not common presenting signs of these disorders in the hospital.

Try to identify whether any of the preceding factors are responsible for the PVCs, and correct them if possible. Hypokalemia, hypoxia, and acid-base disturbances usually can be identified and corrected in the patient's room. However, if there is suspicion of myocardial ischemia, cardiomyopathy, digoxin toxicity, or hyperthyroidism, the patient should be transferred to a telemetry ward or the ICU/CCU for continuous ECG monitoring and initiation of antiarrhythmic agents if indicated.

After the PVCs have been treated, the patient may still be left with *sinus tachycardia.* Investigation and management of the underlying sinus tachycardia should be undertaken as subsequently outlined.

Management of Rapid Regular Rhythms

Sinus Tachycardia. There is no specific drug for the treatment of sinus tachycardia. The key is to find the *underlying cause* of this dysrhythmia. The most common causes of persistent sinus tachycardia in hospitalized patients are as follows:

- Hypovolemia
- Hypotension (cardiogenic, hypovolemic, septic, anaphylactic) (Refer to Chapter 18 for the investigation and management of hypotension.)
- Hypoxia of any cause (CHF, pulmonary embolism, pneumonia, bronchospasm [COPD, asthma]) (Refer to Chapter 24 for the investigation and management of SOB.)

- Fever
- Anxiety or pain
- Hyperthyroidism
- Drugs

Management of sinus tachycardia *always* consists of treatment of the underlying causes.

SVT: Atrial Flutter. The treatment of atrial flutter is similar to that of atrial fibrillation. If *unstable,* the patient may require synchronized cardioversion; if *stable,* the patient may be treated with beta blockers, calcium channel blockers, or digoxin IV or PO (see pages 139 to 140). Often, atrial flutter requires higher doses of digoxin than does atrial fibrillation to slow the ventricular rate. Ironically, treatment of atrial flutter sometimes produces atrial fibrillation. Look for causes in the chart that may predispose the patient to atrial flutter; for the most part, these are the same diseases that can cause atrial fibrillation (see page 140).

SVT: AV Nodal Reentry and Ectopic Atrial Tachycardias

UNSTABLE PATIENT. You will undoubtedly be anxious if called to see a patient with paroxysmal atrial tachycardia (PAT) who is unstable, because you know that it may require *electrical cardioversion,* a technique with which you may not be familiar. Stay calm; there is still much you can do.

If the patient is *unstable,* that is, hypotensive or has chest pain (angina) or SOB (CHF), prepare for immediate cardioversion as follows:

- Ask the RN to immediately call for your resident and ananesthetist.
- Ask the RN to bring the cardiac arrest cart into the room. Attach the patient to the ECG monitor. Set the defibrillator to 25 J, in the *Synchronize* mode.
- Give the patient 100% O_2 by mask (28% for those with COPD).
- Ensure that an IV line is in place.
- Ask the RN to have available *midazolam* 5 mg IV.

    Premedication to alleviate the pain of electrical shocks is required whenever possible. Your anesthesia team may have its own protocols or preferences for conscious sedation. Unless you are faced with a life-threatening situation, it is best to await the arrival of your resident and the anesthetist before administering premedication or proceeding to electrical cardioversion.

- Ask the RN to draw *adenosine* 6 mg IV into a syringe.

    Adenosine has a very brief half-life, may be given to an unstable patient, and may terminate an SVT such as AV nodal reentry without the need for cardioversion. This **should not be given,** however, without the guidance of your resident.

- If the patient has an SVT, you may attempt Valsalva's maneuvers or carotid sinus massage (see below) while you await the arrival of more experienced help.

  > Occasionally, these maneuvers "break" an SVT, obviating the need for pharmacologic or electrical conversion of the arrhythmia. If these maneuvers are unsuccessful, you need to proceed to pharmacologic or electrical cardioversion.

- While waiting for your resident to arrive, try nonelectrical means to convert the rhythm, such as Valsalva's maneuver or carotid sinus massage (see later).

STABLE PATIENT. If the patient is hemodynamically stable, you may try one or more of the following measures to break the tachycardia:

- *Valsalva's maneuver.* Ask the patient to hold his or her breath and to "bear down as if you are going to have a bowel movement."

  > This maneuver increases vagal tone and may terminate an SVT.

- *Carotid sinus massage*

  This maneuver is an effective form of vagal stimulation and may thereby terminate some SVTs. It should always be performed with IV atropine available and with continuous ECG monitoring, both for safety (some patients have developed asystole) and to document the results.

  Listen over the carotid arteries for bruits, and if they are present, do not perform carotid sinus massage. If no bruit is heard, proceed as follows. Turn the patient's head to the left. Locate the carotid sinus just anterior to the sternocleidomastoid muscle at the level of the top of the thyroid cartilage (Fig. 15–15). Feel the carotid pulsation at this point, and apply steady pressure to the carotid artery with two fingers for 10 to 15 seconds. Try the right side, and if this is not effective, try the left side. Simultaneous bilateral massage of the carotid sinus should never be done, because you will effectively cut off cerebral blood flow.

  > Carotid sinus massage has resulted, on several occasions, in cerebral embolization of an atherosclerotic plaque from carotid artery compression. Although this is a rare complication, it can be minimized by first listening over the carotid artery for a bruit. If a bruit is heard, forgo carotid sinus massage on that side.

- *Adenosine.* Give 6 mg as a rapid IV bolus, followed by a saline flush. If this is ineffective, increase to 12 mg IV push. A third dose of 18 mg IV push may be given if the first two lower doses were ineffective but well tolerated. Because of the very short half-life of adenosine, the three incremental doses can be administered at intervals of 60 seconds, if required.

  > IV adenosine should be used with caution in patients with asthma and COPD. Lower doses may be required in

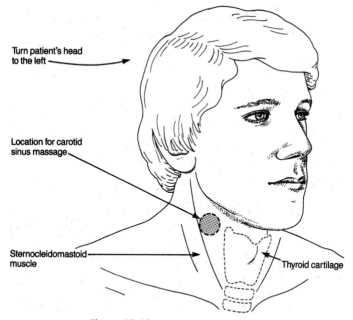

Figure 15–15 Carotid sinus massage.

patients on dipyridamole and in patients who have undergone cardiac transplantation because of supersensitivity to the drug. Common side effects are transient and include facial flushing, dyspnea, and chest pressure. Some SVTs, particularly unifocal atrial tachycardia, may not be responsive to adenosine, in which case IV verapamil may be effective.

- *Verapamil.* Begin with 2.5 to 5 mg IV over 1 to 2 minutes. If there is no effect, the dose may be repeated in 5 to 10 minutes.

  Verapamil increases AV conduction time and may slow ventricular rate. Its advantage over IV digoxin is its more rapid onset of action (1 to 2 minutes for verapamil versus 5 to 30 minutes for digoxin).

  Verapamil may cause hypotension if injected too rapidly. It is essential to give the dose slowly over 2 minutes. Verapamil is also a negative inotropic agent and may precipitate pulmonary edema in a patient predisposed to CHF. Pretreatment or post-treatment with *calcium chloride* (500 to 1000 mg IV over 5 to 10 minutes) may minimize the hypotensive effects of verapamil.

- *Diltiazem.* 0.25 mg/kg IV (usual initial dose, 15 to 20 mg) given slowly over 2 minutes will terminate many reentrant SVTs.

A second dose of 0.35 mg/kg may be given 15 minutes later if the initial dose is ineffective.

> Common side effects of IV diltiazem include bradycardias and hypotension.

- *Digoxin.* Provided that the SVT is not due to digoxin toxicity (i.e., PAT with block), you can use digoxin instead of verapamil. Give *digoxin* 0.25 to 0.5 mg IV, followed by 0.125 to 0.25 mg every 4 to 6 hours until a full loading dose of 1 mg is given. Then a maintenance dose of 0.125 to 0.25 mg PO daily may be given if the patient has normal renal function.

> Digoxin slows AV nodal conduction and may terminate SVT. The common side effects of digoxin (dysrhythmia, heart block, gastrointestinal upset, neuropsychiatric symptoms) are seldom seen acutely when digoxin is prescribed in the regimen as outlined.

- If the patient is known to have WPW syndrome and is having SVT, procainamide or IV amiodarone is a suitable choice.

If the patient is hemodynamically stable and the aforementioned measures have not worked, he or she should be transferred immediately to the ICU/CCU for semielective cardioversion.

Unlike atrial fibrillation and flutter, the reentrant SVTs usually are not secondary to acquired structural cardiac disease or to other illnesses. Of the nonreentrant SVTs, unifocal atrial tachycardia (particularly with 2:1 or 3:1 block) may be a manifestation of *digoxin toxicity,* and junctional tachycardia may be seen with *digoxin toxicity* or after *acute MI* or *aortic or mitral valve surgery.*

Sustained Ventricular Tachycardia. If the patient has no BP or pulse, call for a cardiac arrest cart and proceed with resuscitation as described on page 375.

UNSTABLE PATIENT. If the patient is *unstable* (hypotension, angina, CHF, or impaired mentation), do the following:

- Call for the cardiac arrest cart, your resident, and an anesthetist, and order a 12-lead ECG immediately.
- Attach the patient to the ECG monitor.
- Make sure that an IV line is in place.
- Give the patient 100% O_2 by mask (28% for those with COPD).
- Prepare for *synchronized electrical cardioversion* at 100 J.

STABLE PATIENT. If the patient is *stable* (no hypotension, angina, CHF, or impaired mentation), do the following:

- Call for the cardiac arrest cart, your resident, and an anesthetist, and order a 12-lead ECG immediately.
- Attach the patient to the ECG monitor.
- Make sure that an IV line is in place.
- Give the patient 100% O_2 by mask (28% for those with COPD).

VENTRICULAR TACHYCARDIA IS MONOMORPHIC, CARDIAC FUNCTION IS UNKNOWN OR IMPAIRED. If the ventricular tachycardia is monomorphic and cardiac function is unknown or impaired, order one of the following:

Amiodarone 150 mg IV bolus over 10 minutes
    or
Lidocaine 1 to 1.5 mg/kg IV to be given by syringe as rapidly as possible. At the same time, begin a maintenance infusion of lidocaine at a rate of 1 to 4 mg/min. In elderly patients and in patients with liver disease, CHF, or hypotension, give half the maintenance dose. Additional boluses of lidocaine in doses of 0.5 to 0.75 mg/kg may be given every 5 to 10 minutes after the initial bolus, to a maximum total dose of 3 mg/kg.

> Lidocaine may cause drowsiness, confusion, slurred speech, and seizures, especially in the elderly and in patients with heart failure or liver disease. Once your patient has been transferred to the ICU/CCU, the staff there will need to watch carefully for these signs of lidocaine toxicity.

- Prepare for synchronized cardioversion, if necessary.

VENTRICULAR TACHYCARDIA IS MONOMORPHIC, CARDIAC FUNCTION IS NORMAL. If the ventricular tachycardia is monomorphic and cardiac function is normal, amiodarone or lidocaine can be given in the doses specified earlier; alternatively, *procainamide* 20 mg/min IV (until the arrhythmia is suppressed, hypotension occurs, or the QRS widens by >50) may also be tried. The maximum total dose of procainamide should not exceed 17 mg/kg. This may be followed by a maintenance infusion of 1 to 4 mg/min.

> Although procainamide is often more effective than lidocaine in breaking ventricular tachycardia, the patient will need to be monitored carefully for hypotension.

VENTRICULAR TACHYCARDIA IS POLYMORPHIC, PATIENT IS KNOWN TO HAVE A NORMAL BASELINE QT INTERVAL. If the ventricular tachycardia is polymorphic and the patient is known to have a normal baseline QT interval, IV amiodarone, lidocaine, or beta blockers may be used. If the baseline QT interval is prolonged, torsades de pointes should be suspected (see page 149).

If chemical cardioversion is unsuccessful, electrical cardioversion is usually required. The patient should be continuously monitored, your resident and an anesthetist should be called to the bedside, the patient should be sedated, and *synchronized electrical cardioversion*, beginning at 50 J, should be given.

Ventricular tachycardia with hemodynamic compromise or without a prompt response to lidocaine or procainamide requires cardioversion. A patient with an episode of ventricular tachycardia should be transferred to the ICU/CCU for continuous ECG monitoring.

After immediate resuscitation, look for the following precipitating or potentiating causes of ventricular tachycardia:

- Myocardial ischemia or MI
- Hypoxia

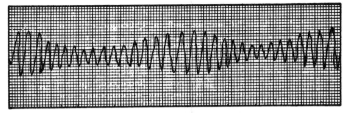

Figure 15-16 Torsades de pointes.

- Electrolyte imbalance (hypokalemia, hypomagnesemia, hypocalcemia)
- Hypovolemia
- Valvular heart disease (mitral valve prolapse)
- Acidemia
- Cardiomyopathy, CHF
- Drugs
  - Quinidine
  - Procainamide
  - Disopyramide
  - Phenothiazines
  - Tricyclic antidepressants
  - Sotalol
  - Amiodarone
  - Cisapride

The drugs listed (and others) may prolong the QT interval to produce a characteristic type of ventricular tachycardia known as torsades de pointes, which resembles a corkscrew pattern in the ECG rhythm strip, with complexes rotating above and below the baseline (Fig. 15-16). These drugs should be discontinued if such a rhythm develops. *Magnesium sulfate* 1 to 2 g IV is often effective in terminating this type of ventricular tachycardia, but overdrive pacing, isoproterenol, phenytoin, or lidocaine can also be tried.

SLOW HEART RATES

PHONE CALL

Questions

1. What is the HR?
2. What is the BP?
3. Is the patient on digoxin, a beta blocker, a calcium channel blocker, or other antiarrhythmic drug?

   Drugs such as digoxin, beta blockers, diltiazem, and verapamil possess both sinus and AV nodal suppressant properties and may result in profound sinus bradycardias or heart blocks.

Other antiarrhythmics such as sotalol or amiodarone possess beta-blocking properties and may also cause bradycardias.

Orders

1. If the patient is hypotensive (systolic BP <90 mm Hg), order an IV line to be started immediately and ask the RN to place the patient in the Trendelenburg position (foot of the bed up).

   IV access is essential to deliver medications to increase the heart rate. Placing the patient in the Trendelenburg position achieves an autotransfusion of 200 to 300 mL of blood.

2. If the heart rate is <40 beats/min, ask the RN to have a premixed syringe of *atropine* 1 mg ready at the bedside.

3. Obtain a stat ECG and rhythm strip.

4. Ask the RN to bring the cardiac arrest cart into the room and attach the patient to the ECG monitor.

Inform RN

"I will arrive at the bedside in . . . minutes."

Bradycardia plus hypotension, or any HR <50 beats/min, requires you to see the patient immediately.

ELEVATOR THOUGHTS

What causes slow heart rates?

Sinus Bradycardia (Fig. 15–17)

Drugs	Beta blockers
	Calcium channel blockers
	Digoxin
	Other antiarrhythmic agents (amiodarone, sotalol)
Cardiac	SSS
	Acute MI (usually of inferior wall)
	Vasovagal attack
Misc	Hypothyroidism
	Healthy young athletes
	Increased intracranial pressure in association with hypertension

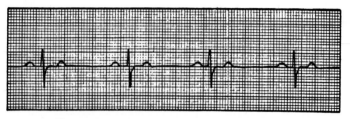

Figure 15–17 Slow heart rate—sinus bradycardia.

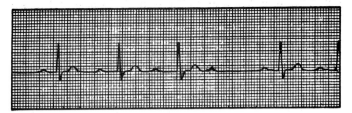

Figure 15–18 Slow heart rate—second-degree atrioventricular block (type I).

Second-Degree Atrioventricular Block: Type I (Wenckebach) (Fig. 15–18) and Type II (Fig. 15–19)

Drugs	Beta blockers
	Digoxin
	Calcium channel blockers
	Other antiarrhythmic agents (amiodarone, sotalol)
Cardiac	Acute MI
	SSS

Third-Degree Atrioventricular Block (Fig. 15–20)

Drugs	Beta blockers
	Calcium channel blockers
	Digoxin
	Other antiarrhythmic agents (amiodarone, sotalol)
Cardiac	Acute MI
	SSS

Atrial Fibrillation with Slow Ventricular Rate (Fig. 15–21)

Drugs	Digoxin
	Beta blockers
	Calcium channel blockers
	Other antiarrhythmic agents (amiodarone, sotalol)
Cardiac	SSS

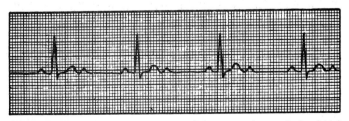

Figure 15–19 Slow heart rate—second-degree atrioventricular block (type II).

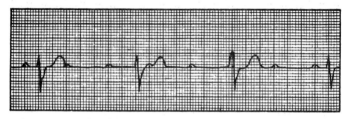

Figure 15–20 Slow heart rate—third-degree atrioventricular block.

Notice that no matter which bradycardia is present, the most common causes are drug related and cardiac.

MAJOR THREAT TO LIFE

- Hypotension
- MI

Two major threats to life exist in a patient with bradycardia. First, if the HR is sufficiently low, it will result in *hypotension* due to inadequate CO, resulting in hypoperfusion of vital organs. Second, if the bradycardia is due to *MI*, the patient will be prone to even more ominous dysrhythmias, such as ventricular tachycardia or fibrillation or asystole.

BEDSIDE

Quick-Look Test

Does the patient look well (comfortable), sick (uncomfortable or distressed), or critical (about to die?)

If the patient looks sick or critical, ask the RN to bring the cardiac arrest cart to the bedside and attach the patient to the ECG monitor. This may provide an instant diagnosis of the patient's

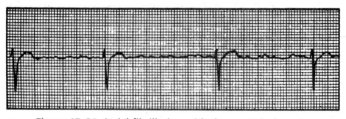

Figure 15–21 Atrial fibrillation with slow ventricular rate.

rhythm, allows continuous monitoring, and provides instant feedback on the effects of your interventions.

Airway and Vital Signs

What is the HR?

Read the ECG to identify which slow rhythm is occurring.

What is the BP?

Most causes of hypotension are accompanied by a compensatory reflex *tachycardia*. If hypotension exists with any of the bradycardias, proceed as follows:

- Notify your resident as soon as possible.
- Elevate the patient's legs.
  > This is a temporary measure that shifts blood volume from the legs to the central circulation.
- Begin a 250- to 500-mL IV bolus of normal saline (NS).
- Give *atropine* 0.5 mg IV as rapidly as possible. If there is no response after 5 minutes, give an additional 0.5 mg atropine IV every 5 minutes, not to exceed a total dose of 0.04 mg/kg. If there is still no improvement, begin transcutaneous pacing, if available, or try *dopamine* 5 to 10 µg/kg per minute IV infusion (must be given through a central line) or *epinephrine* 2 to 10 µg/min IV infusion (must be given through a central line). The patient should be transferred to the ICU/CCU for further monitoring and possible transvenous pacemaker placement.

Selective History and Chart Review

Look for the cause of bradycardia.

Drugs	Beta blockers
	Calcium channel blockers
	Digoxin
	Other antiarrhythmic agents (amiodarone, sotalol)
Cardiac ischemia	Does the patient have a history of angina or previous MI?
	Has there been any hint (chest pain, SOB, nausea, vomiting) that a cardiac ischemic event occurred within the past few days?
	Does the patient have other evidence of atherosclerosis (previous stroke, transient ischemic attacks [TIAs], peripheral vascular disease) that may be a clue to the concomitant presence of coronary artery disease?
	Does the patient have current risk factors (hypertension, diabetes mellitus, smoking, hypercholesterolemia, family history of coronary artery disease) that may suggest that this is the first episode of cardiac ischemia?

	If there is any evidence that the bradycardia is due to an acute MI, the patient should go to the ICU/CCU for ECG monitoring.
Vasovagal attack	Is there a history of pain, straining, or other Valsalva-like maneuver immediately before the occurrence of the bradycardia?

Selective Physical Examination

Look for a cause of bradycardia.

Vitals	Bradypnea (hypothyroidism)
	Hypothermia (hypothyroidism)
	Hypertension (risk factor for coronary artery disease)
HEENT	Coarse facial features (hypothyroidism)
	Loss of lateral third of eyebrows (hypothyroidism)
	Periorbital xanthomas (coronary artery disease)
	Fundi with hypertensive or diabetic changes (coronary artery disease)
	Carotid bruits (cerebrovascular disease with concomitant coronary artery disease)
CVS	New S_3, S_4, or mitral regurgitant murmur (nonspecific but common findings in acute MI)
ABD	Renal, aortic, or femoral bruits (concomitant coronary artery disease)
Ext	Poor peripheral pulses (peripheral vascular disease with concomitant coronary artery disease)
Neuro	Delayed return phase of deep tendon reflexes (hypothyroidism)

Management

Sinus Bradycardia

- No immediate treatment is required if the patient is not hypotensive.
- If the patient is on digoxin with a HR <60 beats/min, further digoxin doses should be held until the HR is >60 beats/min.
- If the patient is on medications that depress conduction, no immediate treatment is required, as long as the patient is not hypotensive. However, with very slow HRs (<40 beats/min), subsequent doses of these medications should be held until the HR is >60 beats/min. Further maintenance doses can be determined in consultation with the attending physician.

Second-Degree Atrioventricular Block (Types I and II) and Third-Degree Block

Patients with either second- or third-degree AV block should be temporarily taken off any drugs that are known to prolong AV conduction and transferred to a bed where continuous ECG monitoring is available.

Atrial Fibrillation with Slow Ventricular Response

This dysrhythmia does not require treatment unless the patient is hypotensive or has symptoms (syncope, confusion, angina, CHF) suggestive of vital organ hypoperfusion. Definitive treatment includes discontinuation of drugs that depress conduction and, in some cases, transfer to the ICU/CCU for pacemaker placement.

REMEMBER

1. Abrupt discontinuation of some beta blockers may result in rebound hypertension, angina, or MI. Observe the patient closely over the next several days. When the HR rises to >60 beats/min, the beta blocker may be reinstituted at a lower dosage. When treated in this manner, rebound hypertension or cardiac ischemia is seldom a problem.
2. Occasionally, digoxin overdose results in life-threatening dysrhythmias that are unresponsive to conventional measures. In these instances, *digoxin-specific antibodies* may be effective in reversing the toxic effects of digoxin.

High Blood Pressure

Calls concerning high blood pressure (BP) are frequent at night. They rarely require the use of drugs that rapidly reduce the pressure. The level of the BP itself is of less importance than the rate of the rise and the setting in which the high BP is occurring.

PHONE CALL

Questions

1. **Why is the patient in the hospital?**
2. **Is the patient pregnant?**
   Hypertension in a pregnant patient may indicate the development of preeclampsia or eclampsia and should be assessed immediately.
3. **Is the patient taking antidepressant drugs?**
   Hypertension occurring in a patient receiving monoamine oxidase (MAO) inhibitors or tricyclic antidepressants suggests the possibility of a catecholamine crisis due to food or drug interaction.
4. **Is the patient in the emergency department?**
   Hypertension in a young individual presenting in the emergency department may be caused by catecholamine hypertension due to cocaine or amphetamine abuse.
5. **How high is the BP, and what has the BP been previously?**
6. **Does the patient have symptoms suggestive of a hypertensive emergency?**
   a. Back and chest pain (aortic dissection)
   b. Chest pain (myocardial ischemia)
   c. Shortness of breath (pulmonary edema)
   d. Headache, neck stiffness (subarachnoid hemorrhage)
   e. Headache, vomiting, confusion, seizures (hypertensive encephalopathy)
7. **What antihypertensive medication has the patient been taking?**

Orders

If the patient has any symptoms of a hypertensive emergency, order intravenous (IV) 5% dextrose in water (D5W) to keep the vein open (TKVO) immediately.

Inform RN

"I will be at the bedside in . . . minutes."

Situations requiring immediate assessment and possibly prompt lowering of BP include the following:

- Eclampsia
- Aortic dissection
- Pulmonary edema resistant to other emergency treatment (see Chapter 24, pages 270 to 272)
- Myocardial ischemia
- Catecholamine crisis
- Hypertensive encephalopathy
- Uncontrolled bleeding anywhere, including worsening vision secondary to retinal hemorrhage

ELEVATOR THOUGHTS

The diagnosis of *preeclampsia* can be made in an obstetric patient with hypertension, edema, and proteinuria. This syndrome usually occurs in the third trimester of pregnancy, at which stage hypertension is defined as BP ≥140/85 mm Hg for longer than 4 to 6 hours or as an increase of ≥30 mm Hg in systolic BP or ≥15 mm Hg in diastolic BP, compared with pregestational values.

Aortic dissection is potentiated by high shearing forces determined by the rate of rise of the intraventricular pressure as well as the systolic pressure.

Elevation of afterload (increased systemic vascular resistance and elevated BP) may be a readily correctable detrimental factor in *myocardial ischemia* and *pulmonary edema*.

Catecholamine crisis can be caused by the following:

Drug overdose	Cocaine, amphetamines
Drug interaction	MAO inhibitors, indirect-acting catechols (wine, cheese, ephedrine)
	Tricyclics, direct-acting catechols (epinephrine, pseudoephedrine, norepinephrine)
Drug withdrawal	Abrupt withdrawal from antihypertensive agents such as beta blockers, centrally acting alpha agonists, and angiotensin-converting enzyme (ACE) inhibitors may result in a rebound hypertensive crisis

Pheochromocytoma	May produce a hypertensive crisis through overproduction of epinephrine or norepinephrine
Burns	Some patients with second- or third-degree burns develop a transient hypertensive crisis, usually resolving within 2 weeks, due to high circulating levels of catecholamines, renin, and angiotensin II

Hypertensive encephalopathy is a rare complication of hypertension and is unusual in hospitalized patients. Vomiting developing over several days, and headache, lethargy, and confusion are suggestive symptoms. Focal neurologic deficits are uncommon in the early course of encephalopathy.

BP fluctuates in normal individuals and more so in hypertensive individuals. Excitement, fear, and anxiety from unrelated medical conditions or procedures can cause marked transient increases in BP. BP measurements require care with regard to proper cuff size and placement and should be repeated to confirm the readings.

MAJOR THREAT TO LIFE

The major immediate threat to life is a marked increase in BP with the following:
- Eclampsia
- Aortic dissection
- Pulmonary edema
- Myocardial infarction (MI)
- Hypertensive encephalopathy

BEDSIDE

Quick-Look Test

Does the patient look well (comfortable), sick (uncomfortable or distressed), or critical (about to die)?

Unless the patient is having seizures (eclampsia, hypertensive encephalopathy) or is markedly short of breath (pulmonary edema), the severity of the situation cannot be assessed by the initial appearance. The patient may have hypertensive encephalopathy yet look deceptively well.

Airway and Vital Signs

What is the BP?

Retake the BP in both arms.

Accompanying arteriosclerosis may unilaterally reduce brachial artery flow and give an artifactually low BP reading. A lower pressure in one arm may be a clue to aortic dissection. Too small a cuff on an obese patient or a patient with rigid arteriosclerotic peripheral vessels may give readings that are factitiously high in relation to the intra-arterial pressure.

What is the heart rate?

Bradycardia and hypertension in a patient not receiving beta blockers may indicate increasing intracranial pressure.

Tachycardia and hypertension can be seen in catecholamine crisis.

Selective History

Can the patient further elucidate the duration of hypertension?

Does the patient have any symptoms suggestive of a hypertensive emergency?

- Headache (an occipital headache or neck ache, lethargy, or blurred vision suggests hypertensive encephalopathy)
- Chest pain (myocardial ischemia)
- Shortness of breath (pulmonary edema)
- Back or chest pain (aortic dissection)
- Unilateral weakness or sensory symptoms (suggests a cerebro-vascular accident); such an episode in a previously hypertensive patient may be associated with a transient increase in BP

Selective Physical Examination

Does the patient have evidence of a hypertensive emergency?

HEENT	Assess the fundi for hypertensive changes (generalized or focal arteriolar narrowing, flame-shaped hemorrhages near the disk, dot-and-blot hemorrhages, exudates)
	Papilledema is an ominous finding in patients with hypertension and is seen in malignant hypertension and hypertensive encephalopathy (Fig. 16–1); hypertensive encephalopathy can occur without papilledema, but retinal hemorrhages and exudates are almost always present
Resp	Crackles, pleural effusion (CHF)
CVS	Elevated JVP, S_3 (CHF)
Neuro	Confusion, delirium, agitation, or lethargy (hypertensive encephalopathy)
	Localized deficits (stroke)

Management

Most often, elevated BP is an isolated finding in an asymptomatic patient known to have hypertension. Although long-term control of

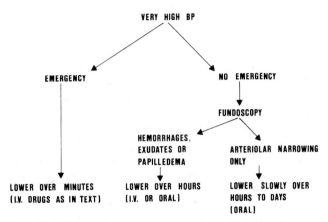

Figure 16–1 Approach to management of very high blood pressure.

hypertension in such patients is of proved benefit, acute lowering of BP is not. Remember, there is a risk of overshooting the mark when acutely reducing BP in patients with long-standing hypertension and a decreased ability to autoregulate cerebral blood flow. Do not treat the BP reading. Treat the condition associated with it.

True emergencies require special management. These include the following:

- Hypertensive encephalopathy
- Malignant hypertension (marked elevation of diastolic BP with fundal hemorrhages and exudates and usually some compromise in renal function)
- Eclampsia
- Subarachnoid or cerebral hemorrhage
- Aortic dissection
- Hypertension and pulmonary edema or myocardial ischemia
- Catecholamine crisis

Call your resident for help if you are unfamiliar with the management of these conditions.

Hypertensive Encephalopathy

This is almost always accompanied by retinal exudates and hemorrhages and is often accompanied by papilledema. Focal neurologic deficits are unusual early on and suggest that the elevated pressure is most likely associated with a stroke. Remember the risk of lowering pressure too quickly in patients with atherothrombotic cerebrovascular disease; you can precipitate a stroke!

1. Transfer the patient to the intensive care unit/cardiac care unit (ICU/CCU) for electrocardiogram (ECG) monitoring and intra-arterial BP monitoring.

2. Because transfer to the ICU/CCU often takes >30 minutes, you can temporarily achieve BP control by giving the patient a single oral tablet of one of the following:

   a. *Nifedipine* 5 to 10 mg PO for one dose. In patients with long-standing hypertension, an abrupt reduction in BP may compromise coronary and cerebral blood flow, and in the presence of atherosclerosis, this can result in MI or stroke. This risk can be reduced if an intact nifedipine capsule is given orally in an initial dose of 5 to 10 mg. The effect of this dose is usually apparent within 30 minutes, and a repeat dose of 5 to 10 mg may be given if there is insufficient BP lowering. Few situations require the more rapid (by 5 to 10 minutes) but less predictable response that occurs after biting and swallowing the capsule. The sublingual route should not be used because nifedipine is not absorbed by the oral mucosa. Aim for diastolic BP levels around 100 mm Hg.

   b. *Captopril* 25 mg PO

   c. *Labetalol* 200 mg PO

   d. *Atenolol* 25 mg PO or *nadolol* 20 mg PO

3. *Labetalol* is a combined alpha- and beta-blocking agent that may be given IV without intra-arterial monitoring. It may be given in repeated incremental doses, beginning at 20 mg IV, every 10 to 15 minutes (e.g., 20 mg, 20 mg, 40 mg, 40 mg) to a maximum of 300 mg. Alternatively, a labetalol infusion beginning at 2 mg/min and titrating to a BP response may be given. Labetalol is not as useful in lowering BP if the patient is already on a beta blocker.

4. A *nitroprusside infusion* may be required. In most medical situations, IV nitroprusside cannot be given to patients in general medical units because of the requirement for intra-arterial BP monitoring. However, you can expedite treatment by informing the ICU/CCU staff in advance that a patient will require IV nitroprusside infusion. The usual dose is 0.10 to 5 µg/kg per minute.

5. Once BP control is achieved through parenteral means, the patient should be started on an appropriate oral regimen to maintain satisfactory BP control.

Malignant Hypertension

Unless this is accompanied by another feature (e.g., encephalopathy, pulmonary edema), there is more time to gain control of the BP. Control can be achieved by using a combination of orally effective antihypertensive drugs. Review the patient's current antihypertensive treatment, and increase to the maximum effective dose or add other agents. More aggressive approaches can wait until morning.

Preeclampsia and Eclampsia

Treatment in these patients is complicated by the risk to the fetus and the mother from both the disorder and the treatment. The treatment of choice near term is magnesium sulfate until delivery of the baby can be effected. Treatment should be initiated only in consultation with the patient's obstetrician. *Magnesium sulfate* is given as an IV infusion: mix 16 g of magnesium sulfate in 1 L of D5W and give a loading dose of 250 mL (4 g) IV over 20 minutes. The maintenance dose is 1 to 2 g (62.5 to 125 mL)/hr or more, as required. Order a serum magnesium level every 4 hours, aiming for a serum magnesium level of 6 to 8 mmol/L.

Note that magnesium sulfate does not lower BP. Local practice may include giving other drugs, such as labetalol, hydralazine, or nitroprusside. Diuretics should be avoided, because these patients are usually already volume depleted, with an activated renin-angiotensin system.

Subarachnoid or Cerebral Hemorrhage

Although there is no proof that lowering pressure alters the outcome, many neurologists administer drugs to control elevated pressure in these situations. Unless you are familiar with the local practice, a neurologist should be consulted.

Aortic Dissection

1. Transfer the patient to the ICU/CCU immediately for intra-arterial BP monitoring and control of BP with parenteral drugs.
2. *Nitroprusside* 0.10 to 5 µg/kg per minute is useful in the management of aortic dissection but should not be used without an accompanying beta blocker, which reduces the rate of rise of intraventricular pressure and hence the shearing force. These beta blockers should be given parenterally, and high doses may be required, as follows:
   a. *Propranolol* 0.1 mg/kg by slow IV push, divided into three equal doses at 2- to 3- minute intervals. Repeat after 2 minutes if necessary. Do not exceed 1 mg/min.
   b. *Esmolol* 0.5 mg/kg for 1 minute, followed by a continuous infusion of 0.05 mg/kg per minute (maximum 0.3 mg/kg per minute). The only advantage of esmolol is its short half-life, providing a rapid onset and offset of action.
3. *Labetalol* alone may be used for aortic dissection in the same regimen as for hypertensive encephalopathy (see page 161).

Hypertension and Pulmonary Edema or Myocardial Ischemia

1. In addition to BP control, pulmonary edema should be treated with the measures outlined in Chapter 24, pages 270 to 272.
2. Transfer the patient to the ICU/CCU for continuous ECG and intra-arterial BP monitoring.
3. Notify the ICU/CCU staff that the patient will require an IV *nitroglycerin infusion.* Experimental evidence suggests that IV

nitroglycerin is preferable to IV nitroprusside for the control of BP in a patient with myocardial ischemia because nitroprusside may cause a coronary steal phenomenon, resulting in extension of the ischemic zone. It is therefore preferable to attempt BP control in a cardiac patient with IV nitroglycerin; if unsuccessful, nitroprusside can be used.

4. If the patient is hypertensive and tachycardic and has myocardial ischemia but no evidence of pulmonary edema, beta blockade is helpful in addition to IV nitroglycerin. Any of the following agents may be used acutely:

   a. *Propranolol* 0.1 mg/kg by slow IV push, divided into three equal doses at 2- to 3-minute intervals. Repeat after 2 minutes if necessary. Do not exceed 1 mg/min.
   b. *Esmolol* 0.5 mg/kg for 1 minute, followed by a continuous infusion of 0.05 mg/kg per minute (maximum 0.3 mg/kg per minute).
   c. *Metoprolol* 5 to 15 mg IV.
   d. *Atenolol* 5 mg IV.

Catecholamine Crisis

Pheochromocytoma (pallor, palpitations, perspiration) is the classic condition associated with intermittent and alarmingly high BP. Other conditions associated with sudden and severe increases in BP include *cocaine* and *amphetamine* abuse; major second- or third-degree *burns*; abrupt antihypertensive *drug withdrawal*; and food (cheese), drug (ephedrine), and drink (wine) interactions with *MAO inhibitors* (antidepressants). Currently used MAO inhibitors include tranylcypromine sulfate (Parnate), phenelzine sulfate (Nardil), and isocarboxazid (Marplan). If sudden increases in pressure are observed in patients on these drugs, the most likely cause is an interaction with a substance that is releasing catecholamine stores, which are overabundant because of inhibition of one of the catecholamine-metabolizing enzymes (MAO).

1. Transfer the patient to the ICU/CCU for ECG and intra-arterial BP monitoring.
2. Notify the ICU/CCU staff that the patient will require special parenteral antihypertensive drugs.
3. In cases of known or suspected **pheochromocytoma,** *phentolamine mesilate,* a direct alpha blocker, may be given IV for marked elevation of BP. This drug causes a decrease in peripheral resistance and an increase in venous capacity due to a direct action on vascular smooth muscle. This effect may be accompanied by cardiac stimulation, with tachycardia greater than can be explained by a reflex response to peripheral vasodilatation. In an emergency, 2.5 to 5 mg IV may be given. However, if time permits and for continuous control, *phentolamine mesilate* should be given at an initial dosage of 5 to 10 µg/kg per minute by continuous IV infusion.

Alternatively, *labetalol* or *nitroprusside* can be used in the same dosages as described previously.

4. In **cocaine-induced hypertension,** *labetalol, phentolamine,* or *nitroprusside* may be used in the same dosages as described previously. Propranolol and beta blockers other than labetalol should be avoided because of the risk of unopposed alpha stimulation.[1]

5. In **amphetamine-induced hypertension,** *chlorpromazine* 1 mg/kg IM can reverse hypertension and hyperactivity. *Nitroprusside* may be used in the same dosages as described previously. Propranolol and beta blockers should be avoided because of the risk of unopposed alpha stimulation.

   Ecstasy is structurally related to methamphetamine, with hallucinogenic and amphetamine-like effects, but it has greater central stimulatory effects than amphetamine does. Its cardiovascular effects include an increase in systolic and diastolic pressure and a reflex slowing of heart rate. Nitroprusside or an alpha-adrenergic-blocking drug are the agents of choice to control BP; chlorpromazine may be helpful to reduce the central stimulatory effects.

6. In **catecholamine crisis** associated with **MAO inhibitors,** phentolamine, labetalol, or nitroprusside may be effective.

Reference

1. Lange RA, Cigarroa RG, Flores ED, et al: Potentiation of cocaine-induced coronary vasoconstriction by beta-adrenergic blockade. Ann Intern Med 1990;112:897-903.

Hypnotics, Laxatives, Analgesics, and Antipyretics

Telephone calls regarding the reordering of hypnotic, laxative, analgesic, and antipyretic medications are frequent. The majority of these requests can be managed over the telephone.

HYPNOTICS

PHONE CALL

Questions

1. **Why is a hypnotic being requested?**
   The majority of requests for nighttime sedation are due to insomnia. Sleeping pills should not be prescribed for restless or agitated patients who have not been examined.
2. **Has the patient received hypnotics before?**
3. **What are the vital signs?**
4. **What was the reason for admission?**
5. **Does the patient have any of the following conditions in which hypnotics are contraindicated?**
   a. Depression—an antidepressant is the drug of choice if insomnia is a manifestation of depression
   b. Confusion
   c. Hepatic or respiratory insufficiency
   d. Sleep apnea
   e. Myasthenia gravis
6. **Is the patient receiving other centrally active drugs that may interact, such as alcohol, antidepressants, antihistamines, and narcotics?**
7. **Does the patient have any drug allergies?**
   The major contraindication to a specific hypnotic is a known allergy to the drug.

165

Orders

A benzodiazepine is the drug of choice for short-term treatment of insomnia. Sedative effects are comparable among all benzodiazepines; only the onset and duration of effect differ. Table 17–1 lists the drug doses of various benzodiazepines.

Inform RN

"I will arrive at the bedside in . . . minutes."

Agitated, restless patients should be assessed before hypnotics are prescribed.

REMEMBER

1. The biologic half-lives of benzodiazepines vary from 4 hours for oxazepam to 50 to 100 hours for diazepam. Accumulation can occur if the second and subsequent doses are given before the previous dose has been metabolized and excreted. Diazepam and flurazepam have active metabolites; the half-lives (see Table 17–1) include the active metabolites. When a drug is prescribed once or twice, the half-life of the drug is of

TABLE 17–1 **Characteristics of Selected Benzodiazepines**

Drug	Usual Adult Dose (mg)	Time of Peak Effect	Biologic Half-life (hr)
Short Acting			
Midazolam (Versed)	0.035–0.1/kg IV	1.5–5 min	1–4
Triazolam (Halcion)	0.125–0.25 PO	1–2 hr	1.5–5
Hypnotic			
Temazepam (Restoril)	30 PO HS	0.8–1.4 hr	8–10
Nitrazepam (Mogadon)	5–10 PO HS	2 hr	26
Flurazepam (Dalmane)	15–30 PO HS	1 hr	50–100
Zaleplon (Sonata, Starnoc)*	5–10 PO HS	1 hr	?
Antianxiety			
Oxazepam (Serax)	30–120/day	1–4 hr	4–13
Alprazolam (Xanax)	0.5–1.5/day	1–2 hr	6–20
Lorazepam (Ativan)	0.5–2/day	1–6 hr	12–15
Chlordiazepoxide (Librium)	15–75/day	2–4 hr	20–24
Clorazepate (Traxene)	30/day	1–2 hr	48
Diazepam (Valium)	4–40/day	2 hr	50–100

*Zaleplon is not structurally related to the benzodiazepines but binds to the same receptors.

no great concern, because diffusion out of the brain, rather than the rate of elimination from the body, is the major factor responsible for the duration of effect. However, with repeated use of benzodiazepines, the drug half-life must be taken into account; the rates of metabolism then become more important in determining the duration of effect. For example, flurazepam given repeatedly causes a daytime hangover, whereas oxazepam does not. However, the shortest-acting drugs may be associated with early-morning insomnia and rebound daytime anxiety.

2. Benzodiazepines should not be prescribed on a nightly basis; they should be discontinued temporarily once one or two nights of acceptable sleep have been achieved. The use of benzodiazepines for less than 14 consecutive nights helps prevent the development of drug tolerance and dependence.

3. Be aware of the adverse effects of any drug you prescribe. The adverse effects of benzodiazepines are central nervous system (CNS) depression (tiredness, drowsiness, detached feeling), headache, dizziness, ataxia, confusion, disorientation in the elderly, and psychological dependence.

4. Barbiturates and nonbarbiturate hypnotics other than benzodiazepines usually carry more risks than advantages and should be avoided.

LAXATIVES

Constipation is frequently aggravated or caused by drugs (e.g., iron supplements, calcium entry blockers, aluminum-containing antacids) or medical conditions (e.g., hypothyroidism, diabetes mellitus, Parkinson's disease, diverticular disease). Hospitalized patients commonly require laxatives, particularly after acute myocardial infarction to limit straining, during the administration of narcotics, during prolonged bed rest, and during evacuation of the bowels before abdominal surgery and some gastrointestinal (GI) diagnostic procedures. The solutions used in *enemas* have either hypertonic properties to stimulate rectal peristalsis or surfactant properties to soften impacted feces.

PHONE CALL

Questions

1. **Why is a laxative being requested?**
    The frequency of bowel movements is highly variable in the normal population, ranging from twice daily to once every 3 days. Make certain you know what this patient's normal bowel pattern is before prescribing a laxative.
2. **Has the patient received laxatives before? If so, which ones have been tried so far?**

3. **What are the vital signs?**
4. **What was the reason for admission?**
5. **When was a rectal examination last performed?**
    Fecal impaction, which requires a rectal examination for diagnosis (and sometimes for treatment), is a relative contra-indication to oral laxative use.
6. **Does the patient have nausea, vomiting, or abdominal pain?**
    These symptoms suggest an acute GI disorder.

Orders

Table 17–2 lists the drug doses of selected laxatives, and Table 17–3 lists the drug doses of enemas. Bowel movements can be increased

TABLE 17–2 **Characteristics of Selected Laxatives**

Drug	Dose	Comments
Bulk Forming		
Psyllium hydrophilic mucilloid (Metamucil and others)	3–6.5 g PO once to TID	Cellulose binds drugs (e.g., digoxin); not useful for acute constipation
Surface Active		
Docusate (sodium dioctyl sulfo-succinate; Colace)	100 mg PO TID; 50 mg/90 mL enema fluid	Stool softener; lowers surface tension
Lubricant		
Mineral oil	Emulsion 15 mL BID	Impairs the absorption of fat-soluble vitamins
Osmotic		
Lactulose	15–30 mL PO	
Glycerin	2.67-g suppository	Onset in 30 min
Milk of magnesia	15–30 mL PO	Do not use Mg preparations in renal impairment
Magnesium citrate oral solution	15 g/300 mL solution, or 7–21 mL of a 70% solution	
Stimulant		
Anthraquinones (cascara, senna)	Variable	Onset in 6 hr; urine may be brown
Diphenylmethanes (e.g., bisacodyl)	5–15 mg PO or 10 mg PR	See page 453
Castor oil	15–60 mL	May give profound evacuation

TABLE 17-3 Characteristics of Selected Enemas

Preparation	Onset	Caution	Usual Adult Dose	Use
Sodium phosphate and sodium biphosphate (Fleet)	Immediate	Do not use when nausea, vomiting, or abdominal pain is present	60–120 mL (6 g sodium phosphate and 16 g sodium biphosphate/100 mL)*	Acute evacuation of the bowel before diagnostic procedures; acute constipation
Bisacodyl (Fleet Bisacodyl)	Immediate	Do not use when nausea, vomiting, or abdominal pain is present; avoid in pregnancy and myocardial infarction; may worsen orthostatic hypotension, weakness, and incoordination in the elderly	37.5 mL (10 mg/30 mL)*	Acute evacuation of the bowel before diagnostic procedures; acute constipation
Mineral oil (Fleet Mineral Oil)	Immediate	Do not use when nausea, vomiting, or abdominal pain is present	60–120 mL*	Impacted feces
Microlax (sodium citrate 450 mg, sodium alkylsulfoacetate 45 mg, sorbic acid 5 mg)	5–15 min	Do not use when nausea, vomiting, or abdominal pain is present	5 mL	Fecal impaction when hard stool is present in the rectum; not useful if rectum is empty

*Available in disposable plastic containers.

in frequency by liquefying the stool. Both bulk and osmotic laxatives increase the water content in the intestine. An increase in the frequency of bowel movements can also be induced by stool softeners and colon-irritating drugs that increase peristalsis.

Inform RN

"I will arrive at the bedside in . . . minutes."

When a laxative has been requested, you need to assess the patient only when there is associated nausea, vomiting, or abdominal pain or when fecal impaction is suspected. (See Chapter 5 for the assessment and management of abdominal pain.)

REMEMBER

1. When a patient is constipated (unless there is fecal impaction), an oral laxative is the treatment of choice. If the oral laxative fails, a stronger-acting laxative can be used; if this is not effective, a suppository is prescribed. Finally, enemas can be used as follows: first, a hypertonic enema solution (e.g., Fleet); if unsuccessful, an oil-retention enema can be tried.
2. When there is fecal impaction, an oil-based enema is the treatment of choice.
3. Soapsuds enemas are used primarily for preoperative bowel cleansing. They are quite uncomfortable because of the large volumes used and are rarely required in the treatment of constipation.

ANALGESICS

Most hospital pharmacies do not allow narcotic medication orders to stand indefinitely. Narcotic medications need to be reordered every 3 to 5 days, depending on the individual medical institution. Consequently, if the house staff fails to reorder these medications during the day, you may be called to do so at night.

PHONE CALL

Questions

1. **Why is an analgesic being requested?**
   The majority of requests are for reordering of medications.
2. **How severe is the pain?**
   This question helps determine whether a non-narcotic analgesic may be sufficient.
3. **Is this a new problem?**
   The new onset of undiagnosed pain requires you to assess the patient at the bedside before ordering an analgesic medication.

4. **What are the vital signs?**
    The onset of fever in association with pain suggests a localized infectious process.
5. **What was the reason for admission?**
6. **Does the patient have any drug allergies?**

Orders

Tables 17–4 and 17–5 provide the drug dosages of selected analgesics.

Inform RN

"I will arrive at the bedside in . . . minutes."
    Any undiagnosed pain, new onset of severe pain, or change in character of previous pain requires you to assess the patient at the bedside before ordering an analgesic.

REMEMBER

If reversal of a narcotic overdose is required, the following are recommended:
1. *Reversal of postoperative narcotic depression.* Give *naloxone* (Narcan) 0.2 to 2 mg IV every 5 minutes until the desired improved level of consciousness is achieved (maximum total dose, 10 mg). Doses every 1 to 2 hours may be required to maintain reversal of CNS depression.
2. *Reversal of suspected narcotic overdose.* If the patient is comatose, intubation for airway protection should be undertaken before reversal. Abrupt reversal may induce nausea and vomiting, with the attendant risk of aspiration pneumonia. Give *naloxone* 0.2 mg IV, SC, or IM every 5 minutes for several doses. If the initial dosages are ineffective, the dose may be increased incrementally to a maximum total dose of 10 mg.
3. *Adverse effects of abrupt narcotic reversal.* Nausea and vomiting, if provoked in a patient with an unprotected airway, may result in aspiration pneumonia. Hypertension and tachycardia can occur during narcotic reversal and may result in congestive heart failure in a patient with poor left ventricular function.

ANTIPYRETICS

Antipyretics should not be prescribed in an adult patient with fever unless the cause of the fever is known or the patient is symptomatic from the fever itself. (Refer to Chapter 12 for the approach to the febrile patient. See Table 17–4 for the dosages and side effects of acetaminophen and aspirin.)

TABLE 17-4 Characteristics of Commonly Used Analgesics for Mild to Moderate Pain

Drug	Duration of Effect (hr)	Usual Adult PO Dose	Comments
Acetaminophen, paracetamol (Tylenol)	4	325–975 mg q4h	Has practically no anti-inflammatory or platelet effects
Aspirin, acetylsalicylic acid	4	650–975 mg q4h	Equal analgesia to acetaminophen, except more effective in inflammatory arthritis; has an irreversible platelet effect
Diflunisal (Dolobid)	8–12	1000 mg, then 500 mg q12h	Salicylate derivative, but has no antiplatelet effect at lower doses
Ibuprofen (Motrin, Advil)	4	400 mg q4–6h	More effective than 650 mg of aspirin as an analgesic
Naproxen (Naprosyn)	6	500 mg, then 250 mg q6–8h	
Indomethacin (Indocin)	8–12	25–50 mg q8–12h	High incidence of gastrointestinal and renal side effects; not indicated for routine use as an analgesic
Diclofenac (Voltaren)	6–8	25–50 mg q6–8h	Can cause an increase in hepatic enzymes
Codeine	2–4	30–60 mg q4–6h	More effective than propoxyphene and less addicting than oxycodone
Oxycodone with acetaminophen or aspirin (Percocet, Percodan)	2–4	—	Not recommended because of high abuse potential
Propoxyphene (Darvon)	2–4	100 mg q4–6h	Equipotent to 650 mg aspirin

TABLE 17-5 **Characteristics of Selected Narcotic Drugs**

Drug	Usual Adult Dose		Comments
	Oral (mg)	SC/IM (mg)	
Morphine Sulfate Preparations			
MSIR (immediate release)	5–30 q4–6h*		Available in oral solution or tablet form
MS Contin (sustained release)	15–120 q12h		Because it is difficult to titrate sustained-release doses, it is best to initiate morphine treatment with an immediate-release preparation
Morphine injection		5–15 q4–6h*	
Other Drugs			
Anileridine (Leritine)	25–50 q4–6h*	25–50 q4–6h*	
Hydromorphone (Dilaudid)	2–4 q4h*	2 q4h*	
Meperidine (Demerol)	50–150 q4h*	50–150 q4h*	

*The duration of action tends to be longer with oral than with parenteral administration.

Hypotension and Shock

Hypotension is a common problem requiring attention at night. Do not panic. Remember that hypotension does not become shock until there is evidence of inadequate tissue perfusion. An adequate blood pressure (BP) is required to perfuse three vital organs—*brain, heart,* and *kidneys.* Some patients normally have systolic BPs in the range of 85 to 100 mm Hg. The BP is usually adequate as long as the patient is not confused, disoriented, or unconscious; is not having angina; and is passing urine. However, a BP of 105/70 mm Hg may result in serious hypoperfusion in a patient who is normally hypertensive.

PHONE CALL

Questions

1. What is the BP?
2. What is the heart rate (HR)?
3. What is the temperature?
    Fever plus hypotension suggests impending septic shock.
4. Is the patient conscious?
5. Is the patient having chest pain?
6. Is there evidence of bleeding?
7. Has the patient been given intravenous (IV) contrast material or an antibiotic within the last 6 hours?
    If you are called to see a hypotensive patient in the x-ray department or a patient who has recently returned to the room after undergoing an x-ray procedure involving the administration of IV contrast material, your primary thought should be that the patient might be having an anaphylactic reaction.
8. What was the admitting diagnosis?

Orders

1. If the information provided over the telephone supports the possibility of impending or established shock, order the

following:

a. Two large-bore (size 16 if possible) IV lines immediately, if not already in place.

> IV access is a high priority in a hypotensive patient.

b. Place the patient in the reverse Trendelenburg position (i.e., head of the bed down and foot of the bed up). Although hypotension should be assessed immediately, if you are unable to get to the bedside for 10 to 15 minutes, also ask the nurse to give 500 mL normal saline (NS) IV as rapidly as possible.

c. Have an arterial blood gas (ABG) tray at the bedside.

> Identification and correction of hypoxia and acidemia are essential in the management of shock.

d. Administer oxygen at a rate of 4 to 10 L by facemask while awaiting the results of the ABG.

2. If there is a suspicion of *anaphylaxis*, ask the RN to have available a premixed syringe of IV epinephrine from the cardiac arrest cart.

3. If the admitting diagnosis is *gastrointestinal (GI) bleed*, or if there is visible evidence of blood loss

a. Ensure that there is blood on hold for the patient. If not, order a stat crossmatch for 2, 4, or 6 units of packed red blood cells (RBCs), depending on your estimate of blood loss.

b. Order a hemoglobin (Hb) stat.

> *Caution*: The Hb may be normal during an acute hemorrhage and drop only with correction of the intravascular volume by a shift of fluid from the interstitial and intracellular spaces, or by fluid therapy. (Refer to Chapter 13 for further investigation and management of GI bleeds.)

4. If an arrhythmia or ischemic myocardial event is suspected, order a stat electrocardiogram (ECG) and rhythm strip.

These may help you identify a rapid heart rhythm or an acute myocardial infarction (MI), which may be responsible for hypotension.

Inform RN

"I will arrive at the bedside in . . . minutes."

Hypotension requires you to see the patient immediately.

ELEVATOR THOUGHTS

What causes hypotension or shock?

- Cardiogenic causes
- Hypovolemia
- Sepsis
- Anaphylaxis

Two formulas are useful to remember when considering the causes of hypotension:

$$BP = \text{cardiac output (CO)} \times \text{total peripheral resistance (TPR)}$$
$$CO = HR \times \text{stroke volume (SV)}$$

From these formulas, it can be seen that hypotension results from a fall in either CO or TPR. *Cardiogenic causes* result from a fall in CO due to either a fall in HR (e.g., heart block) or a fall in SV (e.g., acute MI, cardiac tamponade, massive pulmonary embolism, superior vena cava obstruction, tension pneumothorax). *Hypovolemia* reduces SV; hence CO falls. *Sepsis* and *anaphylaxis* cause hypotension by lowering TPR.

MAJOR THREAT TO LIFE

- Shock

  Remember that hypotension does not become shock until there is evidence of inadequate tissue perfusion. Shock is a relatively easy diagnosis to make. Your goal is to identify and correct the cause of hypotension before it results in hypoperfusion of vital organs.

BEDSIDE

Quick-Look Test

Does the patient look well (comfortable), sick (uncomfortable or distressed), or critical (about to die)?

A patient with hypotension but adequate tissue perfusion usually looks well. However, once perfusion of vital organs is compromised, the patient looks sick or critical.

Airway and Vital Signs

Is the airway clear?

If the patient is obtunded and cannot protect his or her airway, endotracheal intubation is required. Ask the RN to notify the intensive care unit/cardiac care unit (ICU/CCU) immediately. Roll the patient onto the left side to avoid aspiration until intubation is achieved.

Is the patient breathing?

Assess respiration by checking the respiratory rate, the position of the trachea, and chest expansion and by performing auscultation. All patients in shock should receive high-flow oxygen. If acute respiratory distress and marked respiratory effort accompany shock, intubation and ventilation may be necessary.

What is the status of the circulation?

1. If hypotension is not severe, examine for postural changes.

On standing, a postural rise in HR of >15 beats/min, a fall in systolic BP of >15 mm Hg, or any fall in diastolic BP indicates significant hypovolemia.

2. Measure the HR. Most causes of hypotension are accompanied by a compensatory reflex sinus tachycardia. If the patient is experiencing bradycardia or if you suspect a rhythm other than sinus tachycardia, refer to the discussion of bradycardia (later in this chapter) for further evaluation and management.

3. Determine whether the patient is in *shock*. This should take <20 seconds.

Vitals	Repeat now
CVS	Pulse volume, JVP
	Skin temperature and color
	Capillary refill (normal, <2 seconds)
Neuro	Mental status

> Shock is a clinical diagnosis: systolic BP <90 mm Hg with evidence of inadequate tissue perfusion, such as inadequate perfusion of the skin (cold, clammy, cyanotic) and of the central nervous system (agitation, confusion, lethargy, coma). In fact, the kidney is a sensitive indicator of shock (urine output <20 mL/hr), but the immediate placement of a Foley catheter should not take priority over resuscitation measures.

What is the temperature?

An elevated temperature or hypothermia (<36°C) suggests sepsis. However, remember that sepsis may occur in some patients, especially the elderly, with a normal temperature. Hence, the absence of fever does not rule out the possibility of septic shock.

What do the patient's pulse and ECG reveal?

1. **Bradycardia.** If the resting HR is <50 beats/min in the presence of hypotension, suspect one of three things:

    a. *Vasovagal attack.* If this is the case, the patient is usually normotensive by the time you arrive. Look for retrospective evidence of straining, Valsalva's maneuver, pain, or some other stimulus to vagal outflow. If vasovagal attack is suspected and there is persistent bradycardia despite leg elevation, give *atropine* 0.5 to 1 mg IV every 3 to 5 minutes as needed, not to exceed a total dose of 0.04 mg/kg.

    b. *Autonomic dysfunction.* The patient may have been given too much of a prescribed beta blocker or calcium channel blocker, resulting in hypotension, or the patient may be hypotensive for some other reason but is unable to generate a tachycardia because of beta blockade, calcium channel blockade, underlying sick sinus syndrome, or autonomic neuropathy. If the systolic BP is <90 mm Hg,

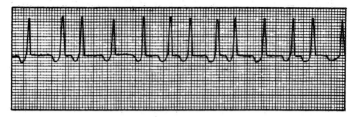

Figure 18–1 Atrial fibrillation with rapid ventricular response.

administer *atropine* 0.5 to 1 mg IV every 3 to 5 minutes as needed, not to exceed a total dose of 0.04 mg/kg.

c. *Heart block.* The patient may have a heart block (e.g., after acute MI). Obtain a stat ECG to document the dysrhythmia. If systolic BP is <90 mm Hg, atropine may be helpful, provided the atrioventricular (AV) block is at the level of the AV node, but it is usually ineffective in infra-nodal (e.g., Mobitz type II) block. The dose is *atropine* 0.5 to 1 mg IV every 3 to 5 minutes as needed, not to exceed a total dose of 0.04 mg/kg. Refer to Chapter 15 for further investigation and management of heart block.

2. **Tachycardia.** A compensatory sinus tachycardia is an expected, appropriate response in a hypotensive patient. Look at the ECG to ensure that the patient does not have one of the following three rapid heart rhythms, which may cause hypotension due to inadequate diastolic filling with or without loss of the atrial kick:

a. Atrial fibrillation with rapid ventricular response (Fig. 18–1)
b. Supraventricular tachycardia (Fig. 18–2)
c. Ventricular tachycardia (Fig. 18–3)

If any one of these three rhythms is present in a hypotensive patient, emergency electrical cardioversion may be required. Prepare by doing the following:

d. Ask the RN to notify your resident and an anesthetist immediately.

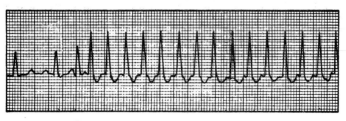

Figure 18–2 Supraventricular tachycardia.

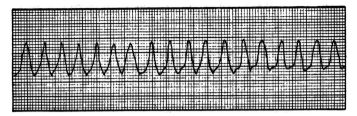

Figure 18–3 Ventricular tachycardia.

   e. Ask the RN to bring the cardiac arrest cart into the room.
   f. Attach the patient to the ECG monitor.
   g. Ask the RN to draw *midazolam* 5 mg IV into a syringe.
   h. Ensure that an IV line is in place. (Refer to Chapter 15, page 135, for further treatment of rapid heart rates associated with hypotension.)
   i. If the patient has a supraventricular tachycardia, also ask the RN to draw *adenosine* 6 mg IV into a syringe. IV adenosine may terminate some supraventricular tachycardias, obviating the need to electrically cardiovert the patient.

Selective Physical Examination

Determine the cause of hypotension or shock by *assessing the volume status.*

Only cardiogenic shock results in a clinical picture of volume overload. Hypovolemic, septic, or anaphylactic shock results in a clinical picture of volume depletion.

Vitals	Repeat now
HEENT	Elevated JVP (CHF), flat neck veins (volume depletion)
Resp	Stridor (anaphylaxis)
	Crackles, pleural effusions (CHF)
	Wheezes (anaphylaxis, CHF)
CVS	Cardiac apex displaced laterally, S_3 (CHF)
ABD	Hepatomegaly with positive HJR (CHF)
Ext	Presacral or ankle edema (CHF)
Skin	Urticaria (anaphylaxis)
Rectal	Melena or hematochezia (GI bleed)

Remember that *wheezing* may be seen in both congestive heart failure (CHF) and anaphylaxis. The administration of epinephrine may save the life of someone with anaphylaxis but may kill someone with CHF. Anaphylactic shock comes on relatively suddenly, and an inciting factor (e.g., IV contrast material, penicillin) can almost always be identified. Usually, other clues, such as angioedema or urticaria, are present.

Management

What immediate measures need to be taken to correct shock or prevent it from occurring?

Normalize the intravascular volume. In the case of *cardiogenic shock* due to suspected MI, stop the IV NS bolus (ordered over the telephone) and replace with 5% dextrose in water (D5W) to keep the vein open (TKVO). Proper management also requires preload and afterload reduction and further investigation, as outlined in Chapter 24.

All other forms of shock require volume expansion. This can be achieved quickly through elevation of the legs (i.e., reverse Trendelenburg) and the administration of repeated small volumes (200 to 300 mL over 15 to 30 minutes) of an IV fluid that will at least temporarily remain in the intravascular space, such as NS or Ringer's lactate. Reassess volume status after each bolus of IV fluid, aiming for a jugular venous pressure (JVP) of 2 to 3 cm H_2O above the sternal angle and concomitant normalization of HR, BP, and tissue perfusion.

If the patient is in *anaphylactic shock,* treat rapidly, as follows[1]:

1. IV NS wide open until normotensive
2. *Epinephrine*

   Two strengths of epinephrine are available for injection. *Make sure that you are using the right strength.*

   For *profound anaphylactic shock* that is immediately life threatening, use the IV route: *epinephrine* 1:10,000, 20 μg (0.2 mL)/min, up to a total dose of 300 μg (3 mL) in 15 minutes. Repeat every 15 minutes if indicated.

   For *less severe situations,* epinephrine can be given IM (note the different concentration): *epinephrine* 1:1000, 500 μg (0.5 mL) IM, repeated after 5 minutes in the absence of improvement or if deterioration occurs. Several doses may be necessary.

   Epinephrine is the most important drug for any anaphylactic reaction. Through its α-adrenergic action, it reverses peripheral vasodilatation; through its β-adrenergic action, it reduces bronchoconstriction and increases the force of cardiac contraction. In addition, it suppresses histamine and leukotriene release.
3. *Hydrocortisone* 500 mg by slow IV or IM injection or PO, followed by 100 mg IV, IM, or PO every 6 hours to help avert late sequelae

   This is particularly necessary in asthmatics who have been treated previously with corticosteroids.
4. *Salbutamol* 2.5 mg/3 mL NS by nebulizer

   This is an adjunctive measure if bronchospasm is a major feature.

5. *Diphenhydramine* 50 to 75 mg by slow IV or IM injection
    The benefits of antihistamines in anaphylactic shock are controversial.

Correct hypoxia and acidemia. If the patient is in shock, obtain ABGs and administer oxygen. If the arterial pH is <7.2 in the absence of respiratory acidosis, order $NaHCO_3$ 0.5 to 1 amp (44.6 mmol) IV. Monitor the effects of treatment by repeat ABGs every 30 minutes until the patient is stabilized.

What is the specific cause of hypotension or shock? (determined while restoring the intravascular volume)

Cardiogenic shock. This is commonly a result of acute MI. Order a stat ECG, portable chest x-ray (CXR), and cardiac enzyme tests. However, any of the causative factors of CHF listed on page 272 may be operative.

Be certain that the patient is in CHF. Four other conditions can cause hypotension and elevated JVP:

1. *Cardiac tamponade* may cause elevated JVP, arterial hypotension, and soft heart sounds (Beck's triad). Suspect this as the diagnosis if there is a pulsus paradoxus of >10 mm Hg during relaxed respirations (see page 266).
2. A massive *pulmonary embolus* can cause hypotension, elevated JVP, and cyanosis and may be accompanied by additional evidence of acute right ventricular overload (e.g., positive hepatojugular reflux [HJR], right ventricular heave, loud P_2, right-sided S_3, murmur of tricuspid insufficiency). If pulmonary embolism is suspected, call your resident immediately, and treat as outlined in Chapter 24, pages 275 to 276.
3. *Superior vena cava obstruction* may cause hypotension and elevated JVP that does not vary with respiration. Additional features may include headache, facial plethora, conjunctival injection, and dilatation of collateral veins in the upper thorax and neck.
4. *Tension pneumothorax* can also cause hypotension and elevated JVP due to positive intrathoracic pressure that decreases venous return to the heart. Look for severe dyspnea, unilateral hyperresonance, and decreased air entry, with tracheal shift *away* from the involved side. If a tension pneumothorax is suspected, do not wait for x-ray confirmation. Call for your resident and get a 14- to 16-gauge needle ready to aspirate the pleural space at the second intercostal space in the midclavicular line on the affected side. This is a medical emergency!

Hypovolemia. If there is suspicion that a *GI bleed* or other *acute blood loss* (e.g., ruptured abdominal aortic aneurysm) is responsible for hypotension, consult a surgeon immediately.

Excess fluid losses via sweating, vomiting, diarrhea, and polyuria and *third space losses* (e.g., pancreatitis, peritonitis) will respond to simple intravascular volume expansion with NS or Ringer's lactate and correction of the underlying problem.

Drugs are common causes of hypotension, resulting from relative hypovolemia with or without bradycardias due to their effects on the heart and peripheral circulation. Common offenders are morphine, meperidine, quinidine, nitroglycerin, beta blockers, calcium channel blockers, angiotensin-converting enzyme (ACE) inhibitors, and antihypertensive agents. In these instances, hypotension is seldom accompanied by evidence of inadequate tissue perfusion and can usually be avoided by reducing the dose or altering the schedule of drug administration.

In most cases, the reverse Trendelenburg position or a small volume (300 to 500 mL) of NS or Ringer's lactate usually suffices to support the BP until the effect of the drug wears off. The hypotension of narcotics (morphine, meperidine) can be reversed by *naloxone hydrochloride* 0.2 to 2 mg (maximum total dose, 10 mg) IV, SC, or IM every 5 minutes until the desired degree of reversal is seen.

Sepsis. Occasionally, intravascular volume repletion and appropriate antibiotics are sufficient to resolve hypotension associated with septic shock. Continuing hypotension despite intravascular volume repletion, however, requires ICU/CCU admission for vasopressor support.

Anaphylactic shock. This must be recognized and treated immediately to prevent fatal laryngeal edema. Treat as described on page 180.

REMEMBER

1. Consider *toxic shock syndrome* in any hypotensive premenopausal female. Ask about tampon use, or if the patient is obtunded, perform a pelvic examination and remove the tampon, if present.
2. The skin is not a vital organ but gives valuable evidence of tissue perfusion. Remember that during the early stage of septic shock, the skin may be warm and dry due to abnormal peripheral vasodilatation.
3. Adequate BP is required to perfuse three vital organs—*brain, heart,* and *kidneys.* After you have successfully rescued your patient from an episode of hypotension, look out for hypotensive sequelae during the next few days. Not surprisingly, the common sequelae involve these three vital organs.
   a. *Brain*—thrombotic stroke in a patient with underlying cerebrovascular disease
   b. *Heart*—MI in a patient with preexisting atherosclerosis

   c. *Kidney*—acute tubular necrosis; monitor urine output and check urea and creatinine levels in a few days

4. Centrilobular hepatic necrosis (manifested by jaundice and elevated liver enzymes) and bowel ischemia or infarction may be sequelae of hypotension in a critically ill patient.

Reference

1. Resuscitation Council (UK): The emergency medical treatment of anaphylactic reactions for first medical responders. 2002. Available at http://www.resus.org.uk/pages/reaction.htm.

Leg Pain

The easiest approach to leg pain at night is to identify which part of the leg hurts. Most leg pain originates from the muscles, joints, bones, or vascular supply to the legs; however, there are also several referred causes of leg pain.

PHONE CALL

Questions

1. Which part of the leg hurts? Is the leg swollen or discolored?
2. What are the vital signs?
3. Was the pain sudden in onset, or is it chronic?
4. What was the reason for admission?
5. Has there been a recent leg injury or fracture? Does the patient have a leg cast on?
   Leg pain after a leg injury, fracture, or casting raises the possibility of a compartment syndrome.

Orders

None.

Inform RN

"I will arrive at the bedside in . . . minutes."

An acute pulseless limb, fever, or severe leg pain of any cause requires you to see the patient immediately. Increasing leg pain 24 to 48 hours after casting also requires you to see the patient immediately.

ELEVATOR THOUGHTS

What causes leg pain?

Bone and Joint Disease

1. Lumbar disk disease (sciatica)
2. Arthritis

a. Septic (*Staphylococcus aureus, Neisseria gonorrhoeae, Streptococcus pneumoniae, Haemophilus influenzae,* and gram-negative bacilli)
b. Inflammatory (gout, pseudogout, rheumatoid arthritis [RA], systemic lupus erythematosus [SLE])
c. Degenerative (osteoarthritis)
3. Osteomyelitis
4. Ruptured Baker's cyst
5. Skeletal tumor

Vascular Disease

1. Arterial disease
   a. Acute arterial insufficiency (e.g., thromboembolism, cholesterol embolism)
   b. Arteriosclerosis obliterans (chronic arterial insufficiency)
   c. Thromboangiitis obliterans (Buerger's disease)
2. Venous disease
   a. Deep venous thrombosis (DVT)
   b. Superficial thrombophlebitis

Muscle, Soft Tissue, or Nerve Pain

1. Fasciitis, pyomyositis, myonecrosis
2. Compartment syndrome
3. Cellulitis
4. Neuropathies (diabetes)
5. Reflex sympathetic dystrophy syndrome
6. Erythema nodosum
7. Nodular liquefying panniculitis
8. Benign nocturnal leg cramps

MAJOR THREAT TO LIFE

- Loss of limb from arterial insufficiency
- Pulmonary embolism from DVT
- Septic arthritis
- Fasciitis, pyomyositis, myonecrosis
- Compartment syndrome

Acute arterial occlusion of the lower extremity, if left untreated, may result in gangrene in as little as 6 hours. *DVT* may result in severe respiratory insufficiency or death if pulmonary embolism occurs. Although *septic arthritis* is not likely to result in loss of life overnight, its prompt recognition and management are essential to avoid permanent joint damage. Anaerobic infections resulting in *fasciitis, pyomyositis,* or *myonecrosis* may lead to septic shock. An unrecognized *compartment syndrome* can result in permanent ischemic muscle contractures within hours.

BEDSIDE

Although the list of possible diagnoses of leg pain is long, only the five major threats to life require emergency treatment at night. You should perform a systematic inspection, looking for evidence of each of these in a patient with leg pain.

Quick-Look Test

Does the patient look well (comfortable), sick (uncomfortable or distressed), or critical (about to die)?
    Most patients with significant leg pain lie still, appear apprehensive, and are reluctant to move the affected extremity.

Airway and Vital Signs

Leg pain should not compromise the vital signs; however, abnormalities in the vital signs may provide clues to the cause of leg pain.

What is the heart rate (HR)? Is it regular or irregular?
    Pain from any cause may result in tachycardia. However, an irregular rhythm suggests atrial fibrillation, raising the possibility of an embolic event.

What is the blood pressure (BP)?
    Pain or anxiety from any cause may raise the BP.

What is the temperature?
    Fever suggests infection or inflammation, as may be seen with DVT, septic arthritis, fasciitis, pyomyositis, or myonecrosis.

Acute Arterial Insufficiency

Selective History

Was the pain sudden in onset, suggesting an arterial embolism?

Is there a history of underlying cardiac disease (e.g., atrial fibrillation, mitral stenosis, ventricular aneurysm, prosthetic heart valve) that might predispose to arterial embolization?

Is there a history of intermittent claudication, which suggests long-standing chronic arterial insufficiency?

Is the patient receiving heparin?
    Heparin-induced thrombocytopenia (platelet count $\leq 150,000/\text{mm}^3$) may result in acute intravascular thrombosis due to platelet aggregation by heparin-dependent immunoglobulin G (IgG) antibodies. This usually occurs after about 5 days of heparin therapy, but it may be seen earlier in patients with a prior history of receiving heparin.

Selective Physical Examination

Look for the four Ps:
1. Pain
2. Pallor
3. Pulselessness
4. Paresthesias

The following findings suggest a major arterial embolism:

Skin	Pallor
	Focal areas of gangrene
	Bilateral brawny discoloration (arteriosclerosis obliterans)
	Diminished temperature, especially if unilateral
CVS	Check the femoral, popliteal, and pedal pulses
	In acute or chronic arterial occlusion, pulses are absent distal to the site of occlusion
Neuro	Paresthesias, diminished light touch in a stocking distribution

An *acute arterial embolism* tends to cause unilateral pain, pallor, paresthesias, and pulselessness (the four Ps), whereas *chronic arterial insufficiency* due to arteriosclerosis obliterans usually involves both lower limbs to a variable extent, with bilateral diminished pulses, trophic skin changes, loss of limb hair, and dependent rubor. Do not be fooled, however—although the presentation of arteriosclerosis obliterans is almost always chronic and progressive, fresh thrombosis on top of a fixed atherosclerotic plaque may completely obstruct arterial flow, resulting in an acute-on-chronic presentation.

Management

Acute arterial insufficiency is a surgical emergency. If you suspect that an arterial embolism has occluded a major artery, take the following steps:
1. Immediately notify your resident and a vascular surgeon.
2. Draw a stat blood sample for a complete blood cell count (CBC) and activated partial thromboplastin time (aPTT).
3. If there are no contraindications, begin *heparin* 100 U/kg IV bolus, followed by a maintenance infusion of 1000 to 1600 U/hr, with the lower range selected for patients with a higher risk of bleeding. (See page 275 for precautions in the use of heparin.)
4. If limb viability is threatened, the patient may require emergency thrombectomy or bypass. If limb viability is not a concern, direct intra-arterial streptokinase may achieve lysis of a thrombus, but this should be initiated *only* under the guidance of a vascular surgeon.

Acute arterial insufficiency due to *heparin-induced thrombocytopenia* is a complex situation; notify your resident and a hematologist for help. Most cases require immediate discontinuation of heparin. If continued intravenous (IV) anticoagulation is necessary (i.e., for the original indication for which heparin was prescribed), ancrod (Arvin) may be substituted for heparin. Ancrod is a thrombin-like enzyme obtained from the venom of the Malayan pit viper and achieves anticoagulation through defibrinogenation.

Chronic arterial insufficiency due to arteriosclerosis obliterans is not usually an emergency unless an acute thrombosis occurs on top of a long-standing fixed plaque. In this case, direct intra-arterial streptokinase or urokinase may result in clot lysis, but this should be administered *only* under the guidance of a vascular surgeon. The more common scenario is a complaint of pain at rest in a patient with chronic intermittent claudication. If there is no immediate concern about limb viability, rest pain can be treated with non-narcotic analgesics, such as *acetaminophen* 325 to 650 mg PO every 4 hours as needed, and placement of the affected extremity in the dependent position. More definitive therapy, including lumbar sympathectomy or direct arterial surgery, is seldom required on an emergency basis.

Deep Venous Thrombosis

Selective History

Look for predisposing causes:
1. Stasis
   a. Prolonged bed rest
   b. Immobilized limb
   c. Congestive heart failure (CHF)
   b. Pregnancy (particularly post partum)
2. Vein injury
   a. Trauma (especially hip fracture)
   b. Surgery (especially abdominal, pelvic, and orthopedic procedures)
3. Hypercoagulability
   a. Malignancy
   b. Inflammatory bowel disease
   c. Nephrotic syndrome
   d. Polycythemia vera
   e. Antiphospholipid syndrome
   f. Deficiencies of antithrombin III or protein C or S
   g. Factor V Leiden mutation
4. Older age (>50 years)
5. Recent abdominal, orthopedic, or neurologic surgery
6. Recent general anesthesia

Selective Physical Examination

Look for the following signs involving the calf or thigh:
1. Tenderness
2. Erythema

3. Edema: subtle degrees of swelling may be appreciated by measuring and comparing the circumferences of both calves and thighs at several different levels
4. Warmth
5. Distention of the overlying superficial veins
6. Homans' sign: with the patient supine, flex the knee and then sharply dorsiflex the ankle; pain in the calf during ankle dorsiflexion is supportive evidence of a calf DVT, but its absence does not exclude the diagnosis

Management

DVT should be recognized and treated immediately to prevent embolization and pulmonary infarction. If your suspicion of DVT is high, you are obligated to begin anticoagulation without further confirmation of the diagnosis at this point. Heparin will inhibit further growth and promote resolution of the thrombus. However, before ordering heparin, ensure that the patient has no history of bleeding disorders; peptic ulcer; intracranial disease, such as recent stroke, subarachnoid hemorrhage, or tumor; or recent surgery. All are contraindications to anticoagulation. These patients require confirmation of DVT by an imaging modality and, if DVT is documented, consultation for possible interruption of the inferior vena cava by the insertion of a transvenous caval device or, occasionally, inferior vena cava ligation.

Draw a blood sample for CBC, aPTT, prothrombin time (PT), and platelet count immediately. If there are no contraindications, begin heparin by one of these two methods:

1. *Heparin* 100 U/kg IV bolus (usual dose, 5000 to 10,000 U IV), followed by a maintenance infusion of 1000 to 1600 U/hr, with the lower range selected for patients with a higher risk of bleeding.

   > Heparin should be delivered by infusion pump, with maintenance dosing ordered as in the following example: heparin 25,000 U/500 mL 5% dextrose in water (D5W) to run at 20 mL/hr = 1000 U/hr. It is dangerous to put large doses of heparin in small-volume IV bags, because runaway IV lines filled with heparin can result in a serious overdose.
   >
   > Heparin and warfarin are dangerous drugs because of their potential for causing bleeding disorders. Write and double-check your heparin orders carefully. Also, measure platelet counts once or twice a week to detect reversible heparin-induced thrombocytopenia, which may occur at any time while a patient is on heparin.

2. *Low-molecular-weight heparin (LMWH).* Several formulations of LMWH exist (Table 19–1), with the different distributions of molecular weight resulting in differences in inhibitory activities against factor Xa and thrombin, the extent of plasma

TABLE 19–1 **Recommended Doses of Low-Molecular-Weight Heparin for the Treatment of Deep Vein Thrombosis**

Product	Dose
Dalteparin	200 IU/kg by deep SC injection once daily
	For patients with an increased risk of bleeding, 100 IU/kg q12h or 100 IU/kg by continuous IV infusion over 12 hr
Enoxaparin	1.5 mg/kg by deep SC injection once daily or 1 mg/kg SC q12h
	Dose should not exceed 180 mg daily
Nadroparin	171 IU/kg by deep SC injection once daily or 86 IU/kg SC q12h
	Dose should not exceed 17,000 IU daily
Tinzaparin	175 IU/kg by deep SC injection once daily

protein binding, and plasma half-lifes. You should familiarize yourself with the LMWH formulation used in your hospital. Also, be careful to note that the dose of LMWH used in the *treatment* of DVT is considerably higher than that used for *prophylaxis* of DVT.

After starting heparin, the diagnosis should be confirmed in the morning by real-time B-mode or duplex ultrasonography, which is the most sensitive noninvasive test to confirm a symptomatic DVT.[1] If this test is not available, impedance plethysmography, nuclear venography, and contrast venography are other options.

In patients receiving IV unfractionated heparin, monitor the aPTT every 4 to 6 hours, and adjust the heparin maintenance dose until the aPTT is in the therapeutic range (1.5 to 2.5 times normal). After this, daily aPTT measurements are sufficient. Initial measurements of aPTT are made only to ensure adequate anticoagulation. LMWH does not consistently modify aPTT or thrombin clotting time in the usual doses given, so these tests cannot be used to modify doses. Anti–factor Xa activity has been used to assess the activity of LMWH but does not appear to correlate with efficacy.

Continue heparin for approximately 5 days. Add *warfarin* (Coumadin) on the first day, beginning at 10 mg PO and titrating the dose to achieve a PT with an international normalized ratio (INR) of 2.0 to 3.0 (this corresponds to a PT of 1.3 to 1.5 times control, using rabbit brain thromboplastin; if you are unsure of the method used by your laboratory, call and ask). Attainment of a therapeutic INR usually takes 5 days, at which time heparin can be discontinued.

Numerous drugs interfere with warfarin metabolism to increase or decrease the PT. Before prescribing any drug to a patient on warfarin, look up its effect on warfarin metabolism and monitor PT carefully if an interaction is anticipated.

Write an order that the patient should receive no aspirin-containing drugs, sulfinpyrazone, dipyridamole, or thrombolytic agents and no IM injections while on anticoagulation.

Ask your patient daily about signs of bleeding or bruising. Instruct your patient that prolonged pressure will be required after venipuncture to prevent local bruising while on anticoagulation.

Septic Arthritis

Selective History

In septic arthritis, the patient most often points to the painful joint involved. Your job is to determine whether the joint in question is infected. Two rules can be helpful: (1) if a single joint is swollen, red, and tender, it should be considered septic until proved otherwise; (2) in a patient with multiple joint involvement (as may be seen with RA or other inflammatory arthritides), if a single joint is inflamed out of proportion to the other joints involved, the joint in question should be considered possibly infected.

Look for predisposing causes:
1. A penetrating wound.
2. Recent arthroscopy or intra-articular injection of steroids.
3. A joint prosthesis or other foreign body in the involved joint.
4. Bacteremia (e.g., endocarditis).
5. New sexual partners recently.

Selective Physical Examination

Fever may be present. The knee joint is most commonly affected. The joint is swollen, tender, restricted in range, and erythematous. These signs may be less marked, however, in an elderly patient or a patient on steroids.

Septic arthritis of the hip is often missed because of the deep location of the hip joint—swelling may not be detected easily. Conditions involving the hip joint sometimes manifest only by referred pain to the groin, buttocks, lateral thigh, or anterior aspect of the knee. The affected extremity is usually held in adduction, flexion, and internal rotation.

Management

Septic arthritis is a medical emergency. Any suspected septic joint should be aspirated without delay. You will need your resident's help or the assistance of a rheumatologist to perform joint aspiration. The diagnosis of septic arthritis is made by demonstrating microorganisms on Gram stain of synovial fluid. Prompt treatment with appropriate antibiotics is required; this should not await confirmation by culture and should be directed by the results of the Gram stain. When microorganisms are not seen on the synovial fluid sample, empirical antibiotics should be administered. The choice of antibiotics depends on the clinical setting (Table 19–2).

Synovial fluid should be sent for the following:

- White blood cell (WBC) count and differential
- Glucose determination
- Gram stain
- Aerobic and anaerobic cultures
- Gonococcal culture
- Tuberculosis (TB) stain and culture

Blood samples should be sent for the following:

- Simultaneous serum glucose determination
- Aerobic and anaerobic cultures
- Gonococcal culture

In septic arthritis, the synovial fluid is usually cloudy or purulent, with a WBC count ≥10,000/mm^3 with ≥90% neutrophils. Synovial glucose is ≤50% of a simultaneously drawn serum glucose.

Necrotizing Fasciitis, Pyomyositis, and Myonecrosis

This group of infections is usually caused by a mixture of organisms, including anaerobes, most often involving *Clostridium perfringens*.

TABLE 19–2 **Usual Causative Organisms and Recommended Antibiotics for the Empirical Treatment of Septic Arthritis**

Clinical Setting	Usual Organism	Recommended Antibiotics before Culture and Sensitivity Results
Recent new sexual partner	*Neisseria gonorrhoeae*	Ceftriaxone 1 g IV q24h or Ciprofloxacin 500 mg IV q12h or Doxycycline 100 mg PO q12h
Adult	*Staphylococccus aureus* Group A streptococcus Gram-negative aerobes	Ceftriaxone 1 g IV q24h with Gentamicin 1 mg/kg IV or IM q8h
With prosthesis	*Staphylococcus epidermidis* *Staphylococcus aureus* Gram-negative aerobes	Ceftriaxone 1 g IV q24h with vancomycin 30 mg/kg/day in 2–4 divided doses if there is a risk of methicillin-resistant staphylococci

Selective History

These infections usually result as a complication of surgery or deep traumatic wounds. The diagnosis may be more elusive in cases that arise spontaneously without a history of obvious injury. Heroin addicts are predisposed to a localized form of pyomyositis that may involve the thigh.

Selective Physical Examination

Look for the following:
1. Pus or gas formation in soft tissues
2. Subcutaneous crepitance
3. Local swelling and edema over a wound site, sometimes with a "frothy" wound exudate
4. Dark patches of cutaneous gangrene (a late finding)
5. In patients with clostridial myonecrosis, the development of systemic toxemia, with tachycardia, hypotension, renal failure, and feelings of impending doom, followed by toxic delirium and coma

Management

These infections are surgical emergencies. If you think the patient has fasciitis, pyomyositis, or myonecrosis, consult a surgeon immediately. Systemic antibiotics (usually including high-dose penicillin) are also indicated in the treatment of these clostridial infections.

Compartment Syndrome

Some muscle groups in the leg are surrounded by well-fitted fascial sheaths, leaving no space for swelling should an injury occur. An increase in pressure within these sheaths may interfere with the circulation to the nerves and muscles within the compartment, resulting in a compartment syndrome.

Selective History

Look for predisposing causes:
1. Recent fractures of the tibia and fibula
2. Overly tight pressure bandages or casts
3. Blunt leg trauma
4. Prolonged, unaccustomed, vigorous exertion
5. Anticoagulant medication

   Patients receiving heparin or warfarin are at risk for developing compartment syndrome due to bleeding within the enclosed fascial sheath, sometimes after relatively minor trauma.[2]

Selective Physical Examination

The anterior compartment of the leg is affected most commonly. It contains the anterior tibial, extensor hallucis longus, and extensor digitorum longus muscles.

Look for the following:

- Pain and tenderness over the involved compartment
- Overlying skin that is possibly erythematous, glossy, and edematous
- Sensory loss on the dorsum of the foot between the first and second toes
- Increasing pain on passive stretching of the involved muscle groups
- Weakness of dorsiflexion of the ankles and toes (footdrop)

Caution: Do not be fooled by the pulses. The pedal pulses are rarely obliterated by the compartment swelling and may be easy to feel despite progressive muscle and nerve damage within the compartment.

If the patient has a tibial fracture that has been casted, it may be difficult to properly examine the affected extremity. Any such patient who develops increasing pain 24 to 48 hours after casting should be suspected of having a compartment syndrome, and the cast should be removed so that the leg can be properly examined.

Management

Once the diagnosis of compartment syndrome is confirmed, a *decompressing fasciotomy* must be performed immediately by a surgeon. A delay of >12 hours may lead to irreversible muscle necrosis and contracture formation. Conservative measures are only temporizing and may involve ice packs and elevation. Pressure dressings should be removed.

Less Urgent Conditions

If the five major threats to life have been excluded, a more leisurely approach to the diagnosis can be taken, looking for other, less urgent conditions.

Selective Physical Examination

Skin   Localized skin and subcutaneous erythema, swelling, and warmth (cellulitis)

Painful subcutaneous red nodules (erythema nodosum, nodular liquefying panniculitis)

Tender superficial vein with surrounding erythema and edema (superficial thrombophlebitis)

"Blue toe syndrome" or livedo reticularis (cholesterol emboli)

Focal areas of gangrene from cholesterol emboli (usually from the thoracic or abdominal aorta) may give one or more toes a bluish discoloration. Livedo reticularis refers to cyanotic mottling of the skin in a fishnet-like pattern.

	Erythema, swelling, dysesthesias, increased hair growth of one foot (reflex sympathetic dystrophy syndrome)
MSS	Posterior knee joint swelling (Baker's cyst)
	Joint inflammation (RA, SLE, gout, pseudogout)
	Hip palpation and ROM (hip joint pathology may cause leg pain with little or no evidence of inflammation)
Neuro	If no visible abnormality is found, a complete neurologic examination is required to look for lumbar disk disease (sciatica) or peripheral neuropathy (e.g., diabetes)

Benign nocturnal leg cramps often occur in the absence of physical findings

Management

Acute Gout

Acute gout results from the sudden release of monosodium urate crystals from the cartilage and synovial membranes into the joint space. The diagnosis is made by synovial fluid aspiration and demonstration of negatively birefringent monosodium urate crystals with the use of polarizing microscopy.

At night, your main goal is to terminate the acute attack as quickly as possible. This can be done by administering *indomethacin* (Indocin) 100 mg PO, followed by 50 mg PO every 6 hours until pain relief occurs. *Colchicine* is a good alternative and can be administered 1 mg PO initially, followed by 0.5 mg PO every 2 hours until the pain improves, abdominal discomfort or diarrhea occurs, or a total of 8 mg is given. Intra-articular *triamcinolone hexacetonide* (15 to 30 mg) or *methylprednisolone acetate* (Depo-Medrol) (20 to 40 mg) is occasionally required.

Pseudogout

Pseudogout is a result of the release of calcium pyrophosphate dihydrate crystals from the joint cartilage into the joint space. Diagnosis is made by joint aspiration and demonstration of weakly positive birefringent rods when viewed under polarized light. Acute inflammation usually responds to *indomethacin* (Indocin) 25 to 50 mg PO three times daily for 10 to 14 days, aspiration of fluid, and steroid injection.

Lumbar Disk Disease

Initially, lumbar disk disease can be treated conservatively with bed rest, analgesics, and muscle relaxants.

Thromboangiitis Obliterans (Buerger's Disease)

The only known effective treatment for this condition is complete abstinence from tobacco.

Erythema Nodosum

Erythema nodosum should be considered a symptom of some other underlying disorder, including drug reaction (oral contraceptives, penicillin, sulfonamides, bromides), inflammatory bowel disease, TB, fungal infection, and sarcoidosis. Treatment of the underlying condition is required.

Nodular Liquefying Panniculitis

The appearance of these nodules can be differentiated from erythema nodosum by their mobility with palpation. They are seen in association with acute pancreatitis or pancreatic neoplasms. Treatment of the underlying condition is required.

Reflex Sympathetic Dystrophy Syndrome

This disorder is often precipitated by a myocardial infarction, stroke, or local trauma occurring weeks to months before characteristic redness, swelling (usually of the entire foot), and burning pain occur. Increased sweating and hair growth of the involved extremity also may occur. The condition may respond to analgesic agents and physical therapy. Occasionally, surgical sympathectomy or a short course of steroids is required.

Baker's Cyst

A Baker's cyst is caused by extension of inflamed synovial tissue into the popliteal space, resulting in pain and swelling behind the knee. A well-known complication is rupture of the synovial sac into the adjacent tissues. This may mimic a calf DVT with tenderness, swelling, and a positive Homans' sign. The diagnosis can be confirmed with a popliteal ultrasonogram or arthrogram. Treatment involves drainage of the cyst or intra-articular steroid injection. Occasionally, surgical synovectomy is required.

Superficial Thrombophlebitis

This condition presents with a tender lower extremity vein with surrounding edema and erythema. Often fever is present. Superficial venous thrombosis seldom propagates into the deep venous system, and anticoagulation therapy is not recommended. Treatment involves local measures, such as leg elevation, heat, and nonsteroidal anti-inflammatory drugs (NSAIDs), such as *indomethacin* (Indocin) 25 to 50 mg PO three times daily.

Cellulitis

Cellulitis is most often caused by *Staphylococcus* or *Streptococcus*. Because it can be difficult to determine which is responsible, treatment to cover both organisms is usual. Small, localized areas of cellulitis with intact skin can be treated with *cloxacillin, cephalexin,* or *erythromycin,* all at doses of 250 to 500 mg PO four times daily. If the patient is febrile, if the area of cellulitis is extensive, or if the patient is diabetic, IV antibiotics should be considered.

Cellulitis associated with skin ulcers in a diabetic patient should be swabbed for Gram stain, culture, and sensitivity. In a diabetic patient, such infections are commonly caused by multiple organisms.

Benign Nocturnal Leg Cramps

The cause of this condition is unknown. They frequently respond to *quinine sulfate* 300 mg PO at bedtime PRN.

References

1. Weinmann E, Salzman EW: Deep-vein thrombosis. N Engl J Med 1994;331:1630-1641.
2. Hay SM, Allen MJ, Barnes MR: Acute compartment syndromes resulting from anticoagulant treatment. BMJ 1992;305:1474-1475.

Lines, Tubes, and Drains

Almost every patient admitted to the hospital will have some form of intravenous (IV) line, tube, or drain inserted during his or her stay. These devices are useful in the care of patients, but on occasion they can clog, leak, or otherwise malfunction, requiring your expertise and common sense to remedy the problem.

Because the corrective measures required to deal with problematic lines, tubes, and drains carry the risk of contact with blood and body fluids, make sure that you are familiar with and follow your institution's infection control guidelines.

This chapter describes some of the problems that can occur with commonly used lines, tubes, and drains.

Nasogastric and Enteral Feeding Tubes

1. Blocked nasogastric (NG) and enteral tubes (page 236)
2. Dislodged NG and enteral feeding tubes (page 237)

CENTRAL LINES

Blocked Central Lines

PHONE CALL

Questions

1. **How long has the line been blocked?**
2. **What are the vital signs?**
3. **What was the reason for admission?**

Orders

Ask the RN to have a dressing set, two pairs of sterile gloves in your size, chlorhexidine (Hibitane) skin disinfectant, a 5-mL syringe, and a 20- or 21-gauge needle at the bedside.

You will probably have to remove the dressing that is securing the central line, and you must keep the site sterile. A second pair of sterile gloves is useful because gloves are easily contaminated.

Inform RN

"I will arrive at the bedside in . . . minutes."

A blocked central line requires you to see the patient immediately.

ELEVATOR THOUGHTS

What causes a central line to block? (Fig. 20–1)

- Kinked tubing
- Thrombus at the catheter tip

MAJOR THREAT TO LIFE

- Failure of delivery of medications

Interruption of the delivery of essential medications may temporarily deprive the patient of required treatment.

BEDSIDE

Quick-Look Test

Does the patient look well (comfortable), sick (uncomfortable or distressed), or critical (about to die)?

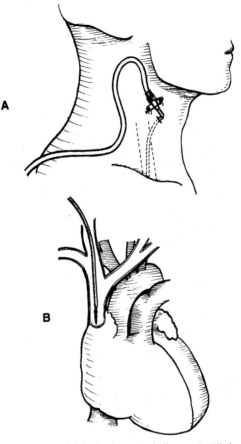

Figure 20–1 Causes of blocked central lines. *A*, Kinked tubing. *B*, Thrombosis at the catheter tip.

A blocked central line by itself should not cause the patient to look sick or critical. If the patient looks unwell, search for another cause.

Airway and Vital Signs

A blocked central line should not compromise the airway or other vital signs.

Selective Physical Examination and Management

1. Inspect the central line. Is the line kinked? If so, remove the dressing securing the line, straighten the line, and see whether there is now a flow of IV fluid. If the problem was a kinked

line, clean the area using sterile technique and secure the line with a plastic occlusive dressing without rekinking it.

2. If there is still no flow of IV fluid with the line wide open, proceed as follows:

    a. Turn off the IV line.

    b. Place the patient in the Trendelenburg position (head down). Take the 5-mL syringe and 20- or 21-gauge capped needle and get ready to disconnect the central line from the IV tubing.

    c. During the expiration phase of respiration, disconnect the central line from the IV tubing. Quickly attach the syringe to the central line and the capped needle to the IV tubing. The latter keeps the tubing sterile.

    > The disconnection must be performed quickly to avoid an air embolus, which may result from air's being sucked into the line due to negative intrathoracic pressure generated during inspiration. The risk of an air embolus is diminished by clamping the IV tubing, placing the patient in the Trendelenburg position, and disconnecting the line only during expiration.

    d. Draw back gently on the syringe, because too much force will collapse the central line tubing. If the line is blocked with a small thrombus, this maneuver will often be sufficient to dislodge the clot.

    e. Draw back 3 mL of blood if possible. During the expiratory phase of respiration, remove the capped needle from the end of the IV tubing, remove the syringe from the central line, and reattach the IV tubing to the central line. Turn the IV on again.

    > Blocked central lines should never be flushed. Flushing may dislodge a clot attached to the catheter tip, causing a pulmonary embolism.

3. If these maneuvers are unsuccessful in unblocking the central line, determine whether the central line is still necessary. Is the patient receiving medications that can be delivered only via a central line (e.g., amphotericin, dopamine, total parenteral nutrition [TPN])? Was the central line started because of lack of peripheral vein access? If so, reexamine the patient to see whether there are now any peripheral veins suitable for IV access.

4. If central venous access is essential, the next step is to insert a new central line at a different site. A new central line should not be inserted over a guidewire placed through the blocked central line, because insertion of the guidewire may also dislodge a clot.

In situations in which central venous access is essential and no alternative sites are available, streptokinase or urokinase has been used to dissolve the obstructing clot. Significant risks accompany the use of these agents, however, and routine use is not recommended.

Bleeding at the Central Line Entry Site

PHONE CALL

Questions

1. What are the vital signs?
2. What was the reason for admission?

Orders

Ask for a dressing set, two pairs of sterile gloves in your size, and chlorhexidine (Hibitane) skin disinfectant to be at the bedside.

> You will probably have to remove the plastic occlusive dressing that is securing the central line, and you must keep the site sterile.

Inform RN

"I will arrive at the bedside in . . . minutes."

Bleeding at the central line site requires you to see the patient immediately.

ELEVATOR THOUGHTS

What causes bleeding at the line insertion site?

1. Oozing of subcutaneous and cutaneous blood vessels (capillaries)
2. Coagulation disorders
   a. Drugs (warfarin, heparin, aspirin, nonsteroidal anti-inflammatory drugs [NSAIDs], streptokinase, tissue plasminogen activator [tPA])
   b. Thrombocytopenia, platelet dysfunction
   c. Clotting factor deficiency

MAJOR THREAT TO LIFE

- Upper airway obstruction

Bleeding into the soft tissues of the neck may cause tracheal compression, resulting in life-threatening upper airway obstruction.

BEDSIDE

Quick-Look Test

Does the patient look well (comfortable), sick (uncomfortable or distressed), or critical (about to die)?

These patients look well unless there is an upper airway obstruction or excessive blood loss has occurred.

Airway and Vital Signs

Is the airway clear?

What is the respiratory rate (RR)?

Check the airway. If there is any evidence of an upper airway obstruction (inspiratory stridor or significant soft tissue swelling of the neck), call your resident for help immediately.

Selective Physical Examination and Management

1. Remove the dressing and try to identify a specific area of bleeding.
2. If you are unable to identify a specific site of bleeding, clean the site using sterile technique and reinspect the area. Usually, generalized oozing of blood is seen at the entry site, with no single skin vessel identified as the culprit.
3. Apply continuous pressure to the entry site for 20 minutes. With a gloved hand, apply a folded, sterile 2- × 2-cm gauze dressing to the site with firm, continuous pressure. Do not release this pressure during the 20 minutes, because the platelet plug you are allowing to form may be broken (Fig. 20–2).
4. Reinspect the entry site. If the bleeding has stopped, clean the area using sterile technique and secure the line with a plastic occlusive dressing. If there is still bleeding at the site, repeat the previous maneuver for an additional 20 minutes. Provided that continuous pressure has been applied, the bleeding should stop. In the unusual circumstance in which the bleeding has not stopped, a coagulation disorder should be suspected. (Refer to Chapter 31 for the management of coagulation problems.) Alternatively, a single suture may be placed at the site of bleeding in an attempt to provide hemostasis.
5. Removal of the central line should be considered if bleeding at the insertion site is excessive and resistant to the previous measures.

Shortness of Breath after Central Line Insertion

PHONE CALL

Questions

1. How long has the patient had SOB?
2. What are the vital signs?
3. What was the reason for admission?

Orders

1. Ask the RN to have a dressing set, two pairs of sterile gloves in your size, chlorhexidine (Hibiclens) skin disinfectant, and a size 16 IV catheter at the bedside.

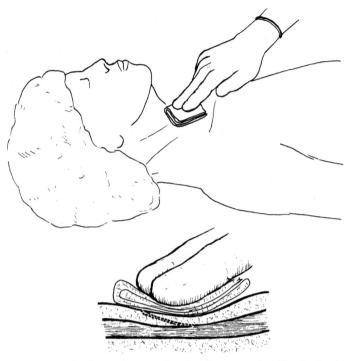

Figure 20–2 Apply continuous, firm local pressure for 20 minutes to stop the oozing of blood from the central line entry site. Make sure the pressure is applied over the puncture site in the vein and not at the skin entry site.

If the patient has a tension pneumothorax, you will need to insert a size 16 IV catheter into the second intercostal space on the hyperresonant side, with your resident's guidance.

2 If you suspect a pneumothorax, order a stat portable chest x-ray (CXR) in the upright position in expiration.

> Hypotension, tachypnea, and pleuritic chest pain after central line insertion are suggestive of a pneumothorax.

3. Order O_2 by mask at 10 L/min.

Inform RN

"I will arrive at the bedside in . . . minutes."

SOB after central line insertion requires you to see the patient immediately.

ELEVATOR THOUGHTS

What causes shortness of breath after central line insertion? (Fig. 20–3)

- Pneumothorax or tension pneumothorax
- Massive soft tissue hematoma from inadvertent carotid artery puncture, resulting in upper airway obstruction
- Cardiac tamponade
- Air embolus
- Pleural effusion

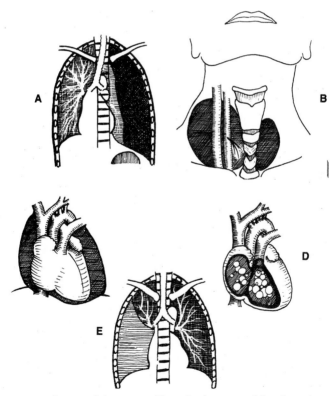

Figure 20–3 Causes of shortness of breath after central line insertion. *A,* Pneumothorax. *B,* Massive soft tissue hematoma from inadvertent carotid artery puncture, resulting in upper airway obstruction. *C,* Cardiac tamponade. *D,* Air embolus. *E,* Pleural effusion.

MAJOR THREAT TO LIFE

- Upper airway obstruction
- Tension pneumothorax
- Cardiac tamponade
- Air embolus

Upper airway obstruction may result from a massive soft tissue hematoma (e.g., from inadvertent carotid artery puncture). A *tension pneumothorax* may develop minutes to days after the insertion of a central line if pleural perforation occurred during insertion. Rarely, *cardiac tamponade* results from perforation of the right atrium or right ventricle by the catheter. Air may inadvertently be introduced if the line is disconnected incorrectly, resulting in an *air embolus*.

BEDSIDE

Quick-Look Test

Does the patient look well (comfortable), sick (uncomfortable or distressed), or critical (about to die)?

A patient with a tension pneumothorax, upper airway obstruction, cardiac tamponade, or air embolus looks sick or critical.

Airway and Vital Signs

Is the airway clear?

Check the airway. If there is any evidence of an upper airway obstruction (i.e., inspiratory stridor or significant soft tissue swelling of the neck), call the intensive care unit/cardiac care unit (ICU/CCU) team immediately for possible intubation.

What are the blood pressure (BP) and RR?

Hypotension and tachypnea in a patient with a recently inserted central line may indicate a tension pneumothorax or cardiac tamponade, inadvertently caused at the time of line insertion. See page 181 for the assessment and page 207 for the management of tension pneumothorax and cardiac tamponade.

Selective Physical Examination

Resp	Tracheal deviation (tension pneumothorax or massive pleural effusion)
	Unilateral hyperresonance to percussion with decreased breath sounds (pneumothorax)
	Stony dullness to percussion, decreased breath sounds, decreased tactile fremitus (pleural effusion)
CVS	Pulsus paradoxus (cardiac tamponade or tension pneumothorax)
	Pulsus paradoxus is present when the decrease in systolic BP with inspiration is >10 mm Hg

(the normal variation in systolic BP with quiet respiration is 0 to 10 mm Hg). A pulsus paradoxus is definitely present if the radial pulse disappears during inspiration.

Elevated JVP (cardiac tamponade or tension pneumothorax)

Distant heart sounds (pericardial effusion or cardiac tamponade)

Mill wheel murmur, hypotension, elevated JVP (major air embolism)

Central line   Check all IV connections to ensure that they are not loose (air embolus)

Management

Tension Pneumothorax

Tension pneumothorax is a medical emergency requiring urgent treatment. You will need supervision by your resident or attending physician.

1. Identify the second intercostal space in the midclavicular line on the affected (hyperresonant) side.
2. Mark this point with the pressure from a capped needle or ballpoint pen.
3. Open the dressing set and pour the chlorhexidine (Hibitane) into the appropriate space.
4. Put on the sterile gloves and clean the identified area.
5. Insert the size 16 IV catheter into the designated site. Remove the inner needle, leaving the plastic cannula in the chest. If a tension pneumothorax is present, there will be a loud sound of air rushing out through the catheter. You do not need to connect the catheter to suction; the lung will decompress itself.
6. Order a chest tube sent to the room immediately. Definitive treatment is insertion of a chest tube.

Pneumothorax Without Tension

Small pneumothoraces usually undergo spontaneous reabsorption over a few days.

Large or *symptomatic pneumothoraces* require chest tube drainage.

Cardiac Tamponade

Cardiac tamponade is a medical emergency.

1. Clamp the IV tubing and turn off the IV line.
2. Call the ICU/CCU team immediately for possible urgent pericardiocentesis. An emergency echocardiogram, if available, will confirm the diagnosis before pericardiocentesis.
3. Volume expansion with normal saline (NS) through a large-bore IV may be a useful temporizing measure to help maintain adequate cardiac output.

Air Embolism

Air embolism may be helped by the following procedure:

1. Place the patient on the right side in Trendelenburg's position (head down) to trap the air bubbles in the right ventricle and prevent them from entering the pulmonary artery. The patient should be kept in this position until the air bubbles have been reabsorbed. (Aspiration of air bubbles from the right ventricle is advocated by some experts.)
2. Reinspect all the IV connections and make sure they are secure.
3. If necessary, a new central line may have to be inserted.

Massive Unilateral Pleural Effusion

Massive unilateral pleural effusion should be managed as follows:

1. Clamp the IV tubing and stop the IV fluid.
2. Perform thoracentesis if the patient has marked SOB.

CHEST TUBES

Chest tubes are inserted to drain air (pneumothoraces), blood (hemothoraces), fluid (pleural effusions), or pus (empyemas) (Fig. 20–4). They should always be connected to an underwater seal. They may be left to straight drainage (no suction) or, more commonly, to suction.

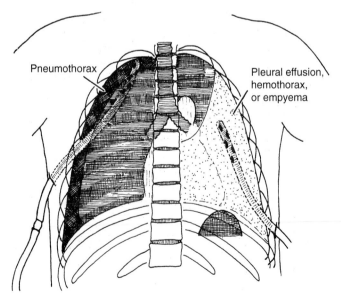

Pneumothorax

Pleural effusion, hemothorax, or empyema

Figure 20–4 Chest tubes are inserted to drain air (pneumothoraces), blood (hemothoraces), fluid (pleural effusions), or pus (empyemas).

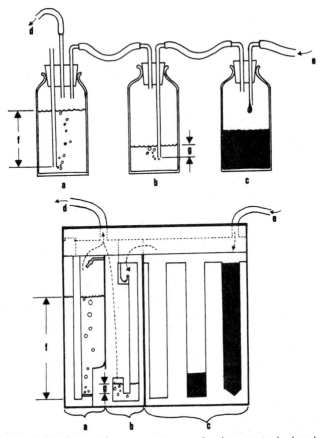

Figure 20–5 Chest tube apparatus. a, Suction control chamber. b, Underwater seal. c, Collection chamber. d, To suction. e, From patient. f, Height equals amount of suction in cm H_2O. g, Height equals underwater seal in cm H_2O.

Figure 20–5 illustrates the various chest tube drainage apparatuses. Common chest tube problems are illustrated in Figure 20–6.

Persistent Bubbling in the Drainage Container (Air Leak)

PHONE CALL

Questions

1. Why was the chest tube inserted?
2. What are the vital signs?

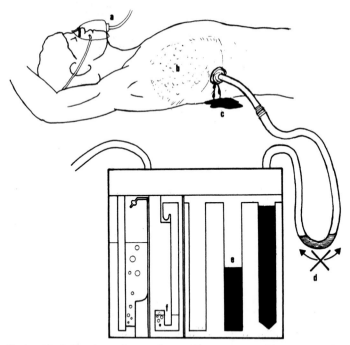

Figure 20–6 Common chest tube problems. a, Shortness of breath. b, Subcutaneous emphysema. c, Bleeding at the entry site. d, Loss of fluctuation. e, Excessive drainage. f, Persistent bubbling.

3. Does the patient have SOB?
4. What was the reason for admission?

Orders

None.

Inform RN

"I will arrive at the bedside in . . . minutes."

Persistent bubbling in the drainage container is a potential emergency, requiring you to see the patient as soon as possible. Any malfunctioning of the chest tube associated with SOB requires you to see the patient immediately.

ELEVATOR THOUGHTS

What causes persistent bubbling in the drainage compartment?

1. Loose tubing connection

2. Air leaking into the chest around the chest tube at the insertion site
3. Traumatic tracheobronchial injury—a large, persistent air leak in a patient with traumatic pneumothorax suggests a concomitant tracheobronchial injury.
4. Persistent bronchopleural air leak
   a. Postlobectomy
   b. Ruptured bleb or bulla (e.g., asthma, emphysema)
   c. After intrathoracic procedures (e.g., needle biopsy, thoracentesis)

MAJOR THREAT TO LIFE

A persistent air leak suggests either a pneumothorax from intrathoracic injury or a loose connection of the drainage apparatus. Hence, the major threat to life is the underlying intrathoracic disease process responsible for the persistent air leak. As long as air continues to bubble through the collection chamber, one can be reasonably certain that excessive intrapleural air will not accumulate.

BEDSIDE

Quick-Look Test

Does the patient look well (comfortable), sick (uncomfortable or distressed), or critical (about to die)?
If a small air leak is the problem, the patient may look well. A patient who looks sick may be developing a larger pneumothorax or may look sick for unrelated reasons.

Airway and Vital Signs

Provided that all tubing connections are snug and the chest tube dressing is airtight, a persistent air leak means that the patient has a pneumothorax. As long as air continues to bubble through the collection chamber, the pneumothorax should drain and thus not result in an alteration of vital signs.

Selective History and Chart Review

Why was the chest tube inserted?
If the chest tube was inserted to drain a pneumothorax, the tube should be bubbling unless the lung is fully expanded and the leak has sealed. If the chest tube was inserted to drain a hemothorax, a pleural effusion, or an empyema with straight drainage (no suction), the new onset of bubbling in the collection chamber represents a loose tubing connection, air leaking into the chest from around the chest tube insertion site, or the development of a pneumothorax.

Selective Physical Examination and Management

Provided that a pneumothorax is not present, a persistent air leak is indicated by air bubbles in the underwater seal section of the Pleur-Evac while the suction is turned off. If the air leak is small, it may be seen only with measures that increase intrapleural pressure (e.g., coughing) (Fig. 20–7).

Clamping of chest tubes before obtaining an x-ray may be dangerous, especially if there is a persistent pneumothorax. *Never leave a patient with a clamped chest tube unattended.* A tension pneumothorax may develop rapidly if a ball-valve mechanism is present.

The following procedure is recommended when there is persistent bubbling in the drainage compartment:

1. Inspect the tubing connections to ensure that all seals are airtight.
2. Remove the dressing at the entry site of the chest tube, listen for sucking sounds, and observe the incision area. If the incision is too large and inadequately closed, insert one or

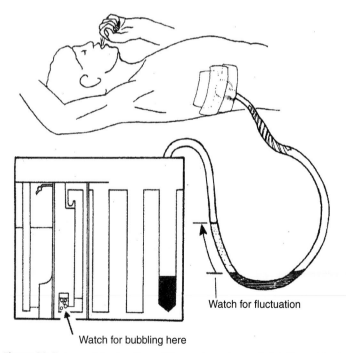

Watch for fluctuation

Watch for bubbling here

Figure 20–7 Loss of fluctuation of the underwater seal. Ask the patient to cough, and observe for any fluctuation or bubbling.

two sterile 2-0 sutures to seal the opening. If the incision is adequately closed with sutures, reapply a pressure dressing, ensuring that the petrolatum (Vaseline) gauze occlusive dressing seals the incision.

3. Disconnect the suction from the Pleur-Evac. Persistent air leak (spontaneous or with coughing) usually means an air leak from the lung (persistent pneumothorax).

4. Obtain a CXR to ensure correct tube placement. The chest tube holes should be inside the thorax, and the tip of the tube should be away from mediastinal and subclavicular structures.

5. If on CXR the lung is not re-expanded, call surgery for possible placement of a second chest tube and for management of the persistent air leak from the lung.

Bleeding Around the Chest Tube Entry Site

PHONE CALL

Questions

1. Why was the chest tube inserted?
2. What are the vital signs?
3. Does the patient have SOB?
4. What was the reason for admission?

Orders

Ask the RN to have a dressing set, two pairs of sterile gloves in your size, and chlorhexidine (Hibiclens) skin cleanser at the bedside. You will have to remove the dressing around the chest tube, and you must keep the site sterile.

Inform RN

"I will arrive at the bedside in . . . minutes."

Bleeding around the chest tube entry site is a potential emergency, requiring you to see the patient as soon as possible. Any malfunctioning chest tube in association with SOB requires you to see the patient immediately.

ELEVATOR THOUGHTS

What causes bleeding around the chest tube entry site?

- Inadequate pressure bandage
- Inadequate closure of the incision with suture
- Coagulation disorders

- Trauma to intercostal vessels or lung during insertion of the chest tube
- Blockage of chest tube or inadequately sized chest tube with drainage of the hemothorax around the entry site

MAJOR THREAT TO LIFE

- Hemorrhagic shock

Continuous oozing, if allowed to progress, may eventually lead to intravascular volume depletion and, in the extreme case, hemorrhagic shock.

BEDSIDE

Quick-Look Test

Does the patient look well (comfortable), sick (uncomfortable or distressed), or critical (about to die)?

If there is only a small amount of bleeding from the chest tube entry site, the patient will probably look well. A patient who has lost more blood may look sick or critical.

Airway and Vital Signs

What are the BP, heart rate (HR), and RR?

Hypotension and tachycardia may indicate major loss of blood. Tachypnea may indicate a large hemothorax.

Selective History and Chart Review

Why was the chest tube inserted?

Check the following recent laboratory results: hemoglobin (Hb), prothrombin time (PT), activated partial thromboplastin time (aPTT), and platelet count.

Selective Physical Examination and Management

Remove the dressing at the chest tube entry site and inspect the incision. If the incision is too large and inadequately closed, insert one or two sutures to seal the opening. If the incision is adequately closed with sutures, reapply a pressure dressing over the site, taking care to ensure that the pressure is maintained. Such maneuvers, when performed adequately, will stop the bleeding in the majority of situations.

If the chest tube is obstructed, resulting in blood draining around the entry site, try milking the chest tube. Reinspect to see if this maneuver has reestablished fluctuation in the underwater seal. The connecting tube is made of rubber and can be carefully stripped using the chest tube strippers. These two maneuvers may help dislodge any blood clots and debris blocking the tube.

If the chest tube is too small, it may be unable to drain a large hemothorax adequately. A larger size chest tube may be required.

Drainage of an Excessive Volume of Blood

PHONE CALL

Questions

1. Why was the chest tube inserted?
2. What are the vital signs?
3. Does the patient have SOB?
4. What was the reason for admission?

Orders

None.

Inform RN

"I will arrive at the bedside in . . . minutes."

Drainage of an excessive volume of blood via the chest tube is a potential emergency and requires you to see the patient immediately. Any malfunctioning chest tube associated with SOB also requires you to see the patient immediately.

ELEVATOR THOUGHTS

What causes excessive blood to drain via the chest tube?

- Intrathoracic bleeding

MAJOR THREAT TO LIFE

- Hemorrhagic shock

Hemorrhagic shock may result from excessive intrathoracic blood loss.

BEDSIDE

Quick-Look Test

Does the patient look well (comfortable), sick (uncomfortable or distressed), or critical (about to die)?

A patient with hemorrhagic shock looks pale, sweaty, and restless.

Airway and Vital Signs

What are the BP and HR?

Hypotension and tachycardia may indicate hemorrhagic shock.

What is the RR?

Tachypnea and hypotension may indicate a tension pneumothorax.

Management I

1. Give supplemental O_2, such as 4 L/min by nasal prongs.
2. If the patient is hypotensive, draw 20 mL of blood and start a large-bore IV (size 16 if possible). Give NS or Ringer's lactate 500 mL IV as fast as possible.
3. Send blood for an immediate crossmatch for 4 to 6 units of packed red blood cells (RBCs) on hold, Hb, PT, aPTT, and platelet count.
4. Order a stat CXR.

Selective Chart Review and Management II

Is the patient receiving anticoagulant medication (heparin, warfarin)?

If so, review the initial indication for anticoagulation. Can the anticoagulant be safely discontinued or reversed? Consult the hematology department for assistance in the management of this difficult and potentially life-threatening situation.

How much blood has the patient lost over the past 48 hours?

Estimate the amount by reviewing the intake-output chart.

- If the patient has lost >500 mL over 8 hours, consultation with a thoracic surgeon is recommended. The patient may need immediate transfer to the operating room for an emergency thoracotomy to localize the site of hemorrhage and achieve hemostasis.
- If the patient has lost <500 mL over 8 hours, order hourly monitoring of the blood lost via the chest tube, noting that a physician needs to be informed if the blood loss is >50 mL/hr.

Loss of Fluctuation of the Underwater Seal

PHONE CALL

Questions

1. Why was the chest tube inserted?
2. What are the vital signs?
3. Does the patient have SOB?
4. What was the reason for admission?

Orders

None.

Inform RN

"I will arrive at the bedside in . . . minutes."

Loss of fluctuation of the underwater seal is a potential emergency and requires you to see the patient as soon as possible. Any malfunctioning chest tube associated with SOB requires you to see the patient immediately.

ELEVATOR THOUGHTS

What causes loss of fluctuation of the underwater seal?

- Kinked chest tube
- Plugged chest tube
- Improper chest tube positioning

The underwater seal is essentially a one-way, low-resistance valve. During expiration, the intrapleural pressure increases, becoming higher than atmospheric pressure, forcing air or fluid that is in the pleural space through the chest tube and underwater seal (see Fig. 20–7).

MAJOR THREAT TO LIFE

- Tension pneumothorax

Inadequate drainage of a pneumothorax because of a blocked chest tube may lead to a tension pneumothorax (Figs. 20–8 and 20–9).

BEDSIDE

Quick-Look Test

Does the patient look well (comfortable), sick (uncomfortable or distressed), or critical (about to die)?

A patient who looks sick may be developing a tension pneumothorax or may look sick for unrelated reasons.

Airway and Vital Signs

What are the BP and RR?

Hypotension and tachypnea may indicate a tension pneumothorax.

Selective History and Chart Review

Why was the chest tube inserted?

How long ago did the chest tube stop fluctuating?

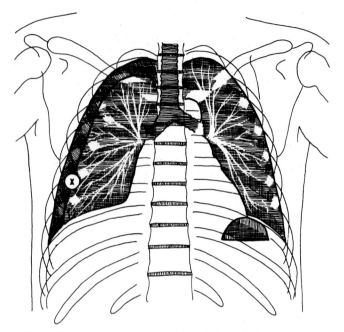

Figure 20–8 Pneumothorax. x, Edge of visceral pleura or lung.

What has been draining from the chest tube? What volume has drained over the past 24 hours?

Selective Physical Examination and Management

1. Inspect the underwater seal. Is there any fluctuation? Ask the patient to cough, and observe the tube for any fluctuation. A chest tube with its distal aperture located within the pleural space fluctuates with respiration.

2. Inspect the chest tube for kinking. You may need to remove the dressing at the chest tube entry site. If the chest tube is kinked, reposition and reinspect it for fluctuation of the underwater seal.

3. Try milking the chest tube. Reinspect it to see if this maneuver reestablishes fluctuation in the underwater seal. The connecting tubing is rubber and can be carefully stripped using chest tube strippers. These two maneuvers help dislodge blood clots and debris that may be blocking the tube.

4. Order a portable CXR. Improper positioning of the chest tube may result in loss of fluctuation of the underwater seal.

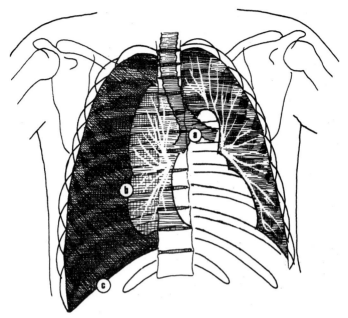

Figure 20–9 Tension pneumothorax. a, Shifted mediastinum. b, Edge of collapsed lung. c, Low, flattened diaphragm.

5. If the tube is not fluctuating after all the aforementioned maneuvers have been attempted, a new chest tube may have to be inserted.

Subcutaneous Emphysema

PHONE CALL

Questions

1. Why was the chest tube inserted?
2. What are the vital signs?
3. Does the patient have SOB?
4. What was the reason for admission?

Orders

Ask the RN to have a dressing set, two pairs of sterile gloves in your size, and chlorhexidine (Hibitane) skin cleanser at the bedside. You will have to remove the dressing around the chest tube, and you must keep the site sterile.

Inform RN

"I will arrive at the bedside in . . . minutes."

Subcutaneous emphysema is a potential emergency requiring you to see the patient immediately. Any malfunctioning chest tube associated with SOB requires you to see the patient immediately.

ELEVATOR THOUGHTS

What causes subcutaneous emphysema?

- Chest tube size too small for the leak
- Inadequate suction
- Chest tube aperture in the chest wall
- Chest tube in the chest wall or abdominal cavity
- Insignificant localized subcutaneous emphysema around the entry site is not uncommon after chest tube insertion

MAJOR THREAT TO LIFE

- Upper airway obstruction

Subcutaneous emphysema extending up into the neck rarely results in tracheal compression.

BEDSIDE

Quick-Look Test

Does the patient look well (comfortable), sick (uncomfortable or distressed), or critical (about to die)?

A patient with upper airway obstruction looks sick or critical, and there may be audible inspiratory stridor.

Airway and Vital Signs

Inspect and palpate the neck for subcutaneous emphysema.

What is the RR?

A patient with upper airway obstruction is tachypneic.

What are the BP and HR?

Subcutaneous emphysema may be accompanied by a tension pneumothorax. If so, the patient will be tachycardic.

Selective History and Chart Review

Why was the chest tube inserted?

Selective Physical Examination and Management

If there is significant upper airway obstruction (palpable subcutaneous emphysema over the trachea, inspiratory stridor, tachypnea), call the

ICU/CCU team immediately for probable intubation and transfer to the ICU/CCU. Cardiothoracic surgery may be required if mediastinal decompression is indicated.

What size chest tube was inserted? Is the tube's diameter too small?

Multifenestrated vinyl chest tubes are available in two sizes: 20F and 36F. The 20F may not be large enough, and air may escape from the pleural cavity into the chest wall, resulting in subcutaneous emphysema. If the chest tube is too small, a larger one must be inserted. Sometimes, two large chest tubes are required for adequate drainage.

Is the chest tube connected to suction?

A large pneumothorax may not be drained adequately if it is connected only to an underwater seal, as opposed to suction.

Remove the dressing at the chest tube site and inspect the chest tube. Are any of the drainage holes in the distal end of the chest tube visible?

None of the drainage lines should be visible. They should all be inside the pleural cavity. Subcutaneous emphysema may be caused by misplacement of the chest tube, with one of the drainage holes inadvertently in the soft tissue of the chest wall. A new chest tube should be inserted. Do not reinsert the partially extruded chest tube, because you may introduce infection into the pleural space.

Shortness of Breath

PHONE CALL

Questions

1. Why was the chest tube inserted?
2. What are the vital signs?
3. What was the reason for admission?

Orders

Ask the RN for a dressing set, two pairs of sterile gloves in your size, chlorhexidine (Hibiclens) skin cleanser, and a size 16 IV catheter.

A tension pneumothorax, if present, is treated most effectively by inserting a size 16 IV catheter into the pleural space on the affected side.

Inform RN

"I will arrive at the bedside in . . . minutes."

SOB in a patient with a chest tube in place is a potential emergency and requires you to see the patient immediately.

ELEVATOR THOUGHTS

What causes shortness of breath in a patient with a chest tube?

Causes Related to the Chest Tube

1. Tension pneumothorax, which may occur because of
   a. Inadequate suction
   b. Misplaced tube (i.e., chest tube not in the pleural cavity)
   c. Blocked or kinked tube
   d. Bronchopulmonary fistula
2. Increasing pneumothorax, which may result from the same causes as tension pneumothorax
3. Subcutaneous emphysema
4. Increasing pleural effusion or hemothorax
5. Re-expansion pulmonary edema (sometimes this occurs after rapid expansion of a pneumothorax, drainage of pleural fluid, or both)

Causes Unrelated to the Chest Tube

See Chapter 24, page 263.

MAJOR THREAT TO LIFE

- Tension pneumothorax
- Upper airway obstruction

Inadequate drainage of a pneumothorax produced through a ball-valve mechanism may result in a life-threatening *tension pneumothorax*. Tracheal compression from interstitial emphysema rarely causes *upper airway obstruction*.

BEDSIDE

Quick-Look Test

Does the patient look well (comfortable), sick (uncomfortable or distressed), or critical (about to die)?
    A sick- or critical-looking patient may have a tension pneumothorax or may have an unrelated reason for SOB (see Chapter 24).

Airway and Vital Signs

Inspect and palpate the neck for subcutaneous emphysema.

What is the RR?
    Rates >20/min suggest hypoxia, pain, or anxiety. Look for thoracoabdominal dissociation, which may indicate impending

respiratory failure. Remember that the rib cage and abdominal wall normally move in the same direction during inspiration and expiration.

What are the BP and HR?

Hypotension and tachycardia may indicate a tension pneumothorax or another unrelated cause of SOB (see Chapter 24).

Selective Physical Examination

Does the patient have a tension pneumothorax?

Vitals	Tachypnea
	Hypotension
HEENT	Tracheal deviation away from the hyperresonant side
Resp	Unilateral hyperresonance
	Decreased air entry on hyperresonant side
CVS	Elevated JVP
Chest tube	Is there bubbling in the collection chamber?
	Absence of bubbling suggests malposition or malfunction of the chest tube

Selective Chart Review

Why was the chest tube inserted?

Management

1. If there is *significant upper airway obstruction* (palpable subcutaneous emphysema over the trachea, inspiratory stridor, tachypnea), call the ICU/CCU team immediately for probable intubation and transfer to the ICU/CCU.
2. *Tension pneumothorax* is a medical emergency requiring urgent treatment. You will need supervision by your resident or attending physician.
   a. Identify the second intercostal space in the midclavicular line on the affected (hyperresonant) side.
   b. Mark this point using pressure from the cap of a needle or ballpoint pen.
   c. Open the dressing set and pour the chlorhexidine (Hibitane) into the appropriate container.
   d. Put on the sterile gloves and clean the identified area.
   e. Insert the size 16 IV catheter into the designated site. Remove the inner needle, leaving the plastic cannula in the chest. If a tension pneumothorax is present, there will be a loud sound of air rushing out through the catheter. You do not need to connect the catheter to suction; the lung space will decompress itself.
   f. Order a chest tube sent to the room immediately. Definitive treatment is insertion of a chest tube.

3. If there is an increasing pneumothorax but no evidence of a tension pneumothorax, order a stat upright CXR in expiration. Meanwhile, look for any correctable causes, such as kinked or blocked tubing, inadequate suction, or a dislodged chest tube.

4. For the management of other causes of SOB (i.e., causes unrelated to chest tubes), see Chapter 24.

URETHRAL CATHETERS

There are five types of urethral catheters (Fig. 20–10).

1. The *Foley* (balloon retention) *catheter* is the most commonly used. It consists of a double-lumen tube. The larger lumen drains

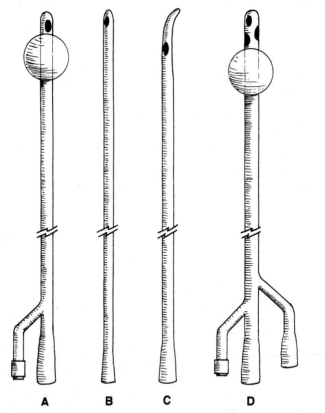

A   **B**   **C**   **D**

Figure 20–10 Urethral catheters. *A*, Foley catheter. *B*, Straight (Robinson) catheter. *C*, Coudé catheter. *D*, Three-way irrigation catheter.

urine, and the smaller lumen admits 5 to 30 mL of water to inflate the balloon tip.

2. *Straight (Robinson) catheters* are used to obtain in-and-out collections of urine, to obtain sterile specimens in patients who are unable to void voluntarily, and to obtain postvoiding residual urine volume measurements.

3. A *coudé catheter* has a curved tip that facilitates insertion when a urethral obstruction (e.g., benign prostatic hypertrophy) makes passage of a Foley catheter difficult.

4. *Three-way irrigation catheters* have, in addition to a lumen for urine drainage and one for balloon inflation, a third lumen for bladder irrigation. These catheters are commonly used after transurethral prostate resection to facilitate bladder irrigation and drainage of blood clots.

5. A *Silastic catheter* is similar to a Foley catheter but is constructed of softer, less reactive plastic. It is used when a urethral catheter is required on a long-term basis.

Blocked Urethral Catheter

PHONE CALL

Questions

1. How long has the catheter been blocked?
2. What are the vital signs?
3. Does the patient have suprapubic pain?
    Urinary retention secondary to a blocked catheter can result in suprapubic pain due to bladder distention.
4. What was the reason for admission?

Orders

Ask the RN to try flushing the catheter with 30 to 40 mL of sterile NS if this has not been done.

Inform RN

"I will arrive at the bedside in . . . minutes."
    Provided that the patient does not have suprapubic pain (bladder distention), assessment of a blocked urinary catheter can wait an hour or two if you have higher-priority problems.

ELEVATOR THOUGHTS

What causes blocked urethral catheters?

- Urinary sediment
- Blood clots

- Kinked catheter (look under the bed sheets)
- Improperly placed or dislodged catheter

MAJOR THREAT TO LIFE

- Bladder rupture
- Progressive renal insufficiency

Bladder rupture may occur if bladder distention progresses without decompression. Because bladder distention is painful, bladder rupture from this cause is usually seen only in an unconscious or paraplegic patient. Persistent lower urinary tract obstruction may lead to hydronephrosis and *renal failure*.

BEDSIDE

Quick-Look Test

Does the patient look well (comfortable), sick (uncomfortable or distressed), or critical (about to die)?

Most patients with blocked urethral catheters look well. However, patients with acute bladder distention may look distressed because of abdominal pain.

Airway and Vital Signs

A blocked urethral catheter is not usually responsible for alterations in vital signs unless pain due to bladder distention causes tachypnea or tachycardia.

Selective Physical Examination and Management

1. Percuss and palpate the abdomen to determine whether the bladder is distended. Suprapubic dullness and tenderness suggest a distended bladder.
2. Examine the tubing for kinking of the catheter, blood clots, or sediment.
3. Order a sterile dressing tray, a 50-mL bulb syringe (or a 50-mL syringe and an adapter), and two pairs of sterile gloves in your size. Aspirate and irrigate the catheter with 30 to 40 mL of sterile NS as follows:
   a. Ask an assistant to hold the distal part of the catheter close to the connection between the tubing and urinary drainage bag.
   b. Wear sterile gloves and clean the distal catheter and the proximal connecting tubing with chlorhexidine.
   c. Disconnect the drainage tubing from the catheter. Ask an assistant to hold the connecting tubing in the air to maintain a sterile tip.

    d. Using a 50-mL syringe, aspirate the catheter vigorously to dislodge and extract any blood clots or sediment. If the maneuver is unsuccessful, flush the catheter with 30 to 40 mL of sterile NS. Several attempts at aspiration should be made before abandoning this technique.

    e. Reconnect the catheter to the connecting tubing, using sterile technique.

    The majority of blocked Foley catheters become unplugged with this maneuver.

4. If flushing of the catheter fails to relieve the obstruction, a new catheter should be inserted if one is still required.

Gross Hematuria

PHONE CALL

Questions

1. Why was the urethral catheter inserted?
2. What are the vital signs?
3. Is the patient receiving anticoagulant drugs or cyclophosphamide?
4. What was the reason for admission?

Orders

None.

Inform RN

"I will arrive at the bedside in . . . minutes."

    Gross hematuria in an anticoagulated patient requires you to see the patient immediately.

ELEVATOR THOUGHTS

What causes gross hematuria in a catheterized patient?

1. Urethral trauma
    a. Inadvertent or partial removal of the catheter with the balloon still inflated
    b. Trauma during catheter insertion (false passage)
2. Drugs
    a. Anticoagulants (heparin, warfarin)
    b. Thrombolytic agents (streptokinase, tPA, urokinase)
    c. Cyclophosphamide
3. Coagulation abnormalities
    a. Disseminated intravascular coagulation (DIC)
    b. Specific factor deficiencies
    c. Thrombocytopenia

4. Unrelated problems
   a. Renal stones
   b. Carcinoma of the kidney, bladder, or prostate
   c. Glomerulonephritis
   d. Prostatitis
   e. Rupture of a bladder vein

MAJOR THREAT TO LIFE

- Hemorrhagic shock

Although gross hematuria is dramatic and distressing to the patient, it is rare for bleeding to be significant enough to result in hemorrhagic shock. Only 1 mL of blood in 1 L of urine will change the color from yellow to red.

BEDSIDE

Quick-Look Test

Does the patient look well (comfortable), sick (uncomfortable or distressed), or critical (about to die)?

It is unusual for a patient with gross hematuria to look other than well. If a patient looks sick or critical, search for a separate unrecognized problem.

Airway and Vital Signs

What is the BP?

Hypotension in a patient with gross hematuria may be a sign of hemorrhagic shock.

What is the HR?

A resting tachycardia, though a nonspecific finding, may indicate hypovolemia if significant blood loss has occurred.

Selective History and Chart Review

Is the patient receiving any of the following medications?
Heparin, warfarin
Streptokinase, tPA, urokinase
Cyclophosphamide

Is there any abnormality in the coagulation profile?
PT
aPTT
Platelet count

Is there a history of urethral trauma?

Recent inadvertent removal of a Foley catheter with the balloon
still inflated (especially in an elderly, confused patient)
Recent genitourinary (GU) surgery
Recent difficulty inserting a urethral catheter

*Has there been a recent decrease in the Hb value? How much blood
has the patient lost?*

Bleeding via the urinary tract is unlikely to cause significant
hemodynamic changes unless there has been recent GU surgery.

Management

1. If the patient is anticoagulated, review the initial indication
   for the anticoagulation. Decide, in consultation with your resident and a hematologist, whether the risk of anticoagulation
   is still warranted.
2. If a coagulation abnormality is identified, refer to Chapter 31
   for a discussion of investigation and management.
3. If there is a history of recent urethral trauma, continued significant blood loss is unlikely. Have the vital signs taken every
   4 to 6 hours for the next 24 hours. Significant bleeding may
   be manifested by tachycardia and orthostatic hypotension.

Inability to Insert a Urethral Catheter

PHONE CALL

Questions

1. Why was the urethral catheter ordered?
2. What are the vital signs?
3. Does the patient have suprapubic pain?
4. How many attempts have been made to catheterize the
   patient?
5. What was the reason for admission?

Orders

Ask the RN to have a catheter insertion set, two pairs of sterile gloves
in your size, and chlorhexidine (Hibiclens) skin disinfectant at the
bedside.

Inform RN

"I will arrive at the bedside in . . . minutes."

Provided that the patient does not have suprapubic pain (bladder
distention), insertion of a urethral catheter can wait an hour or two
if there are higher-priority problems.

ELEVATOR THOUGHTS

What causes difficulty in urethral catheterization?

1. Urethral edema
   a. Multiple insertion attempts
   b. Inadvertent removal of a Foley catheter with the balloon still inflated
2. Urethral obstruction
   a. Benign prostatic hypertrophy
   b. Carcinoma of the prostate
   c. Urethral stricture
   d. Anatomic anomaly (diverticulum, false passage)

MAJOR THREAT TO LIFE

- Bladder rupture
- Progressive renal insufficiency

Bladder rupture may occur if bladder distention is not relieved by placement of a urinary catheter. A suprapubic catheter may be required if urethral catheterization is impossible. Persistent bladder obstruction may lead to hydronephrosis and *renal failure.*

BEDSIDE

Quick-Look Test

Does the patient look well (comfortable), sick (uncomfortable or distressed), or critical (about to die)?

Patients with acute bladder distention may look distressed because of abdominal pain.

Airway and Vital Signs

Inability to insert a urethral catheter should not compromise the vital signs.

Selective History and Chart Review

Is there a history of recent multiple attempts at catheterization or removal of a catheter with the balloon still inflated (urethral edema)?

Is there a history of benign prostatic hypertrophy, carcinoma of the prostate, urethral stricture, or an anatomic abnormality of the urethra?

What was the original indication for urethral catheter placement? Does the indication still exist?

Selective Physical Examination and Management

1. Percuss and palpate the abdomen to determine whether the bladder is distended. Suprapubic tenderness and dullness are suggestive of a distended bladder.

2. If urethral edema is suspected, try inserting a smaller catheter.
3. If there is a history of urethral obstruction, try inserting a coudé catheter.
4. If you are unable to catheterize the patient, consult the urology department for assistance.

T-TUBES, J-TUBES, AND PENROSE DRAINS

T-tubes are usually used for postoperative drainage of the common bile duct after common bile duct exploration or choledochotomy (Fig. 20–11). A T-tube cholangiogram is commonly performed on the 7th to 10th postoperative day. If the cholangiogram is normal, the T-tube is removed. If a blockage (stricture, tumor, retained common duct stones) exists, the T-tube is left in place.

J-tubes, or jejunostomy tubes, are surgically inserted to provide enteral nutrition on a long-term basis. They are particularly useful when gastroesophageal reflux and aspiration are a problem.

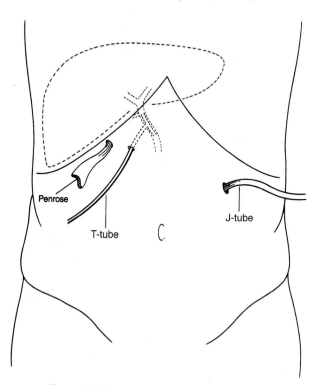

Figure 20–11 T-tube, J-tube, and Penrose drain.

Gastrostomy tubes may be inserted percutaneously under direct vision (e.g., gastroscopy or fluoroscopy) and are used for long-term feeding when there is no gastroesophageal reflux.

Penrose drains are flat rubber drains inserted into wounds or operative sites with potential dead spaces to prevent the accumulation of pus, intestinal contents, blood, bile, or pancreatic juice.

Closed suction (Davon or Jackson-Pratt) *drains* are used in operative sites with large potential dead spaces, where bacterial ingress may contaminate sterile cavities.

Sump drains have filters incorporated to prevent airborne bacteria from entering. They are usually used to drain peripancreatic fluid collections. Interventional radiologists sometimes insert various percutaneous drains into the biliary tree and intra-abdominal abscesses. Problems with these drains should be referred to the radiologist or surgeon.

Blocked T-Tubes and J-Tubes

PHONE CALL

Questions

1. How long has the tube been blocked?
2. What type of tube is in place?
3. Has the tube been dislodged?
4. What operation was performed, and how many days ago?
5. What are the vital signs?
6. What was the reason for admission?

Orders

Ask the RN to have a dressing set, two pairs of gloves in your size, and chlorhexidine (Hibitane) skin disinfectant at the bedside. You will have to remove the dressing around the drainage tube, and you must keep the site sterile.

Inform RN

"I will arrive at the bedside in . . . minutes."

If you are certain that the tube has not been dislodged, assessment of blocked T-tubes and J-tubes can wait an hour or two if higher-priority problems exist.

ELEVATOR THOUGHTS

What causes blocked T-tubes or J-tubes?

- Blood clots in the tube
- Debris in the tube
- Failure to irrigate the tube regularly

MAJOR THREAT TO LIFE

- Sepsis with blocked T-tubes

Blocked T-tubes may lead to postoperative infection, with resultant abscess formation or systemic sepsis. Provided that they are not dislodged, blocked J-tubes present no immediate threat to life. The risk of further surgery exists if the tube must be replaced.

BEDSIDE

Quick-Look Test

Does the patient look well (comfortable), sick (uncomfortable or distressed), or critical (about to die)?

A patient with a blocked T-tube or J-tube looks well unless the underlying problem causes the patient to look sick or critical.

Airway and Vital Signs

A blocked T-tube or J-tube should not compromise the airway or vital signs.

Selective Physical Examination and Management

Aspirate and irrigate the tube as follows:

1. Ask an assistant to hold the distal part of the T-tube or J-tube close to the connection between the tube and the drainage bag.
2. Wear sterile gloves and clean the distal end of the T-tube or J-tube and the proximal connecting tubing with chlorhexidine (Hibitane).
3. Disconnect the tube from the connecting tubing and give the connecting tubing to the assistant to maintain a sterile field.
4. Using a 5-mL syringe, aspirate very gently (i.e., withdraw the syringe plunger) to dislodge and extract the obstruction.
5. If this maneuver is unsuccessful, fill a second 5-mL syringe with 3 mL of sterile NS and *very gently* flush the T-tube or J-tube by applying slow, careful pressure to the syringe plunger. After flushing with saline, attempt to aspirate gently. If this maneuver fails, do not try again.
6. Reconnect the T-tube or J-tube and the drainage bag, maintaining sterile technique.

If aspiration and irrigation are unsuccessful, the surgeon should be informed immediately. A decision between a T-tube cholangiogram to visualize the problem and a closed exploration of the obstructed tube with a Fogarty catheter must be made. Closed exploration should be performed only by someone experienced in the procedure. It can be done only when a large, intact T-tube has been used or when the back wall of the T-limb has been cut away.

An adequately functioning T-tube usually drains 100 to 250 mL over 8 hours.

Dislodged T-Tubes, J-Tubes, and Penrose Drains

PHONE CALL

Questions

1. How long ago was the tube or drain dislodged?
2. What type of tube is in place?
3. What operation was performed, and how many days ago?
4. What are the vital signs?
5. What was the reason for admission?

Orders

Ask the RN to have a dressing set, two pairs of gloves in your size, and chlorhexidine (Hibitane) skin cleanser at the bedside. You will have to remove the dressing around the drainage tube, and you must keep the site sterile.

Inform RN

"I will arrive at the bedside in . . . minutes."

Assessment of dislodged T-tubes and J-tubes requires you to see the patient immediately, because urgent replacement is mandatory if the tube was inserted recently. A delay may result in the patient's requiring emergency surgery to replace the tube.

ELEVATOR THOUGHTS

What causes dislodgment of tubes and drains?

- Failure to secure the tube or drain adequately
- Confused, uncooperative patient

MAJOR THREAT TO LIFE

- Sepsis

Dislodged T-tubes and Penrose drains may lead to postoperative sepsis, with resultant abscess formation or systemic sepsis. Dislodged J-tubes and T-tubes that cannot be replaced early may require surgical replacement, increasing the risk of morbidity and mortality from a second anesthetic.

BEDSIDE

Quick-Look Test

Does the patient look well (comfortable), sick (uncomfortable or distressed), or critical (about to die)?

A patient with a recently dislodged T-tube, J-tube, or Penrose drain looks well unless the underlying problem causes the patient to look sick or critical.

Airway and Vital Signs

A dislodged T-tube, J-tube, or Penrose drain should not compromise the vital signs acutely.

Selective Physical Examination and Management

Dislodged T-Tube

A dislodged T-tube draining the common bile duct is a potentially life-threatening situation, because septic shock can follow rapidly. If dislodgment is suspected, order an immediate T-tube cholangiogram and inform the surgeon. The patient will need surgery to reestablish drainage if dislodgment is confirmed by the cholangiogram.

Dislodged J-Tube

A dislodged J-tube (enterostomy tube) must be reinserted immediately, as follows:

1. Wear sterile gloves, and clean and drape the tube exit site.
2. If the tube is only partially dislodged, carefully clean the exposed tubing and gently advance the tube to the appropriate (previous) depth.
3. If the tube has been completely dislodged, select a similar sterile tube and introduce it gently through the track left by the previous tube. Do not force the tube.
4. If this maneuver is successful, secure the tube well by suturing it in place with a 3-0 suture.
5. Order a water-soluble radiocontrast x-ray to confirm correct positioning of the replaced or repositioned tube.

If replacement of the J-tube is unsuccessful, notify the surgeon, who will decide whether an urgent reoperation is indicated.

Dislodged Penrose Drain

Dislodged Penrose drains should not be reinserted into the wound because doing so would introduce bacteria into the site. Secure the Penrose drain in the position you find it and examine the area daily for abscess formation (heat, tenderness, swelling) for the next few days. Inform the surgeon that the Penrose drain has become dislodged.

NASOGASTRIC AND ENTERAL FEEDING TUBES

Blocked Nasogastric and Enteral Feeding Tubes

PHONE CALL

Questions

1. How long has the tube been blocked?
2. What type of tube is in place?
3. Has the tube been dislodged?
4. What are the vital signs?
5. What was the reason for admission?

Orders

Ask the RN to have a 50-mL syringe, sterile NS, and a bowl at the bedside.

Inform RN

"I will arrive at the bedside in . . . minutes."

A blocked NG or enteral tube is not an emergency. Assessment can wait an hour or two if higher-priority problems exist.

ELEVATOR THOUGHTS

What causes blocked nasogastric or enteral feeding tubes?

- Debris in the tube
- Blood clots in the tube
- Failure to irrigate the tube regularly

MAJOR THREAT TO LIFE

- Aspiration pneumonia

If the NG tube is blocked and thus fails to drain the stomach, gastric contents can be aspirated into the lungs.

BEDSIDE

Quick-Look Test

Does the patient look well (comfortable), sick (uncomfortable or distressed), or critical (about to die)?

If a blocked NG tube fails to drain the gastric contents, the patient may experience nausea and vomiting, thus looking sick.

Airway and Vital Signs

What is the RR?

A blocked NG tube should not compromise the airway unless gastric contents accumulate and are aspirated into the lungs.

Selective Physical Examination and Management

1. Irrigate the tube with 25 to 50 mL of NS. As the tube is being irrigated, listen over the stomach region for the gurgling of fluid, which indicates that the tube is in the stomach.
2. If the previous maneuver is unsuccessful, remove the tube and replace it with a new tube if there is ongoing gastric stasis with the potential for aspiration.
3. Ensure that the usual nursing protocols are being followed for regular irrigation of the tube.

Dislodged Nasogastric and Enteral Feeding Tubes

PHONE CALL

Questions

1. How long has the tube been dislodged?
2. What type of tube is in place?
3. What are the vital signs?
4. What was the reason for admission?

Orders

None.

Inform RN

"I will arrive at the bedside in . . . minutes."

Assessment of a dislodged NG or enteral feeding tube can wait an hour or two if higher-priority problems exist. Be careful, however, not to leave a diabetic patient who has received insulin without caloric intake for too long.

ELEVATOR THOUGHTS

What causes a nasogastric or enteral feeding tube to become dislodged?

- Failure to secure the tube adequately
- Confused, uncooperative patient

MAJOR THREAT TO LIFE

- Aspiration pneumonia

If the NG tube is dislodged and thus fails to drain the stomach, gastric contents may accumulate and can be aspirated into the lung. With a dislodged or misplaced enteral feeding tube, the danger is infusion of the enteral feeding solution into the lung.

BEDSIDE

Quick-Look Test

Does the patient look well (comfortable), sick (uncomfortable or distressed), or critical (about to die)?

Patients who have aspirated because of a dislodged NG tube or a malpositioned feeding tube may appear tachypneic and unwell.

Airway and Vital Signs

A dislodged NG or enteral feeding tube should not compromise the vital signs unless aspiration of gastric contents or enteral feeding solutions has occurred.

Selective Physical Examination and Management

1. Inspect the tube, looking for markings that indicate how far in it is. If you are not familiar with these markings, ask the RN to bring a similar tube so that you can estimate how far in the tube is.
2. Aspirate the tube to see if gastric contents can be obtained. Instill 25 to 50 mL of air using the 50-mL syringe while listening over the stomach region with your stethoscope. If the tube is properly positioned, you should hear a gurgling swoosh as air is introduced into the stomach.
3. A small-bore enteral feeding tube should not be pushed farther down if it has been dislodged. Do *not* insert the guidewire down the tube blindly, because laceration or perforation of the esophagus, stomach, or duodenum may occur if the tip of the guidewire exits from one of the distal apertures in the tube. Dislodged enteral feeding tubes must be removed and replaced. The same tube can be reused, with the guidewire inserted into the tube under direct vision ex vivo. The tube, stiffened by the guidewire, can then be reinserted.
4. Ensure that the usual nursing protocols are being followed for regular irrigation of the tube.

Polyuria, Frequency, and Incontinence

You will receive many calls at night regarding patients' urinary volume; they may be voiding either too much or too little. It is often difficult for a patient to differentiate between problems of *polyuria* and *frequency*, and for many elderly patients, either of these problems may present as *incontinence*. Once you clarify which of these three problems is present, the rest is easy.

PHONE CALL

Questions

1. **Which problem is present?**

   Polyuria refers to a urine output >3 L/day. This usually comes to the attention of the nurse when reviewing the fluid balance record or when the urinary drainage bag requires frequent emptying.

   Frequency of urination refers to the frequent passage of urine, whether of large or small volume, and may occur in concert with polyuria or urinary incontinence.

   Urinary incontinence refers to the involuntary loss of urine.

2. **What are the vital signs?**
3. **What was the admitting diagnosis?**

Orders

Polyuria, frequency, and incontinence are seldom urgent problems. Urinary incontinence is a common problem in hospitalized elderly patients and is a frequent source of frustration for nurses. Avoid ordering a Foley catheter as the first line of treatment.

Inform RN

"I will arrive at the bedside in . . . minutes."

If the patient's vital signs are stable and other sick patients require assessment, a patient with polyuria, frequency, or incontinence need not be seen immediately.

ELEVATOR THOUGHTS

What causes polyuria?

- Diabetes mellitus
- Diabetes insipidus (central, nephrogenic)
- Psychogenic polydipsia
- Large volumes of oral or intravenous (IV) fluids
- Diuretics
- Diuretic phase of acute tubular necrosis
- Postobstructive diuresis
- Salt-losing nephritis
- Hypercalcemia

What causes frequency?

- Urinary tract infection (UTI)
- Partial bladder outlet obstruction (e.g., prostatism)
- Bladder irritation (tumor, stone, infection)

What causes incontinence?

- Urge incontinence: caused by UTI, diabetes mellitus, urolithiasis, dementia, stroke, normal pressure hydrocephalus, benign prostatic hypertrophy (BPH), pelvic tumor, depression, anxiety
- Stress incontinence: in multiparous women, caused by lax pelvic bladder support; in men, occurs after prostate surgery
- Overflow incontinence: caused by bladder outlet obstruction, as in BPH, urethral stricture; spinal cord disease; autonomic neuropathy; fecal impaction
- Environmental factors: inaccessible call bell, obstacles to the bathroom
- Iatrogenic factors: diuretics, sedatives, anticholinergics, alpha blockers, calcium channel blockers, angiotensin-converting enzyme (ACE) inhibitors

MAJOR THREAT TO LIFE

- Polyuria: intravascular volume depletion. If polyuria is not due to fluid excess and continues without adequate fluid replacement, the intravascular volume will drop, and the patient may become hypotensive.
- Frequency or incontinence: sepsis. Frequency or incontinence does not pose a major threat to life unless an underlying UTI goes unchecked and progresses to pyelonephritis or sepsis.

BEDSIDE

Quick-Look Test

Does the patient look well (comfortable), sick (uncomfortable or distressed), or critical (about to die)?

Most often, patients with polyuria, frequency, or incontinence look well. If the patient looks sick or critical, search for a previously unrecognized problem. For example, if polyuria is due to previously undetected diabetes mellitus, the patient may be ketoacidotic and appear sick. Similarly, frequency or incontinence may be the presenting manifestation of UTI in a patient who appears sick.

Airway and Vital Signs

Are there postural changes?

A rise in heart rate (HR) >15 beats/min, a fall in systolic blood pressure (BP) >5 mm Hg, or any fall in diastolic BP indicates significant hypovolemia. *Caution:* A resting tachycardia alone may indicate decreased intravascular volume.

Does the patient have a fever?

Fever suggests possible UTI.

Selective Physical Examination I

Is the patient volume depleted?

CVS	Pulse volume, JVP
	Skin temperature and color
Neuro	Level of consciousness

Management I

What immediate measure must be taken to correct or prevent intravascular volume depletion?

Replace intravascular volume. If the patient is volume depleted, give IV normal saline (NS) or Ringer's lactate, aiming for a jugular venous pressure (JVP) of 2 to 3 cm H_2O above the sternal angle and normalization of the vital signs.

> Remember that aggressive fluid repletion in a patient with a history of congestive heart failure may compromise cardiac function. Do not overshoot the mark.

Selective History and Chart Review

Identify the specific problem.

Polyuria

Polyuria may be suspected by the history but can be confirmed only through scrutiny of meticulously kept fluid balance sheets. If these are not available, order strict intake-output monitoring. It is worthwhile to document polyuria (>3 L/day) before embarking on an exhaustive workup of a possibly nonexistent problem.

1. Ask about associated symptoms. "Polyuria + polydipsia" suggests diabetes mellitus, diabetes insipidus, or compulsive water drinking (psychogenic polydipsia). Of these, diabetes mellitus is the most common.
2. Check the chart for recent laboratory results.
   a. Blood glucose (diabetes mellitus)
   b. Potassium
   c. Calcium
      Hypokalemia and hypercalcemia are important reversible causes of nephrogenic diabetes insipidus. (Refer to Chapter 33 for management of hypokalemia and Chapter 30 for management of hypercalcemia.)
3. Make sure that the patient is not on any drugs that may cause either nephrogenic diabetes insipidus (lithium carbonate, demeclocycline) or diuresis (diuretics, mannitol).

Frequency

Frequency can be assessed by questioning the patient. Estimate from the nursing notes or fluid balance sheets whether the patient is a reliable historian. Ask about associated symptoms. Fever, dysuria, hematuria, and foul-smelling urine suggest UTI. Poor stream, hesitancy, dribbling, or nocturia suggests prostatism.

Incontinence

Incontinence is obvious when it occurs and is often embarrassing to the patient. You need an honest history from the patient to make a proper diagnosis. Address the subject nonjudgmentally. Review the patient's medications to ensure that he or she is not receiving medications that may cause incontinence.

Selective Physical Examination II

Look for specific causes and complications of polyuria, frequency, or incontinence.

Vitals	Fever (UTI)
HEENT	Visual fields (pituitary neoplasm)
Resp	Kussmaul's respiration (diabetic ketoacidosis)
	Kussmaul's respiration is characterized by deep, pauseless breathing at a rate of 25 to 30 breaths/min.
ABD	Enlarged bladder (neurogenic bladder, bladder outlet obstruction with overflow incontinence)
	Suprapubic tenderness (cystitis)
Neuro	Level of consciousness
	Localizing findings

An alert, conscious person with polyuria and with free access to fluids and salt will not become volume depleted. If volume depletion is present, suspect metabolic or structural neurologic abnormalities impairing the normal response to thirst. Perform a complete neurologic examination, looking for evidence of stroke, subdural hemorrhage, or metabolic abnormalities.

Skin   Perineal skin breakdown (a complication of repeated incontinence and a source of infection)

Rectal   Enlarged prostate (bladder outlet obstruction)
Perineal sensation, resting tone of anal sphincter, anal wink

An anal wink is elicited by gently stroking the perineal mucosa with a tongue depressor. A normal response is manifested by contraction of the external sphincter.

If abnormalities in perineal sensation, anal sphincter tone, or anal wink are discovered in a male patient, the bulbocavernosus reflex should also be tested. To elicit this reflex, the index finger of the examining hand is introduced into the rectum, and the patient is asked to relax the sphincter as much as possible. The glans penis is then squeezed with the opposite hand, which normally results in involuntary contraction of the anal sphincter. Innervation of the anus is similar to that of the lower urinary tract; therefore, abnormalities in perineal sensation or in the sacral reflexes may be a clue that a spinal cord lesion is responsible for the incontinence.

Management II

What more needs to be done tonight?

Polyuria

1. Once intravascular volume is restored, ensure adequate continuing replacement fluid (usually IV) as estimated by urinary, insensible (400 to 800 mL/day), and other (nasogastric suction, vomiting, diarrhea) losses. Recheck the volume status periodically to ensure that your mathematic estimates for replacement correlate with an appropriate clinical response.
2. Order that strict intake-output records be kept.
3. Order serum glucose or finger-prick blood glucose testing.

This will identify diabetes mellitus before it progresses to ketoacidosis (type 1 diabetes) or hyperosmolar coma (type 2 diabetes). The presence of glycosuria on urinalysis provides more rapid evidence of hyperglycemia as a possible cause of polyuria. Random blood glucose levels of ≤11 mmol/L are seldom accompanied by osmotic diuresis. If hyperglycemia of >11 mmol/L exists, refer to Chapter 32, pages 349 to 353, for further management.

4. It may not be standard practice to measure the serum calcium level as a stat test at night, but if there is a strong suspicion of hypercalcemia (polyuria or lethargy in a patient with malignancy, hyperparathyroidism, or sarcoidosis), contact the laboratory for permission to perform this test on an urgent basis.

5. Maximal urine concentrating ability measured by the water deprivation test can help differentiate among central diabetes insipidus, nephrogenic diabetes insipidus, and psychogenic polydipsia. This test can be arranged on an elective basis in the morning.

Frequency

1. If other symptoms (urgency, dysuria, low-grade fever, suprapubic tenderness) of UTI (cystitis) are present, empirical treatment with antibiotics may be warranted, pending urine culture and sensitivity results, which usually take 48 hours to complete. Scrutiny of the patient's chart may reveal a previous urine culture or previous antibacterial therapy that may affect the selection of empirical treatment.

    Any of the following may be effective therapy in an uncomplicated case of cystitis (i.e., no evidence of upper UTI, no evidence of prostatitis, no renal disease, and no recent urinary tract instrumentation). The usual infecting organisms are *Escherichia coli* and *Staphylococcus saprophyticus*. The condition may resolve spontaneously. Antibiotics are generally used for 3 days in women and for 7 days in men. However, women with diabetes, a structural urinary tract abnormality, or a recently treated UTI should receive a 7-day course.

    a. *Trimethoprim-sulfamethoxazole* (160 mg/800 mg) 1 tablet PO twice daily
    b. *Trimethoprim* 100 mg PO twice daily
    c. *Nitrofurantoin* 100 mg PO twice daily
    d. *Cephalexin* 500 mg PO every 6 hours
    e. *Ciprofloxacin* 250 mg PO every 12 hours

2. If the history and physical examination suggest partial bladder outlet obstruction, examine the abdomen carefully for an enlarged bladder. If the patient has urinary retention, a Foley catheter should be placed. (Refer to Chapter 9 for further investigation and management of urinary retention.)

    Always check for heart murmurs before catheterizing a patient. Patients with cardiac valvular abnormalities are at risk for the development of infective endocarditis after genitourinary procedures, including Foley catheterization. High-risk patients (those with prosthetic heart valves, previous endocarditis, cyanotic congenital heart disease) should receive *ampicillin* 2 g IV or IM plus gentamicin 1.5 mg/kg IV or IM. Both antibiotics should be given 30 minutes before catheterization. Then, 6 hours later, give *ampicillin* 1 g IV or IM or *amoxicillin* 1 g PO. Moderate-risk patients (those with mitral valve prolapse with regurgitation, hypertrophic cardiomyopathy, acquired valvular dysfunction, most noncyanotic congenital cardiac malformations) should receive *amoxicillin* 2 g PO 1 hour before catheterization or *ampicillin* 2 g IV or IM 30 minutes before catheterization. High-risk patients allergic to ampicillin or amoxicillin can be given *vancomycin* 1 g IV over 1 to 2 hours plus *gentamicin* 1.5 mg/kg IV or IM. In moderate-risk patients allergic to ampicillin or amoxicillin, vancomycin should be given, but the gentamicin can be omitted.[1]

A brief in-and-out catheterization, in the presence of sterile urine, may not require antibiotic prophylaxis. If, however, the patient has a prosthetic cardiac valve, you may want to err on the safe side and administer prophylactic antibiotics. Ask your resident or the patient's cardiologist for advice in this situation.

3. Other causes of frequency, such as bladder irritation by stones or tumors, can be addressed by urologic consultation in the morning. You may be able to expedite the diagnosis of bladder tumor by ordering a collection of urine for cytologic study.

Incontinence

1. Even if incontinence is the only symptom, order a urinalysis and urine culture to ensure that a UTI is not contributing to the patient's symptoms.
2. Check for hyperglycemia, hypokalemia, and hypercalcemia if there is a question of polyuria. These conditions may present as incontinence in an elderly or bedridden patient, and specific treatment may alleviate the incontinence.
3. If the neurologic examination (e.g., abnormal sacral reflexes, diminished perineal sensation, lower limb weakness or spasticity) suggests the presence of a *spinal cord lesion*, consultation should be arranged with a neurologist.
4. In the case of *overflow incontinence*, one must differentiate between overflow due to bladder outlet obstruction (e.g., BPH, uterine prolapse) and that due to impaired ability of detrusor contraction (e.g., lower motor neuron bladder). This is best done in the morning by assessment of urinary bladder dynamics under the direction of a urologist. If the bladder is palpably enlarged and the patient is distressed, bladder

catheterization may be attempted. Forceful attempts at catheterization should be avoided, however, and a urologist should be called for assistance if the catheter does not pass easily (see Chapter 20, page 229). If no correctable obstruction is found, long-term treatment may involve intermittent straight catheterization, which is less likely to cause infection than a chronic indwelling Foley catheter. Aim for a urine volume <400 mL every 4 to 6 hours. Greater volumes result in ureterovesical reflux, which promotes ascending UTI. A young, motivated patient with a neurogenic bladder can be taught to self-catheterize. In these cases, a silicone elastomer (Silastic) Foley catheter should be used. This type is less predisposed to calcification and encrustation and may be kept in place for up to 6 weeks at a time.

5. *Urge incontinence* (detrusor instability) is a condition in which the bladder escapes central inhibition, resulting in reflex contractions. It is the most common cause of incontinence in the elderly population and is often manifested by involuntary micturition preceded by a warning of a few seconds or minutes. Ensure that there are no physical barriers preventing the patient from reaching the bathroom or commode in time. Is there easy access to the call bell? Are the nurses responding promptly? Are the bed rails kept up or down? Does the patient have a medical condition (e.g., Parkinson's disease, stroke, arthritis) that prevents easy mobilization when the urge to void occurs? If there is no evidence of perineal skin breakdown, *urinary incontinence pads* with frequent checks and changes by the nursing staff are adequate. (Babies exist for years in such a state.) If perineal skin breakdown or ulceration is present, a Foley or condom catheter is justified to allow skin healing. Long-term treatment involves regular toileting every 2 to 3 hours while awake and limiting the evening fluid intake.

6. Urinary spillage with coughing or straining suggests *stress incontinence*. Again, if there is no evidence of perineal skin breakdown, urinary incontinence pads are adequate until urologic consultation can assess the need for medical versus surgical management.

REMEMBER

Urinary incontinence is an understandable source of frustration for nurses. Listen to the concerns of the nurses looking after your patients and discuss with them the reasons for your actions.

Reference

1. Prevention of bacterial endocarditis. JAMA 1997;277:1794-1801.

Pronouncing Death

One of the required duties of medical students and residents on call at night is to pronounce death in recently deceased patients. This situation is seldom addressed in medical school, but you need to know what must be done to pronounce a patient dead. Unfortunately, there has long been uncertainty surrounding what constitutes the medical and legal definitions of death.

Traditionally, the determination of death has been solely a medical decision. In the United States, legislation on the criteria for death falls within state jurisdiction. Many states have opted to follow the recommendations set forth by the Harvard Medical School Ad Hoc Committee,[1] Capron and Kass,[2] or the Kansas legislation of 1971.[3] It is best to be familiar with the medical and legal criteria accepted for the determination of death in the state in which you work.

The recommended criteria for death issued by the Law Reform Commission of Canada[4] in 1981, and used for all purposes within the jurisdiction of the Parliament of Canada, were as follows:

1. A person is dead when an irreversible cessation of all that person's brain function has occurred.
2. The irreversible cessation of brain function can be determined by the prolonged absence of spontaneous circulatory and respiratory functions.
3. When the determination of the prolonged absence of spontaneous circulatory and respiratory functions is made impossible by the use of artificial means of support, the irreversible cessation of brain function can be determined by any means recognized by the ordinary standards of current medical practice.

Although criterion 1 alone may imply that a complete neurologic examination is required for the pronouncement of death, we know that this is neither practical nor necessary. Criterion 2 accounts for this by assuming that when "prolonged absence of spontaneous circulatory and respiratory functions" exists, irreversible cessation of the patient's brain function has occurred. Hence, in the majority of cases, there will be no question that the patients you are asked to pronounce dead are indeed medically and legally dead, because they fulfill criterion 2. Thus, in most cases, all that is legally required for you to pronounce a patient dead is to verify that there has been a prolonged absence of spontaneous circulatory and respiratory functions. A slightly more detailed assessment is recommended, however, and takes only a few minutes to complete.

The RN will page you and inform you of the death of the patient, requesting that you come to the unit and pronounce the patient dead.

1. Identify the patient by the hospital identification tag worn on the wrist.

2. Ascertain that the patient does not rouse to verbal or tactile stimuli.

3. Listen for heart sounds, and feel for the carotid pulse.
   | A deceased patient is pulseless and without heart sounds.

4. Look at and listen to the patient's chest for evidence of spontaneous respirations.
   | A deceased patient shows no evidence of breathing movements or of air entry on examination.

5. Record the position of the pupils and their reactions to light.
   | A deceased patient shows no evidence of pupillary reaction to light. Although the pupils are usually dilated, this is not invariable.

6. Record the time at which your assessment was completed.
   | Although other emergencies take precedence over pronouncing a patient dead, try not to postpone this task too long, since the time of death is legally the time at which you pronounce the patient dead.

7. Document your findings on the chart. A typical chart entry may read as follows: "Called to pronounce Mr. Doe dead. Patient unresponsive to verbal or tactile stimuli. No heart sounds heard, no pulse felt. Not breathing, no air entry heard. Pupils fixed and dilated. Patient pronounced dead at 2030 hours, December 7, 2003."

8. Notify the family physician, attending physician, or both if the nurses have not already done so. Decide together with the attending physician whether an autopsy would be useful and appropriate in this patient's case.

9. Notify relatives. Next of kin should be notified as soon as possible. Normally, it is the responsibility of the family physician to notify the relatives once he or she has been told of the patient's death. Occasionally, the family physician may have signed over his or her nighttime calls to a partner or to another physician who does not know the patient or family. In this situation, it is best to inform the physician on call, and if he or she is uncomfortable speaking to the family, a member of the house staff who knows the patient or the family well should notify the next of kin. The family will appreciate hearing the news from a familiar voice. If neither

the family physician on call nor the house staff knows the patient, spend a few minutes familiarizing yourself with the patient's medical history and mode of death. If you are appointed to deliver the news to the family, the following guidelines may be helpful.

- Identify yourself: "This is Dr. Jones calling from St. Paul's Hospital."
- Ask for the next of kin: "May I speak with Mrs. Doe, please?"
- Deliver the message: "Mrs. Doe, I am sorry to inform you that your husband died at 8:30 this evening."
- You may find that in many instances the news is not unexpected. It is, however, always comforting to know that a relative has died peacefully: "As you know, your husband was suffering from a terminal illness. Although I was not with your husband at the time of his death, the nurses looking after him assure me that he was very comfortable and that he passed away peacefully."
- If an autopsy is desired by one of the medical staff, this question should be broached now: "Your husband had an unusual illness, and if you are agreeable, it would be very useful to us to perform an autopsy. Although it obviously cannot change the course of events in your husband's illness, it may provide some valuable information for other patients suffering from similar problems." If there is any hesitation by the next of kin, emphasize that he or she is under no obligation to grant permission for an autopsy to be performed if it is against the perceived wishes of the patient or the family. If the next of kin refuses, do not argue, no matter how interested you may be in the outcome of the case. Accept the family's decision graciously: "We understand completely, and of course we will respect your wishes."
- Ask the next of kin if he or she would like to come to the hospital to see the patient one last time. Inform the nurses of this decision. Questions pertaining to funeral homes and the patient's personal belongings are best referred to the nurse in charge.

SPECIAL SITUATIONS

Medical technology has introduced two other scenarios in the pronouncement of a patient's death.

The Mechanically Ventilated Patient without Circulatory Function

There is a general understanding that those patients whose hearts have stopped beating despite being mechanically ventilated meet the criteria for legal death through a lack of spontaneous ventilation once the ventilator is turned off. Thus, it is reasonable practice to do the following:

1. Ensure that connections are intact and properly attached if the patient is on the electrocardiogram monitor. (This ensures that the absence of cardiac electrical activity is not due to faulty electrical connections.)
2. Follow the usual procedure for pronouncing death.
3. Discuss your findings with the attending physician *before* disconnecting the ventilator.
4. After agreement with the attending physician, disconnect the ventilator. Observe the patient for 3 minutes for evidence of spontaneous respiration.
5. Document your findings in the chart: "Called to pronounce Mr. Doe dead. Patient unresponsive to verbal or tactile stimuli. No heart sounds heard, no pulse felt. Pupils fixed and dilated. Patient being mechanically ventilated. Ventilator disconnected at 2030 hours after discussion with attending physician, Dr. Smith. No spontaneous respirations noted for 3 minutes. Patient pronounced dead at 2033 hours, December 7, 2003."

The Mechanically Ventilated Patient with Circulatory Function Intact

This type of patient is usually being cared for in the intensive care unit. A variety of controversial criteria exists for the determination of brain death,[5-8] and criteria may differ between geographic locations. The task of pronouncing a mechanically ventilated patient dead and the discussion of organ procurement are best left to the intensive care unit staff and associated subspecialists in consultation with the patient's family.

References

1. Report of the Ad Hoc Committee of the Harvard Medical School to Examine the Definition of Brain Death. JAMA 1968;205:337.
2. Capron, Kass: A statutory definition of the standards for determining human death. 121 U Pa L Rev 87 (1972).
3. Kan Stat Ann 77-202 (Supp 1974).
4. Report on the Criteria for the Determination of Death. Law Reform Commission of Canada, 1981.
5. Conference of Royal College and Faculties of the United Kingdom: Diagnosis of brain death. Lancet 1976;2:1069-1070.
6. Guidelines for the diagnosis of brain death. Can Med Assoc J 1987; 136:200A-200B.
7. Halevy A, Brody B: Brain death: Reconciling definitions, criteria, and tests. Ann Intern Med 1993;119:519-525.
8. Spoor MT, Sutherland FR: The evolution of the concept of brain death. Ann R Coll Physians Surg Can 1995;28:30-32.

Seizures

A seizure is one of the more dramatic events you may witness while on call. Usually, everyone around will be in a panic. The key to controlling the situation is to remain calm.

PHONE CALL

Questions

1. **Is the patient still seizing?**
2. **What type of seizure was witnessed?**
   Was the seizure generalized tonic-clonic, or was it focal?
3. **What is the patient's level of consciousness?**
4. **Has there been any obvious injury?**
5. **What was the reason for admission?**
6. **Does the patient have diabetes mellitus?**

Orders

1. Ask the RN to make sure that the patient is positioned on his or her side.
   During both the seizure and the postictal state, the patient should be kept in the lateral decubitus position to prevent aspiration of gastric contents.
2. Ask the RN to have the following available at the bedside:
   a. Oral airway
   b. Intravenous (IV) setup with normal saline (NS) (flushed through and ready for immediate use)
   c. Two blood tubes (one for chemistry and one for hematology)
   d. *Diazepam* 20 mg
   e. *Thiamine* 100 mg
   f. 50% dextrose in water (D50W) 50 mL (1 ampule)
   g. Chart
3. If the patient is postictal, ask the RN to remove any dentures, suction the oropharynx, and insert an oral airway.
4. Order a stat finger-prick blood glucose (FPBG) reading if the patient is in the postictal state (unconscious).

Inform RN

"I will arrive at the bedside in . . . minutes."

A seizure requires you to see the patient immediately.

ELEVATOR THOUGHTS

What causes seizures?

1. Drugs
   a. Drug withdrawal
      (1) Antiepileptic medication inadvertently discontinued or nontherapeutic level
      (2) Alcohol withdrawal. *Caution:* Does the patient have delirium tremens in addition to seizures?
      (3) Benzodiazepine or barbiturate withdrawal
   b. Drug toxicity (does not necessarily imply "overdose")
      (1) Meperidine overdose (an easily missed diagnosis in an elderly postoperative patient)
      (2) Penicillin at high doses
      (3) Theophylline toxicity
      (4) Lidocaine HCl infusion
      (5) Isoniazid
      (6) Lithium carbonate
      (7) Neuroleptics (e.g., chlorpromazine)
      (8) Cocaine, amphetamines
2. Central nervous system (CNS)
   a. Tumor
   b. Previous stroke
   c. Previous head injury
   d. Meningitis/encephalitis
   e. Idiopathic epilepsy
3. Endocrine: the four "hypos"
   a. Hypoglycemia
   b. Hyponatremia
   c. Hypocalcemia
   d. Hypomagnesemia
4. Miscellaneous
   a. Uremia
   b. CNS vasculitis
   c. Hypertensive encephalopathy
   d. Hypoxia/hypercapnia
   e. Pseudoseizure
5. In patients with acquired immunodeficiency syndrome (AIDS)
   a. Mass lesions (toxoplasmosis, CNS lymphoma)
   b. Human immunodeficiency virus (HIV) encephalopathy
   c. Meningitis (cryptococcal, herpes zoster, toxoplasmosis, aseptic)

d. Any of the usual causes of seizures seen in immunocompetent hosts

MAJOR THREAT TO LIFE

- Aspiration
- Hypoxia

The patient should be lying in the lateral decubitus position to prevent the tongue from falling posteriorly and blocking the airway and to minimize the risk of aspiration of gastric contents while in the postictal state. Patients usually keep breathing throughout seizure activity. Most patients can be in status epilepticus for 30 minutes with no subsequent neurologic damage.

IF THE SEIZURE HAS STOPPED

The majority of seizures will have stopped by the time you arrive at the bedside. The procedures and protocols to follow if the seizure has stopped are discussed here. The procedures and protocols to follow if the seizure persists begin on page 258.

BEDSIDE

Quick-Look Test

Does the patient look well (comfortable), sick (uncomfortable or distressed), or critical (about to die)?

Most patients after a generalized tonic-clonic seizure are unconscious (the postictal state).

Airway, Vital Signs, and Blood Glucose Results

In what position is the patient lying?

The patient should be positioned in the lateral decubitus position to prevent aspiration of gastric contents (Fig. 23–1).

Remove any dentures and suction the airway. Insert an oral airway if one is not already in place (Fig. 23–2). The patient is not out of danger yet. He or she might experience another seizure, so make sure the airway is protected.

Give oxygen by facemask or nasal prongs.

What is the FPBG result?

Hypoglycemia needs to be treated immediately to prevent further seizures.

Management I

Draw blood (20 mL) and establish IV access. Send the blood for the following tests.

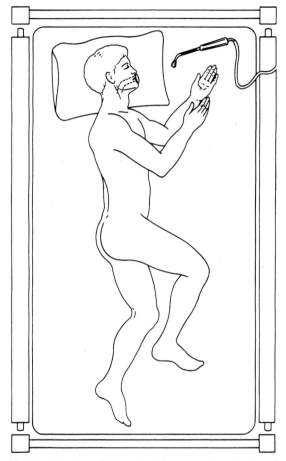

Figure 23–1 Positioning of the patient to prevent aspiration of gastric contents.

- *Chemistry tube:* electrolytes, urea, creatinine, random blood glucose, calcium, magnesium, albumin, and antiepileptic drug levels (if the patient is receiving these medications). If the patient is undergoing a 3-day fast for investigation of possible hypoglycemia, order an insulin level as well.
- *Hematology tube:* complete blood cell count (CBC) and manual differential.

Once the IV is established, keep the line open with NS. NS is the IV fluid of choice because phenytoin is not compatible with dextrose-containing solutions.

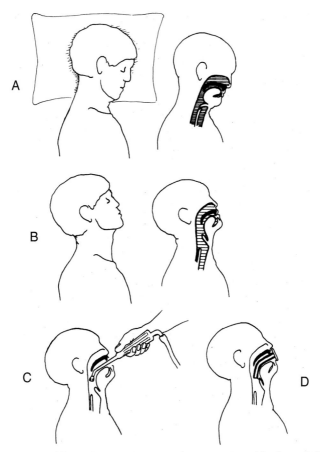

Figure 23–2 Airway management requires correct positioning of the head, correct suctioning, and correct insertion of an oral airway. *A,* Neck flexion closes the airway. *B,* Neck extension to the sniffing position opens the airway. *C,* Suctioning. *D,* Placement of the airway.

If the FPBG reading reveals hypoglycemia, give *thiamine* 100 mg IV by slow, direct injection over 3 to 5 minutes, followed by D50W 50 mL IV by slow, direct injection.

> Thiamine is given before the administration of glucose to prevent an exacerbation of Wernicke's encephalopathy.

Draw arterial blood gases (ABGs) if the patient appears cyanotic.

Selective Physical Examination I

Assess the patient's level of consciousness.

Does the patient respond to verbal or painful stimuli? Is the patient in a postictal state (i.e., decreased level of consciousness)?

Remember: If the patient does not regain consciousness between seizures, after 30 minutes the diagnosis becomes *status epilepticus.*

Selective History and Chart Review

1. Ask any witnesses the following details about the seizure:
   a. Duration?
   b. Generalized tonic-clonic or focal?
   c. Generalized or focal onset?
   > A focal onset of a generalized tonic-clonic seizure suggests structural brain disease, which may be old or new.
   d. Any injury observed during the seizure?
2. Is there a history of epilepsy, alcohol or sedative withdrawal, head injury (e.g., recent fall while in the hospital), stroke, CNS tumor (primary or secondary), or diabetes mellitus?
3. Is the patient receiving any of the following medications, which may induce seizures?
   a. Penicillin
   b. Meperidine
   c. Insulin
   d. Oral hypoglycemics
   e. Antidepressants, lithium carbonate
   f. Isoniazid
   g. Lidocaine
   h. Neuroleptics (e.g., chlorpromazine)
   i. Theophylline
4. Is the patient HIV positive or otherwise immunosuppressed?
   > Seizures are a common manifestation of CNS disease in HIV-positive patients.
5. What are the most recent laboratory results?
   a. Glucose
   b. Sodium
   c. Calcium
   d. Albumin
   e. Magnesium
   f. Antiepileptic drug levels
   g. Urea
   h. Creatinine

The chart is reviewed before the more detailed physical examination is performed because an immediate, treatable cause (e.g., insulin or meperidine overdose, hyponatremia) is more likely to be found in the chart.

Selective Physical Examination II

Vitals	Repeat now
HEENT	Tongue or cheek lacerations, nuchal rigidity

Resp	Signs of aspiration
Neuro	Complete CNS examination within the limits of level of consciousness
	Can the patient speak, follow commands?
	Is there any asymmetry of pupils, visual fields, reflexes, or plantar responses?
	Asymmetry suggests structural brain disease.
MSS	Palpate skull and face, spine, and ribs
	Passive ROM of all four limbs
	Are there any lacerations, hematomas, or fractures?

Management II

Establish the *provisional* and *differential diagnoses* of the seizure—this must be a causally defined diagnosis (e.g., "generalized tonic-clonic seizure secondary to hypoglycemia").

Are there any complications of the seizure giving rise to a second diagnosis?
> For example, if a head injury has been sustained, the provisional diagnosis might be forehead hematoma, and the differential diagnosis would include subdural hematoma and frontal bone fracture.

Treat the underlying cause. Seizure is a sign, not a diagnosis.

Maintain IV access for 24 hours with NS. If there is concern about volume overloading, use a heparin lock instead of keeping the IV line open with NS.

Patients with a Single Seizure. In most patients with a single seizure, it is not necessary to administer antiepileptic medications, particularly if a rapidly correctable metabolic cause is found. Exceptions include patients already on antiepileptic medications but with inadequate serum concentrations, patients with suspected structural CNS abnormalities, and HIV-positive patients (in whom seizures tend to be recurrent). If further seizures are anticipated, a long-acting antiepileptic drug (e.g., phenytoin rather than diazepam) is recommended (see page 260 for dosage). Although diazepam is useful as an anticonvulsant to halt seizures, it is not useful as a prophylactic. The antiepileptic medication of choice is phenytoin.

Elderly and Other Patients Suspected of Having Structural CNS Disease as a Cause of Their Seizures. These patients should have a computed tomography (CT) head scan performed.

HIV-Positive Patients. HIV-positive patients should have a CT head scan (because of the high incidence of CNS mass lesions) and, if there is no risk of herniation, a lumbar puncture. Occasionally, cryptococcal meningitis may coexist in an HIV-positive patient who has a mass lesion on CT head scan.

Seizure precautions should be instituted for the next 48 hours and then reviewed (Box 23–1).

IF THE PATIENT IS STILL SEIZING

Don't panic (almost everybody else will). Most seizures resolve without treatment within 2 minutes.

BEDSIDE

Quick-Look Test

Does the patient look well (comfortable), sick (uncomfortable or distressed), or critical (about to die)?

A patient having a generalized tonic-clonic seizure often engenders anxiety in observers. Remember, if the patient is seizing, you can be sure that he or she has both a blood pressure (BP) and a pulse.

Ask the RN to notify your resident of the situation—a seizure is a medical emergency.

Airway, Vital Signs, and Blood Glucose Result

In what position is the patient lying?

The patient should be positioned and maintained in the lateral decubitus position to prevent aspiration of gastric contents. One or two assistants may be required to hold the patient in this position if the seizure is violent.

Suction the airway. Do not insert an oral airway or attempt to remove dentures if force is required; you might break the patient's teeth.

Give oxygen by facemask or nasal prongs.

BOX 23–1 Seizure Precautions

1. Place the bed in the lowest position.
2. Provide an oral airway at the head of the bed.
3. Keep the side rails up when the patient is in bed. In the case of generalized tonic-clonic seizures, pad the side rails.
4. Provide the patient with a firm pillow.
5. Provide suction at the bedside.
6. Provide oxygen at the bedside.
7. Allow bathroom use only with supervision.
8. Allow baths or showers only with a nurse in attendance.
9. Take the axillary temperature only.
10. Provide direct supervision when the patient uses sharp objects such as a straight razor or nail scissors.

What is the patient's BP?

It is virtually impossible to take a BP during a generalized tonic-clonic seizure, so palpate the femoral pulse. (You may need an assistant to hold the patient's knee against the bed.) A palpable femoral pulse usually indicates a systolic BP >60 mm Hg.

What is the FPBG result?

Hypoglycemia, if present, needs to be treated immediately.

Management I

How long has the patient been seizing?

If the seizure has stopped, refer to page 253.

If the seizure has lasted <3 minutes:

- Do not give diazepam yet.
- Recheck the airway.
- Observe the seizure activity.
- Do *not* attempt to start an IV line yet; it will be much easier in 1 or 2 minutes, after the seizure has stopped.
- Ensure that IV tubing is flushed through with NS and that thiamine, D50W, diazepam, and two blood tubes are available at the bedside.

If the seizure has lasted >3 minutes:

- Draw blood (20 mL) and establish IV access.

Tips on Starting the IV Line. If the patient is seizing, it will be very difficult to establish an IV line. Because this is an emergency, it is not the appropriate time for a novice to practice starting an IV. Appoint the most experienced person present to obtain IV access. The patient's arm should be held firmly by one or two assistants (Fig. 23–3) while maintaining the patient on his or her side. It is much easier to start an IV line while sitting rather than standing. Try for the largest vein available, but avoid using the antecubital vein unless necessary, because the elbow will then have to be splinted to avoid losing IV access.

Medications. Order the following medications to be given immediately:

1. *Thiamine* 100 mg IV by slow, direct injection over 3 to 5 minutes.
2. *D50W* 50 mL IV by slow, direct injection. If the patient is hypoglycemic, he or she will abruptly become conscious while receiving the first 30 mL of D50W. Do not proceed with any further medication; change the IV fluid to D5W.

   Thiamine is given before the administration of glucose to protect against an exacerbation of Wernicke's encephalopathy.
3. *Diazepam* at a rate of 2 mg/min IV until the seizure stops or to a maximum dose of 20 mg. It will take 10 minutes to deliver 20 mg of diazepam at this rate. (An Ambu bag should be available at the bedside whenever IV diazepam is being given, because it may cause respiratory depression.) If diazepam is

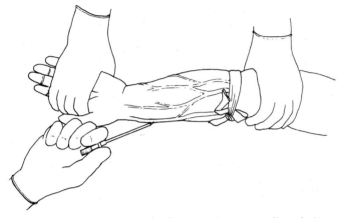

Figure 23–3 Position required when starting an IV line during a generalized tonic-clonic seizure.

not available, a good alternative is *lorazepam* 2 to 4 mg IV over 3 to 5 minutes.

4. Phenytoin. Ask an assistant to do the following:
   - Establish a second IV setup with NS (Fig. 23–4).

     Diazepam and phenytoin are not compatible, so they cannot be given via the same IV line.

   - Have *phenytoin*, loading dose 18 mg/kg (1250 mg for a 70-kg patient), available at the bedside. The phenytoin loading dose can be injected directly via the NS IV line at a rate no faster than 25 to 50 mg/min or given as an infusion (add the loading dose to 100 mL of NS) at a rate no greater than 25 to 50 mg/min. After phenytoin administration, the IV line should be flushed through with NS to avoid local venous irritation due to the drug's alkalinity.

     Phenytoin may cause hypotension and cardiac dysrhythmias. Monitor the femoral pulse for a decrease in volume

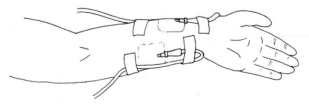

Figure 23–4 Two IV lines are needed if both diazepam and phenytoin are to be administered.

(hypotension) and for rhythm irregularities (Fig. 23–5). If either of these problems occurs, slow the phenytoin infusion rate.

If seizing continues despite administering half the maximum dose of diazepam (10 mg), begin administering the loading dose of phenytoin (no faster than 25 to 50 mg/min), but continue the diazepam until the maximum dose has been given.

If the patient has *already received phenytoin* or has an inadequate level, give *half* the phenytoin loading dose IV.

The most frequent side effects of an extra loading dose are dizziness, nausea, and blurred vision for a few days. These are not major risks.

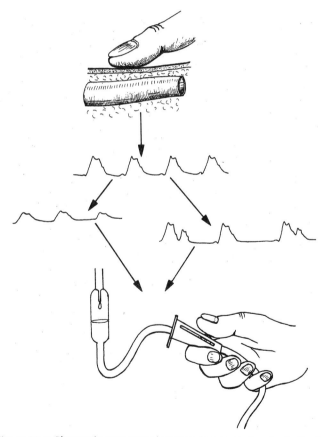

Figure 23–5 Phenytoin may cause hypotension or cardiac dysrhythmias, detectable by palpating the femoral pulse. If either one is present, the phenytoin infusion rate should be slowed.

If the seizure stops, stop giving diazepam but give the full loading dose of phenytoin. It is now practical to arrange for continuous electrocardiographic monitoring and repeated measurements of BP, which are important while the remainder of the phenytoin is being infused. See page 253 for further instructions. Most seizures can be controlled with diazepam and phenytoin. If not, CNS infection or structural brain disease should be considered.

If the seizure has persisted for 30 minutes, the patient is now in *status epilepticus*. This is an emergency. A neurologist, intensivist, or anesthesiologist should be consulted immediately. The patient should be transferred to the intensive care unit/cardiac care unit (ICU/CCU) for management of the airway and probable intubation.

Status epilepticus is rare. It is defined as a single seizure lasting 30 minutes or repetitive seizures without intervening periods of normal consciousness lasting more than 30 minutes.

Additional treatment in the ICU/CCU may include an IV phenobarbital infusion or, rarely, general anesthesia with halothane and neuromuscular blockade.

Shortness of Breath

Calls at night to assess a patient's breathing are common. Do not become overwhelmed by the myriad causes of shortness of breath (SOB) that you learned in medical school. In hospitalized patients, there are only four common causes of SOB: congestive heart failure (CHF), pulmonary embolism, pneumonia, and bronchospasm.

PHONE CALL

Questions

1. **How long has the patient had SOB?**
   The sudden onset of SOB suggests pulmonary embolus or pneumothorax.
2. **Is the patient cyanotic?**
   Clinical cyanosis indicates significant hypoxia and requires you to see the patient immediately.
3. **What are the vital signs?**
4. **What was the reason for admission?**
5. **Does the patient have chronic obstructive pulmonary disease (COPD)?**
   What you need to know is whether the patient is a CO_2 retainer. In most cases, this applies to patients with COPD or with a history of heavy smoking.
6. **Does the patient have O_2 ordered?**

Orders

1. *Oxygen.* If you are certain that the patient is not a CO_2 retainer, you can safely order any concentration of O_2 in the short-term situation. If you are not certain, order O_2 28% by Venturi mask and reassess on arrival at the bedside.
2. If the admitting diagnosis is asthma and the patient has not received an inhaled bronchodilator within the last 2 hours, order nebulized *salbutamol* 2.5 to 5 mg in 3 mL of normal saline (NS) or 180 µg (2 puffs) by metered dose inhaler, immediately.
3. *Arterial blood gas* (ABG) set at the bedside.

Not all patients with SOB require ABG determination, but it is best to have the equipment ready if needed. Alternatively, ask for an urgent measurement of pulse oximetry, if available.

Inform RN

"I will arrive at the bedside in . . . minutes."

SOB requires you to see the patient immediately.

ELEVATOR THOUGHTS

What causes shortness of breath?

1. Cardiovascular causes
   a. CHF
   b. Pulmonary embolism
2. Pulmonary causes
   a. Pneumonia
   b. Bronchospasm (asthma, COPD)
3. Miscellaneous causes
   a. Upper airway obstruction
   b. Anxiety
   c. Pneumothorax
   d. Massive pleural effusions
   e. Massive ascites
   f. Postoperative atelectasis
   g. Cardiac tamponade
   h. Aspiration of gastric contents

MAJOR THREAT TO LIFE

- Hypoxia

Inadequate tissue oxygenation is the most worrisome end result of any process causing SOB. Hence, you must direct your initial assessment toward determining whether *hypoxia* is present.

BEDSIDE

Quick-Look Test

Does the patient look well (comfortable), sick (uncomfortable or distressed), or critical (about to die)?

This simple observation helps determine the necessity of immediate intervention. If the patient looks sick, order ABGs, O$_2$, and an intravenous (IV) line of D5W to keep the vein open (TKVO). Ask the RN to bring the cardiac arrest cart to the bedside, attach the patient to the electrocardiogram (ECG) monitor, and prepare for possible intubation. Consult the intensive care unit immediately.

Airway and Vital Signs

Is the patient adequately ventilating?

To adequately ventilate, a patient must do two things—make adequate breathing efforts and have an open airway.

Is the patient making adequate breathing efforts?

If the patient is no longer breathing or is making inadequate breathing efforts, you must perform a head tilt–chin lift or a jaw thrust to open the airway and begin ventilation with a bag-mask device.

Is the airway open?

If the patient is making adequate breathing efforts (looks tachypneic, is agitated, and is struggling to breathe) but is not ventilating, suspect an upper airway obstruction. In an unconscious patient, upper airway obstruction is usually due to prolapse of the tongue into the posterior pharynx, a situation that can be corrected with the head tilt–chin lift or jaw thrust maneuver. Other causes of upper airway obstruction include a food bolus in the posterior pharynx, tracheal collapse due to loss of tone in the supporting muscles, and laryngospasm due to aspiration of oral secretions. These situations may require a "finger sweep" to clear the airway of foreign material, positive pressure ventilation with a bag-mask device, or endotracheal intubation.

What is the respiratory rate (RR)?

Rates <12/min suggest a central depression of ventilation, which is usually due to a stroke, narcotic overdose, or some other drug overdose. Rates >20/min suggest hypoxia, pain, or anxiety. Look also for thoracoabdominal dissociation, which may indicate impending respiratory failure. Remember that the chest cage and abdominal wall normally move in the same direction.

What is the heart rate?

Sinus tachycardia is an expected accompaniment of hypoxia. This is because vascular beds supplying hypoxic tissue dilate, and a compensatory sinus tachycardia occurs in an effort to increase cardiac output and thereby improve oxygen delivery.

What is the temperature?

An elevated temperature suggests infection (pneumonia, pyothorax, or bronchitis) but is also consistent with pulmonary embolism.

What is the blood pressure (BP)?

Hypotension may indicate CHF, septic shock, massive pulmonary embolism, or tension pneumothorax (see Chapter 18). If you suspect any of these conditions, call your resident for help. Also, measure the amount of pulsus paradoxus, which, in asthmatics, roughly correlates with the degree of airflow obstruction.

Pulsus paradoxus also may be a clue to the presence of cardiac tamponade.

Pulsus paradoxus is an inspiratory fall in systolic BP >10 mm Hg. To determine whether a pulsus paradoxus is present, inflate the BP cuff 20 to 30 mm Hg above the palpable systolic BP. Deflate the cuff slowly. Initially, Korotkoff's sounds will be heard only in expiration. At some point during cuff deflation, Korotkoff's sounds will appear in inspiration as well. The number of millimeters of mercury between the initial appearance of Korotkoff's sounds and their appearance throughout the respiratory cycle represents the degree of pulsus paradoxus (Fig. 24–1).

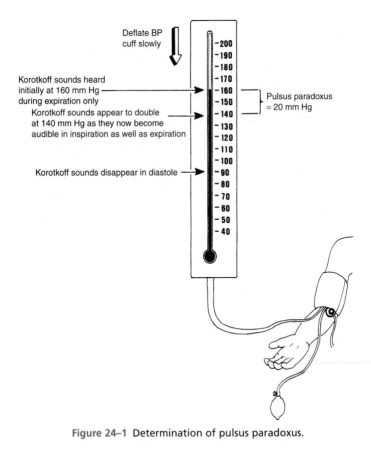

Figure 24–1 Determination of pulsus paradoxus.

Selective Physical Examination

Is the patient hypoxic?

Vitals   Repeat now; again, ensure airway patency

HEENT   Check for central cyanosis (blue tongue and mucous membranes)

> Cyanosis often does not occur until there is severe hemoglobin desaturation and may not occur at all in an anemic patient. If hypoxia is suspected, confirm by ABG measurement. *Remember:* Cyanosis is helpful only if it is present—its absence does not mean that the Po_2 is adequate.

Check that the trachea is midline

Resp   Are breath sounds present and of normal intensity?

Check for crackles, wheezing, consolidation, or pleural effusion

Neuro   Check level of sensorium: is the patient alert, confused, drowsy, or unresponsive?

Management

What immediate measure needs to be taken to correct hypoxia?

Supply adequate O_2.

> The initial concentration of O_2 ordered depends on your judgment of how sick the patient is. An accurate assessment can be made by drawing ABG samples, beginning empirical O_2 treatment, and adjusting Fio_2, depending on the results of subsequent ABGs or pulse oximetry. If pulse oximetry is available, gradually increase the Fio_2 until the O_2 saturation is >94%; then recheck the ABGs. Remember that pulse oximetry tells you nothing about Pco_2, pH, or $(A–a)O_2$ gradient. In most cases, a Po_2 >60 mm Hg or an O_2 saturation of 94% is adequate.

What harm can your treatment cause?

Some patients with COPD are CO_2 retainers and are dependent on mild hypoxia to stimulate the respiratory center. An Fio_2 >0.28 may remove this hypoxic drive to breathe. Unless there is or has been hypercarbia (check the patient's old chart), it is difficult to predict which patients with COPD are CO_2 retainers. It is therefore prudent to assume that all patients with COPD and heavy smoking histories are CO_2 retainers until proved otherwise.

> Administration of 100% O_2 can cause atelectasis or O_2 toxicity if given over a period of days. This is of greater concern in a mechanically ventilated patient, because these Fio_2 levels are impossible to attain unless the patient is intubated.

Why is the patient short of breath or hypoxic?

There are four common causes of SOB in hospitalized patients:

- Cardiovascular causes
    1. CHF
    2. Pulmonary embolism
- Pulmonary causes
    3. Pneumonia
    4. Bronchospasm (asthma, COPD)

In most cases, it is easy to distinguish among these four conditions. Look for specific associated signs and symptoms (Table 24–1) to help you identify which one your patient most likely has, and then treat him or her accordingly. Once you have established which pattern of SOB your patient has, obtain a more thorough selective history and physical examination.

CARDIOVASCULAR CAUSES

Congestive Heart Failure

Selective History

Is there a history of CHF or cardiac disorder?

Is there orthopnea?

Is there paroxysmal nocturnal dyspnea?

Are there trends in daily weight or fluid balance records that heighten your suspicion of fluid retention and hence CHF?

Selective Physical Examination

Assess the volume status.

Is the patient volume overloaded?

Vitals	Tachycardia, tachypnea
HEENT	Elevated JVP
Resp	Inspiratory crackles ± pleural effusions (more often on the right side)
CVS	Cardiac apex displaced laterally
	S_3
	Systolic murmurs (aortic stenosis, mitral regurgitation, VSD, tricuspid regurgitation)
ABD	Hepatomegaly with positive HJR
Ext	Presacral or ankle edema

Crackles and S_3 are the most reliable indication of left-sided heart failure, whereas elevated jugular venous pressure (JVP), enlarged liver, positive hepatojugular reflex (HJR), and peripheral edema

TABLE 24-1 **Discriminating Features in the History and Physical Examination of a Patient with Shortness of Breath**

	CHF	Pulmonary Embolism and Infarction	Pneumonia	Asthma/COPD
History				
Onset	Gradual	Sudden	Gradual	Gradual
Other	Orthopnea	Risk factors (see p 273)	Cough	Previous history
			Fever	
			Sputum production	
Physical Examination				
Temperature	Normal	Normal or slightly elevated	High	Normal
Pulsus paradoxus	No	No	No	Yes
JVP	Elevated	Elevated or normal	Normal	Normal
S_3	Present	Occasional RV S_3 present	Absent	Absent
Respiratory				
Crackles	Bibasal	Unilateral	Unilateral	No
Wheezes	±	±	±	Present
Friction rub	No	Pleural effusions	Consolidation	No
Other			Bronchial breath sounds	
			Whispering pectoriloquy	

CHF, congestive heart failure; COPD, chronic obstructive pulmonary disease; JVP, jugular venous pressure; RV, right ventricular; S_3, third heart sound.

indicate right-sided heart failure. Although right-sided heart failure does not necessarily cause SOB on its own, it is a common accompaniment of left-sided heart failure and pulmonary disorders (cor pulmonale).

Other Investigations

Chest X-ray (Fig. 24–2)

Chest x-ray can reveal the following conditions:
- Cardiomegaly
- Perihilar congestion
- Bilateral interstitial (early) or alveolar (more advanced) infiltrates
- Redistribution of pulmonary vascular markings
- Kerley's B lines
- Pleural effusions

Treatment

General Measures

- IV D5W TKVO
  | IV access is required to deliver medications. Switch to heparin lock when the acute episode has resolved.
- O$_2$
- Restricted-sodium diet
- Bed rest
- *Heparin* (5000 U SC every 8 hours)

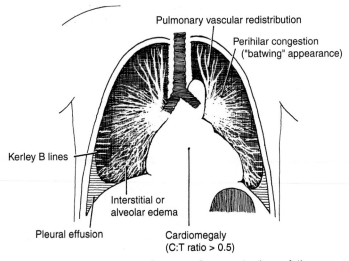

Figure 24–2 Chest x-ray features of congestive heart failure.

| Patients with CHF are predisposed to venous thrombosis and pulmonary emboli and should receive prophylactic SC heparin while on bed rest.

- Fluid balance charting
- Daily weight

Specific Measures

Cardiac function can be improved by altering preload, afterload, or contractility. In the acute situation, intervention initially involves decreasing the preload.

TEMPORARY MEASURES

The following three temporary measures shift the excessive intra-vascular volume from the central veins. Only diuretics actually reduce extracellular volume.

- Sit the patient up.
  | This position pools blood in the legs.
- Give *morphine sulfate* 2 to 4 mg IV every 5 to 10 minutes, up to 10 to 12 mg.
  | This pools blood in the splanchnic circulation. Morphine sulfate may cause hypotension or respiratory depression. Take the BP and RR before and after each dose is given. If necessary, *naloxone hydrochloride* 0.2 to 2 mg IV, IM, or SC can be used to reverse the hypotension or respiratory depression of morphine, up to a total of 10 mg. Nausea or vomiting may occur and usually can be controlled with *dimenhydrinate* 25 mg IV or IM or 50 mg PO every 4 hours PRN.
- Give *nitroglycerin ointment* 2.5 to 5 cm (1 to 2 inches) topically every 6 hours. If nitroglycerin ointment is not readily available, you can give *nitroglycerin* tablets 0.3 to 0.6 mg SL or *nitroglycerin* spray 1 puff SL every 5 minutes until the patient feels less short of breath, as long as the systolic BP remains >90 mm Hg. All nitroglycerin preparations pool blood in the peripheral circulation. Nitroglycerin preparations commonly cause headaches, which can be treated with *acetaminophen* 325 to 650 mg PO every 4 hours PRN.

DIURESIS

- Give *furosemide* 40 mg IV over 2 to 5 minutes. If there is no response (e.g., lessening of the symptoms and signs of CHF, diuresis), double the dose every 1 hour (i.e., 40, 80, and then 160 mg) to a total dose of about 400 mg. Larger initial doses (e.g., 80 to 120 mg) may be required if the patient has renal insufficiency, is in severe CHF, or is already on maintenance furosemide. Doses of furosemide >100 mg should be infused at a rate not exceeding 4 mg/min to avoid ototoxicity. Smaller initial doses (e.g., 10 mg) may suffice for frail, elderly (80- to 90-year-old) patients.

- The addition of a diuretic with a different site of action (e.g., a thiazide) may result in diuresis in patients who are resistant to furosemide alone.

  > The diuretics mentioned may cause hypokalemia, which is of particular concern in a patient receiving digitalis. Monitor the serum potassium level once or twice daily in the acute situation. High doses of these diuretics also may lead to serious sensorineural hearing loss, especially if the patient is also receiving other ototoxic agents, such as aminoglycoside antibiotics.

If diuretics are ineffective, it is unlikely that the patient is going to produce urine. Other methods of removing intravascular volume, such as *phlebotomy* (200 to 300 mL) and *rotating tourniquets*, are seldom required in the hospital setting. If there is a persistent component of bronchospasm (cardiac asthma), an inhaled beta agonist may improve oxygenation.

Digoxin is not of benefit acutely unless the CHF was precipitated by a bout of supraventricular tachycardia (e.g., atrial fibrillation or flutter with rapid ventricular response rates), which can be slowed by digoxin. (Refer to Chapter 15 for the management of tachydysrhythmias.)

Determining the Cause

CHF is a symptom, and a very serious one. After you have treated the symptom, sit down and determine *why* the patient developed CHF. This requires you to identify the *etiologic factor,* of which there are six possibilities:

1. Coronary artery disease
2. Hypertension
3. Valvular heart disease
4. Cardiomyopathy (dilated, restrictive, hypertrophic)
5. Pericardial disease
6. Congenital heart disease

If the patient has a history of CHF, the etiologic factor may already be identified in the patient's chart. However, the job does not end there, for you must also identify a *precipitating factor,* of which the following 10 are most common:

1. Myocardial infarction (MI) or ischemia
2. Fever, infection
3. Dysrhythmia
4. Pulmonary embolism
5. Increased sodium load (dietary, medicinal, parenteral)
6. Cardiac depressant drugs (e.g., beta blockers, disopyramide, calcium entry blockers)
7. Sodium-retaining agents (e.g., nonsteroidal anti-inflammatory drugs [NSAIDs])
8. Noncompliance with diet or medication
9. Renal disease
10. Anemia

Remember that any new etiologic factor may also act as a precipitating factor in a patient with a history of CHF. Document the suspected etiologic and precipitating factors in the chart.

Pulmonary Embolism

The classic triad of SOB, hemoptysis, and chest pain actually occurs in only a minority of cases. The best way to avoid missing this diagnosis is to consider it in every patient with SOB.

Selective History

Look for predisposing causes.

Stasis

- Prolonged bed rest
- Immobilized limb
- Obesity
- CHF
- Pregnancy

Vein Injury

- Trauma (especially hip fractures)
- Surgery (especially abdominal, pelvic, and orthopedic procedures)

Hypercoagulability

- Malignancy
- Inflammatory bowel disease
- Nephrotic syndrome
- Use of birth control pills
- Deficiencies of antithrombin III, protein C or S; antiphospholipid antibodies; factor V Leiden mutation

Selective Physical Examination

Features suggestive of pulmonary embolism include the following:
- Pleural friction rub
- Pulmonary consolidation
- Unilateral or bilateral pleural effusion
- Sudden-onset cor pulmonale
- New-onset tachydysrhythmia
- Simultaneous deep venous thrombosis (DVT)

Other Investigations

Chest X-ray (Fig. 24–3)

If clinically stable, the patient should have an upright posteroanterior and lateral chest x-ray (CXR) rather than a portable CXR to ensure optimal imaging and prevent the masking of pleural fluid,

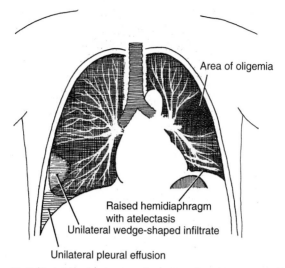

Area of oligemia

Raised hemidiaphragm
with atelectasis
Unilateral wedge-shaped infiltrate

Unilateral pleural effusion

Figure 24–3 Variable chest x-ray features of pulmonary embolism. Positive findings on radiography depend on the presence of pulmonary infarction. An entirely normal chest x-ray in the setting of severe shortness of breath, however, is very suggestive of a pulmonary embolism.

which can occur when images are taken with the patient in the supine position. CXR may reveal the following:

- Atelectasis (loss of volume)
- Unilateral wedge-shaped pulmonary infiltrate
- Unilateral pleural effusion
- Raised hemidiaphragm
- Areas of oligemia
- Normal findings

Electrocardiogram

Only a massive pulmonary embolism causes the classic right ventricular strain pattern of S_1, Q_3, right-axis deviation, and right bundle branch block. The most common ECG finding is a *sinus tachycardia*, but other supraventricular tachycardias also may occur.

Arterial Blood Gases

The most common finding on ABG determination is acute respiratory alkalosis. Of patients with pulmonary embolism, 85% have P_{O_2} <80 mm Hg on room air. If the P_{O_2} is >80 mm Hg and pulmonary embolism is still suspected, look for an elevated $P(A–a)_{O_2}$. (See Appendix E, page 425, for the calculation.)

Management

Thrombolytic Therapy. If your suspicion of pulmonary embolism is high and the patient is hypotensive, *thrombolytic therapy* should be considered.[1] In this case, call your resident now. The aim of thrombolytic therapy is to dissolve the pulmonary embolism; either *streptokinase* 250,000 IU given IV over 30 minutes followed by 100,000 IU/hr for 24 hours or *tissue plasminogen activator* (tPA) 100 mg IV over 2 hours may be given, but streptokinase is less expensive. Pulmonary arteriotomy with embolectomy may also be lifesaving in centers where this procedure is immediately available.[2]

Anticoagulation Therapy. If your suspicion of pulmonary embolism is high and the patient is hemodynamically stable, you are obligated to begin *anticoagulation therapy* without further confirmation of the diagnosis. The aim of anticoagulation is not to dissolve the pulmonary embolism but rather to prevent further embolization from the site of venous thrombosis, which may prove fatal.

> However, before ordering a thrombolytic agent or an anticoagulant, ensure that the patient has no history of bleeding disorders; peptic ulcers; intracranial disease, such as recent stroke, subarachnoid hemorrhage, or tumor; or recent surgery. All are contraindications to anticoagulation. These patients require confirmation of pulmonary embolism with ventilation-perfusion ($\dot{V}/\dot{Q}$) scan or pulmonary angiography; if an embolism is documented, consultation must be obtained for consideration of interruption of the inferior vena cava by inserting a transvenous intracaval device.

Draw a blood sample for complete blood count (CBC), activated partial thromboplastin time (aPTT), prothrombin time (PT), and platelet count immediately. If there are *no contraindications*, begin *heparin* 100 U/kg IV bolus (usual dose, 5000 to 10,000 U IV), followed by a maintenance infusion of 1000 to 1600 U/hr, with the lower range selected for patients with a higher risk of bleeding.

> Heparin should be delivered by infusion pump, with maintenance dosing ordered as in the following example: heparin 25,000 U/500 mL D5W to run at 20 mL/hr = 1000 U/hr. It is dangerous to put large doses of heparin in small-volume IV bags, because runaway IV bags filled with heparin can result in serious overdose.
>
> Heparin and warfarin are dangerous drugs because of their potential for causing bleeding disorders. Write and double-check your heparin orders carefully. Also, measure platelet counts once or twice a week to detect reversible heparin-induced thrombocytopenia, which may occur at any time while a patient is on heparin.

Low-molecular-weight heparin (LMWH) is a safe and effective alternative to IV unfractionated heparin in the treatment of selected patients with pulmonary embolism.[3] Several formulations of LMWH exist, with different distributions of molecular weight resulting in differences in inhibitory activities against factor Xa and thrombin, the extent of plasma protein binding, and plasma half-lives. Familiarize yourself with the LMWH formulation used in your hospital. Also, be careful to note that the dose of LMWH used in the *treatment* of pulmonary embolism is considerably higher than that used for *prophylaxis* of DVT. One formulation used for the *treatment* of pulmonary embolism is *tinzaparin* 175 U/kg SC daily.

After starting heparin, obtain a $\dot{V}/\dot{Q}$ scan as soon as possible to confirm the diagnosis of pulmonary embolism.

- A *high-probability* $\dot{V}/\dot{Q}$ scan indicates an approximately 90% probability of pulmonary embolism[4] and is sufficient evidence to continue anticoagulation.
- A *normal* $\dot{V}/\dot{Q}$ scan rules out clinically important pulmonary embolism.
- A *low-* or *intermediate-probability* $\dot{V}/\dot{Q}$ scan in the presence of high clinical suspicion should be confirmed by pulmonary angiography before committing the patient to long-term anticoagulation. Alternatively, the demonstration of simultaneous DVT by nuclear or contrast venography, impedance plethysmography, or duplex ultrasonography is sufficient evidence to continue anticoagulation.

In patients receiving IV unfractionated heparin, monitor the aPTT every 4 to 6 hours and adjust the heparin maintenance dose until the aPTT is in the therapeutic range (1.5 to 2.5 times normal). After this, daily aPTT measurements are sufficient. Initial measurements of aPTT are made only to ensure adequate anticoagulation. Because of the more predictable anticoagulant response of LMWH, patients receiving this medication do not require monitoring of the aPTT.

Continue IV heparin for 5 days. Add oral *warfarin* on the first day, beginning at 10 mg PO and titrating the dose to achieve a PT with an international normalized ratio (INR) of 2.0 to 3.0. (This corresponds to a PT of 1.3 to 1.5 times control, using rabbit brain thromboplastin. If you are unsure of the method used by your laboratory, call and ask.) Measure aPTT and PT daily during this initial adjustment phase. The attainment of a therapeutic PT usually takes 5 days, at which time the heparin can be discontinued.

> Numerous drugs interfere with warfarin metabolism to increase or decrease the PT. Before prescribing any drug to a patient on warfarin, look up its effect on warfarin metabolism and monitor PT carefully if an interaction is anticipated.
>
> Except in unusual circumstances, a patient receiving heparin should receive no aspirin-containing drugs, sulfinpyrazone, dipyridamole, or thrombolytic agents and no IM injections.

Ask your patient daily about signs of bleeding or bruising. Instruct your patient that prolonged pressure will be required after venipuncture to prevent local bruising while on anticoagulation.

PULMONARY CAUSES

Pneumonia

Selective History and Physical Examination

- Cough: a cough productive of purulent sputum is typical; however, the cough may be dry in the early stages of pneumonia
- Fever, chills
- Pleuritic chest pain
- Is the patient immunocompromised?
- Pulmonary consolidation ± pleural effusion

Other Investigations

Complete Blood Count

A white blood cell count >15,000/mm^3 suggests a bacterial infection. Lower counts, however, do not exclude a bacterial cause of pneumonia. Lymphopenia (absolute lymphocyte count <1000/mm^3) or a low CD4 cell count (<200/mm^3) suggests that you are dealing with pneumonia in a human immunodeficiency virus (HIV)–infected patient.[5]

Chest X-ray

Findings are variable, from patchy diffuse infiltrates to consolidation (pleural effusion). Remember that a volume-depleted patient may not manifest the typical CXR findings of pneumonia until the intravascular volume is restored to normal. Trust your clinical examination.

Identification of the Organism

- Sputum Gram stain and culture. If the patient is unable to spontaneously cough up sputum, you can induce it with ultrasonic nebulization or chest physical therapy. Take a sputum sample to the laboratory yourself and examine the Gram stain. (See Appendix E, page 426, for interpretation of the Gram stain.) Sputum should also be sent for staining and culture for acid-fast bacilli and *Legionella* culture or direct fluorescent antibody test.
- Blood culture (×2)
- Blood for measurement of *Mycoplasma* IgM
- Thoracentesis. Moderate to large pleural effusions should be tapped to exclude empyema. Pleural biopsy is necessary if tuberculosis (TB) is a consideration. Send pleural fluid to the laboratory for the following:
  Gram stain and aerobic and anaerobic cultures
  Ziehl-Neelsen (ZN) stain and TB cultures
  Cell count and differential

Lactate dehydrogenase (LDH)
Protein
Glucose
- If appropriate, send for the following:
  Fungal cultures
  pH
  Cytology
  Amylase
  Triglycerides

A simultaneous serum glucose, protein, and LDH should be drawn immediately after the pleural tap has been completed. These serum determinations are necessary to compare with pleural fluid values in assessing whether the fluid is a transudate or exudate.

Always consider TB in your differential diagnosis. Order ZN stains and sputum for culture if TB is suspected.

Pneumocystis carinii is the most common cause of pneumonia in patients who are positive for HIV. This organism occasionally may be demonstrated by immunofluorescent staining of a sputum sample obtained by inducing sputum production, although bronchoalveolar lavage is the best method of confirming the diagnosis.

Management

General Measures

- O_2
- Chest physical therapy

Specific Measures

- Antimicrobial agents
  Your choice depends on the results of Gram stain or other available stains. However, in the absence of a definitive smear, the choice of antimicrobial agent should be based on the rapidity of progression, the severity of pneumonia, the presence of comorbid conditions, and knowledge of local etiologic organisms and resistance patterns.

Community-Acquired Pneumonia. For community-acquired pneumonia in immunocompetent individuals that is severe enough to require hospitalization, the probable organisms include the following:
- *Streptococcus pneumoniae*
- "Atypical" agents (*Mycoplasma pneumoniae, Chlamydia pneumoniae, Legionella sp.*)
- *Haemophilus influenzae*

A useful antibiotic choice in this situation is *erythromycin* 500 mg PO or IV every 6 hours.

> IV erythromycin is painful, but the pain can be reduced by diluting each 500-mg dose in 500 mL of fluid and giving slowly over 6 hours.

Complex Pneumonias. For complex pneumonias (pneumonia complicating COPD, pneumonia acquired in hospitals or nursing homes, pneumonia in patients with previous antibiotic exposure), the following *additional* organisms are possible:

- Oral anaerobes
- Gram-negative bacilli
- *Staphylococcus aureus*

A useful antibiotic choice in these situations is one of the following:

- *Ceftriaxone* 1 to 2 g IV daily plus erythromycin 500 mg PO or IV every 6 hours
- *Levofloxacin* 250 to 500 mg PO or IV daily
- *Meropenem* 500 to 1000 mg PO or IV every 8 hours

If multiple resistant gram-negative organisms or *Pseudomonas aeruginosa* is a consideration, a combination of two of the following may be helpful:

- *Ceftazidime* 1 to 2 g IV every 8 hours
- *Piperacillin* 6 to 18 g/day in four to six divided doses
- *Imipenem/cilastatin* 500 mg every 6 to 8 hours
- *Meropenem* 500 to 1000 mg PO or IV every 8 hours
- *Gentamicin* 5 to 7 mg/kg IV daily, followed by maintenance doses determined by the creatinine clearance

If methicillin-resistant *S. aureus* is a risk, *vancomycin* or *rifampin* may be necessary.

Aspiration Pneumonia. Aspiration pneumonia should be considered in any situation in which there is a decreased level of consciousness or interference with the cough reflex (e.g., alcoholism, stroke, seizure, postsurgery). Episodes of aspiration do not require antibiotic treatment unless there are clinical signs of bacterial infection (e.g., fever, sputum production, leukocytosis).

Pneumonia in Alcoholic Patients. Alcoholics, as well as patients with aspiration pneumonia, have a high frequency of *Klebsiella pneumoniae*. This should be treated with two drugs—usually a cephalosporin and an aminoglycoside, such as *cefazolin* 1 to 2 g IV every 8 hours and *gentamicin* 5 to 7 mg/kg IV daily if renal function is normal.

> Aminoglycosides can cause nephrotoxicity and ototoxicity. Avoid these side effects by following serum aminoglycoside levels, usually after the third or fourth maintenance dose, and serum creatinine levels. If the patient already has renal insufficiency, *give the same initial dose*, but adjust the maintenance dose or interval according to the creatinine clearance (see Appendix E, page 425).

Pneumonia in HIV-Positive Patients. The most common infecting pulmonary pathogen in HIV-positive patients is *P. carinii*. Urgent diagnostic bronchoscopy is advisable when this organism is suspected, although induced sputum samples sometimes demonstrate the organism. If the patient looks sick and bronchoscopy is not immediately available, the attending physician may want to give one dose of trimethoprim-sulfamethoxazole or pentamidine isethionate and arrange for bronchoscopy as soon as possible. Steroids also may be helpful in patients who are ill with *P. carinii* pneumonia.[6]

Pentamidine has numerous side effects, including hypotension, tachycardia, nausea, vomiting, unpleasant taste, and flushing. Some of these side effects can be minimized by administering the dose in 500 mL D5W over 2 to 4 hours. In addition, biochemical abnormalities may include hyperkalemia, hypocalcemia, megaloblastic anemia, leukopenia, thrombocytopenia, hyperglycemia or hypoglycemia, elevated liver enzyme levels, and dose-related reversible nephrotoxicity.

Patients with HIV infection are also predisposed to bacterial infections, particularly by encapsulated organisms such as *S. pneumoniae* and *H. influenzae*.[7] Pulmonary infection with *Mycobacterium avium* and fungi (cryptococci, *Histoplasma*, *Coccidioides*) is frequently part of disseminated disease involving these organisms. *Mycobacterium tuberculosis* may occur as localized or disseminated disease.

Bronchospasm (Asthma and COPD)

Asthma is a condition characterized by airflow obstruction that varies significantly over time.

COPD may take the form of *chronic bronchitis*, which is a clinical diagnosis (production of mucoid sputum on most days for 3 months of the year in 2 consecutive years), or *emphysema*, which is a pathologic diagnosis (enlargement of airways distal to the terminal bronchioles). Most patients with COPD have features of both.

Selective History

Does the patient smoke cigarettes?

Is the patient on theophylline or steroids?

Has the patient ever required intubation?

Can precipitating factors (e.g., specific allergies, nonspecific irritants, upper respiratory tract infection], pneumonia, beta blocker administration) be identified?

Is the patient having an anaphylactic reaction?

Look for evidence of systemic autocoid (e.g., histamine) release (i.e., wheezing), itch (urticaria), and hypotension. Anaphylactic reactions in hospitalized patients are most commonly seen after the administration of IV dye, penicillin, or aspirin. If there is suspicion of anaphylaxis, refer immediately to Chapter 18, pages 180 to 181, for appropriate management. This is an emergency!

Selective Physical Examination

Is there evidence of obstructive airway disease?

Vitals   Pulsus paradoxus
HEENT   Cyanosis
             Elevated JVP (cor pulmonale):
             > Cor pulmonale is defined as right-sided heart failure secondary to pulmonary disease.

             Position of trachea
             > Pneumothorax may be a complication of asthma or COPD and results in a shift of the trachea away from the affected side.

Resp   Intercostal indrawing
             Use of accessory muscles of respiration
             Increased anteroposterior (AP) diameter
             Hyperinflated lungs with depressed hemidiaphragms
             Wheezing
             > Diffuse wheezing is most often a manifestation of asthma or COPD but may also be seen in CHF (cardiac asthma), pulmonary embolism, pneumonia, or anaphylactic reactions. Ensure that the patient has not undergone IV dye studies within the past 12 hours.

             Prolonged expiratory phase
CVS   Loud P_2
             Right ventricular (RV) heave, RV S_3 (pulmonary hypertension, cor pulmonale)

Other Investigations

Chest X-ray

CXR may reveal the following:
- Hyperinflation of lung fields
- Flattened diaphragms
- Increased AP diameter
- Infiltrates (suggesting concomitant pneumonia), atelectasis (suggesting mucous plugging), pneumothorax, or pneumomediastinum

Spirometry

Spirometry provides an objective measurement of the severity of airflow limitation and is helpful in evaluating the efficacy of therapy in patients with mild to moderate asthma. Some patients with severe asthma are too unwell for the performance of spirometry. The common parameters followed are the forced expiratory volume in 1 second (FEV_1) and the peak expiratory flow rate. The results from the best of three attempts should be recorded.

Management

General Measures

- O_2
- Hydration
- Pulse oximetry monitoring

Specific Measures

STEP 1

Administer inhaled beta agonists, such as *salbutamol* 2.5 to 5 mg in 3 mL of NS by nebulizer or 180 µg (2 puffs) by metered-dose inhaler every 4 hours.

> When delivered properly (Box 24–1) under supervision, therapy given by a metered-dose inhaler is as effective as, and less expensive than, nebulizer treatments.[8] If a patient is too dyspneic and distressed to coordinate the efforts required to allow effective delivery of a beta-2 agonist by metered-dose inhaler, nebulization of the drug may be preferable.

An anticholinergic agent, such as *ipratropium bromide* 250 to 500 µg (1 to 2 mL) in 3 mL of NS by nebulizer, may also improve oxygenation but should always be preceded or followed by an inhaled beta agonist because it occasionally can worsen bronchoconstriction.

> Although standard dosing intervals for beta agonists are every 4 to 6 hours, they may be given almost continuously in severe bronchospasm, as long as you watch closely for potential side effects (supraventricular tachycardias, premature ventricular contractions, muscle tremors).

STEP 2

Administer steroids (most useful in patients with pure asthma). In hospitalized patients, IV steroids have no advantage over oral steroids in hastening the resolution of bronchospasm.[9] The optimal steroid preparation and dosage are controversial. However, because pure asthma is predominantly a response to airway inflammation,

---

BOX 24–1 Technique for Inhalation of Beta-2 Agonists from Metered-Dose Inhalers

1. Shake the canister thoroughly.
2. Hold the mouthpiece of the inhaler 4 cm in front of the open mouth, or use a spacer between the inhaler and the mouth.
3. Breathe out slowly and completely.
4. Discharge the inhaler while taking a slow, deep breath (5 to 6 seconds).
5. Hold the breath at full inspiration for 10 seconds.

From Nelson HS: β-Adrenergic bronchodilators. N Engl J Med 1995; 333:501.

steroids should be used early in the management of exacerbations. In addition, steroids may take 6 hours to work, so they must be given immediately if persistent wheezing is anticipated in the next 6 to 24 hours. *Prednisone* 40 to 60 mg PO daily is recommended. If the patient is unable to swallow or absorb oral medications, *methylprednisolone* 125 mg IV, followed by 40 to 60 mg IV every 6 hours, or *hydrocortisone* 500 mg IV bolus, followed by a maintenance dose of 100 mg IV every 6 hours, may be given. Beclomethasone dipropionate (Beclovent) is not useful in acute bronchospasm.

> Steroids have few side effects in the short-term situation. Sodium retention is of concern in a patient with CHF or hypertension; hyperglycemia may occur in diabetics.
>
> Tapering steroids too rapidly has been a concern. A person on steroids for less than 2 weeks, however, can have the steroids discontinued abruptly without fear of steroid withdrawal. Of more concern is exacerbation of wheezing as steroids are tapered. This may limit the rate at which steroids can be withdrawn.

When a patient develops an exacerbation of bronchospasm, a general rule is to administer medications *beyond* what is usually required as an outpatient. For example, an asthmatic patient normally controlled on a salbutamol inhaler at home probably requires more frequent inhaled beta agonist ± ipratropium as well as steroids during an exacerbation. If a patient with COPD is wheezing despite outpatient treatment with a beta agonist and a theophylline preparation, or if the patient is already on a small dose of prednisone, he or she should be given higher doses of prednisone during the acute attack. Theophylline preparations do not provide more bronchodilation than that achieved by beta-2 agonists in patients with acute severe asthma and are no longer recommended.[10,11]

Look for evidence of bronchitis or pneumonia as the precipitant of bronchospasm. In patients so affected, bronchospasm may persist until appropriate antibiotics are given.

Five Warnings in Asthma

1. Sudden acute deterioration in an asthmatic patient may represent a *pneumothorax.*
2. *Rising* P_{CO_2}. Patients with an acute attack of asthma hyperventilate. A normal P_{CO_2} of 40 mm Hg in the acute situation may signify impending respiratory failure.
3. *Disappearance of wheezing* in the acute situation is an ominous sign, indicating that the patient is not moving sufficient air in and out to generate a wheeze.
4. *Sedatives are contraindicated in asthma and COPD.* The RN may not be aware of this and may unknowingly request a sleeping pill from a colleague while you are off duty. To avoid this pitfall, write clearly in your orders "No sedatives or sleeping pills."

5. Some asthmatic patients have a triad of asthma, nasal polyps, and aspirin sensitivity. When prescribing analgesics in asthmatics, it is best to *avoid NSAIDs*, including aspirin, because fatal anaphylactoid reactions have occurred in some patients given these medications.

RESPIRATORY FAILURE

Any of the four conditions causing SOB and a variety of others may lead to respiratory failure. Suspect that this is occurring if the RR is <12/min or if there is thoracoabdominal dissociation. Confirm the diagnosis of acute respiratory failure by ABG determination. A Po_2 <60 mm Hg or a Pco_2 >50 mm Hg with a pH <7.30 while breathing room air indicates *acute respiratory failure.*

1. Ensure that the patient has not received narcotic analgesics in the past 24 hours, which may depress the RR. Pupillary constriction may provide a clue that a narcotic is the culprit. If a narcotic has been given or if you are uncertain, order *naloxone hydrochloride* 0.2 to 2 mg IV immediately.

2. If there is no response to naloxone, arrange for the patient's transfer to the intensive care unit/cardiac care unit. Acute respiratory acidosis with a pH <7.30 may respond to aggressive treatment of the underlying respiratory or neuromuscular disorder. Noninvasive pressure support ventilation delivered by facemask may be useful for acute exacerbations of COPD (if the RR is >30/min and the pH <7.35) and may prevent the need for intubation.[12] However, if there is no rapid improvement, make arrangements for possible endotracheal intubation. Acute respiratory acidosis with a pH <7.20 usually requires mechanical ventilation until the precipitating cause of respiratory deterioration can be reversed.

REMEMBER

1. Abdominal problems can masquerade as SOB. (In one case, a patient's SOB resolved as soon as urinary retention was relieved by placement of a Foley catheter and 1300 mL of urine was drained.) Massive ascites and obesity may also compromise respiratory function.

2. Do not worry about your inexperience with endotracheal intubation. A patient in respiratory failure can be bagged and masked effectively for hours until someone with intubation experience is available to assist you.

3. Notice that *epinephrine* does not appear in the protocol for the treatment of asthma. There is no need to use epinephrine in an adult with an attack of asthma or COPD unless bronchospasm as a component of an anaphylactic reaction is present.

Epinephrine given inadvertently in cases of cardiac asthma has resulted in fatal MI.

4. An occasional patient has SOB as a manifestation of anxiety. In this instance, SOB is often qualitatively unique, in that the patient describes "shortness of the *deep* breath," with the sensation that he or she cannot get a satisfactory deep breath. Sighing and yawning are common accompaniments.

References

1. Wolfe M, Skibo CK, Goldenhaber SZ: Pulmonary embolic disease: Diagnosis, pathophysiologic aspects, and treatment with thrombolytic therapy. Curr Probl Cardiol 1993;18:625-627, 630.
2. Gulba DC, Schmid C, Borst HG, et al: Medical compared with surgical treatment for massive pulmonary embolism. Lancet 1994;343:576-577.
3. Simonneau G, Sors H, Charbonnrer B, et al: A comparison of low-molecular-weight heparin with unfractionated heparin for acute pulmonary embolism. N Engl J Med 1997;337:663-669.
4. The PIOPED Investigators: Value of the ventilation/perfusion scan in acute pulmonary embolism. JAMA 1990;263:2753-2759.
5. Bartlett JG, Mundy LM: Community acquired pneumonia. N Engl J Med 1995;333:1618-1624.
6. The National Institutes of Health–University of California Expert Panel for Corticosteroids as Adjunctive Therapy for Pneumocystis Pneumonia: Consensus statement on the use of corticosteroids as adjunctive therapy for pneumocystis pneumonia in the acquired immunodeficiency syndrome. N Engl J Med 1990;323:1500-1504.
7. Shelhamer JH, Toews GB, Masur H, et al: NIH conference: Respiratory disease in the immunosuppressed patient. Ann Intern Med 1992;117:415-431.
8. Bowton DL, Goldsmith WM, Haponik EF: Substitution of metered dose inhalers for hand-held nebulizers: Success and cost savings in a large, acute care hospital. Chest 1992;101:305-308.
9. Beveridge RC, et al: Guidelines for the emergency management of asthma in adults. Can Med Assoc J 1996;155:25-36.
10. Kelly HW, Murphy S: Beta-adrenergic agonists for acute, severe asthma. Ann Pharmacother 1992;26:81-91.
11. Siegel D, Sheppard D, Gelb A, Weinberg PF: Aminophylline increases the toxicity but not the efficacy of inhaled beta-adrenergic agonist in the treatment of acute exacerbations of asthma. Am Rev Respir Dis 1985;132:283-286.
12. Brochard L, Mancebo J, Wysocki M, et al: Noninvasive ventilation for acute exacerbations of chronic obstructive pulmonary disease. N Engl J Med 1995;333:817-822.

Skin Rashes and Urticaria

Reading this chapter will not transform you into a dermatologist, able to diagnose any rash with one quick glance. It will, however, help you to accurately describe rashes you are asked to examine while on call at night. This ability will facilitate confirmation of the diagnosis in the morning by more experienced physicians. You may be called because a rash has appeared abruptly (e.g., drug reaction) or because a patient has been admitted with a rash and the nursing staff is concerned that it may be infectious (e.g., scabies or lice). Urticarial rashes are rare in hospitalized patients; however, they are important to recognize because they may be the prodrome of anaphylactic shock.

PHONE CALL

Questions

1. **How long has the patient had the rash?**
   If the rash has appeared abruptly, a drug reaction is most likely.
2. **Is there any urticaria (hives)?**
   Urticaria is often the first sign of an impending anaphylactic reaction. Urticaria of the central part of the face is a common manifestation of angioedema.
3. **Is there any facial swelling, audible wheezing, or shortness of breath (SOB)?**
   These features suggest impending airway obstruction.
4. **What are the vital signs?**
5. **What drugs has the patient received within the past 12 hours? Has the patient received blood products or intravenous (IV) contrast material within the past 12 hours?**
   Remember that patients undergoing computed tomography (CT) scans are often given IV contrast material.
6. **Does the patient have any known allergies?**
7. **What was the reason for admission?**

Orders

If the patient has evidence of anaphylaxis or angioedema (urticaria, wheezing, SOB, or hypotension), order that the following be available at the bedside:

1. IV line to be started immediately with normal saline (NS).
2. *Epinephrine* 1:10,000, 20 μg (0.2 mL) for IV administration (available in a predrawn syringe from the emergency cart). For less severe situations, *epinephrine* 1:1000, 500 μg (0.5 mL) IM can be given. Note the different concentrations and the different routes of administration.

Inform RN

"I will arrive at the bedside in . . . minutes."

Evidence of facial urticaria (which may be the first manifestation of angioedema) or of anaphylaxis (urticaria, wheezing, SOB, or hypotension) requires you to see the patient immediately. Also, if the rash is acute and the patient has been or is receiving systemic medication, blood, or IV contrast material, you should go directly to the bedside. Assessment of a rash with no associated symptoms of anaphylaxis can wait an hour or two if other problems of higher priority exist.

ELEVATOR THOUGHTS

What causes skin rashes?

The majority of calls at night regarding acute-onset skin rashes involve drug reactions. The lesions may be urticarial and occasionally are associated with life-threatening anaphylaxis. Other drug reactions can have widely varied morphology but are usually symmetrical and often start on the buttocks. Early drug reactions are often localized.

1. Urticaria (rare but life threatening)
   a. Drugs
      (1) IV contrast material
      (2) Opiates (codeine, morphine, meperidine)
      (3) Antibiotics (penicillins, cephalosporins, sulfonamides, tetracycline, quinine, polymyxin, isoniazid)
      (4) Anesthetic agents (curare)
      (5) Angiotensin-converting enzyme (ACE) inhibitors (captopril, enalapril, lisinopril, fosinopril)
      (6) Aspirin and other nonsteroidal anti-inflammatory drugs (NSAIDs)
   b. Blood transfusion reaction
   c. Food allergies, especially nuts, fruits, tomatoes, lobster, shrimp
   d. Physical urticarias—cold, heat, pressure, vibration

2. Erythematous maculopapular (morbilliform) rashes
   a. Antibiotics (penicillin, ampicillin, sulfonamides, chloramphenicol)

   > Ampicillin commonly causes a generalized maculopapular eruption 2 to 4 weeks after administration of the first dose; thus, it is important to check not only the current drugs the patient is receiving but also all recently discontinued drugs, because the eruption may appear several weeks after the drug has been stopped.
   >
   > Erythematous maculopapular rashes are common in patients with acquired immunodeficiency syndrome (AIDS) receiving sulfonamides and characteristically occur around day 10 of treatment for *Pneumocystis* pneumonia.

   b. Antiretroviral agents (nelfinavir, abacavir, didanosine, stavudine)

   > Severe allergic reactions consisting of fever, rash, nausea, vomiting, diarrhea, and abdominal pain have been reported in 3% to 5% of people taking abacavir.

   c. Antihistamines
   d. Antidepressants (amitriptyline)
   e. Beta-lactam antibiotics (usually with a raised papular component)
   f. Diuretics (thiazides)
   g. Oral hypoglycemics
   h. Anti-inflammatory drugs (gold, phenylbutazone)
   i. Sedatives (barbiturates)
   j. Sulfonamides (usually morbilliform)
   k. Delavirdine, nevirapine, efavirenz
   l. Scabies and lice

   > These organisms commonly produce excoriated papules. The lesions of scabies are usually present on the finger webs, wrists, waist, axillae, areolae, genitals, and feet. Lesions from lice may occur anywhere on the body but are common on the scalp, pubic area, neck, flanks, waistline, and axillae. Both organisms are associated with intense itching.

3. Vesicobullous rashes
   a. Antibiotics (sulfonamides, dapsone)
   b. Anti-inflammatory drugs (penicillamine)
   c. Sedatives (barbiturates)
   d. Halogens (iodides, bromides)
   e. Herpes zoster
   f. Toxic epidermal necrolysis (sulfonamides, allopurinol)
4. Purpura

   > Drug-induced thrombocytopenia causes nonpalpable purpura, whereas vasculitis causes palpable purpura.

   a. Antibiotics (sulfonamides, chloramphenicol)
   b. Diuretics (thiazides)

   c. Anti-inflammatory drugs (phenylbutazone, indomethacin, salicylates)
5. Exfoliative rashes

> If a drug eruption is not recognized early and the drug is not discontinued, the patient may develop mucosal erosions and profound skin injury, with blistering and extensive loss of epidermis (Stevens-Johnson syndrome or toxic epidermal necrolysis).

   a. Antibiotics (sulfa derivatives, co-trimoxazole, penicillins, streptomycin)
   b. Anti-inflammatory drugs (phenylbutazone, piroxicam)
   c. Antiseizure medication (carbamazepine, phenytoin)
   d. Sedatives/anxiolytics (barbiturates, chlormezanone)
   e. Miscellaneous (allopurinol)
6. Fixed drug eruption

> Certain drugs may produce a skin lesion in a specific area. Repeat administration of the drug reproduces the skin lesion in the same location. The lesion is usually composed of dusky red patches distributed over the trunk or proximal limbs.

   a. Antibiotics (sulfonamides, metronidazole)
   b. Anti-inflammatory drugs (phenylbutazone)
   c. Analgesics (phenacetin)
   d. Sedatives (barbiturates, chlordiazepoxide)
   e. Laxatives (phenolphthalein)

MAJOR THREAT TO LIFE

- Upper airway obstruction due to angioedema
- Anaphylactic shock
- Toxic epidermal necrolysis

Urticarial skin rash may be a prodrome of *angioedema* or *anaphylaxis*, whereas other types of skin rashes are not. Drugs and IV contrast material are the usual causes of anaphylactic shock in hospitalized patients—unless the allergic patient happened to be stung by a wasp or ate shrimp.

A patient with *toxic epidermal necrolysis* looks scalded, with peeling of the outer surface of the skin. Frequently, fever is difficult to control. If you suspect toxic epidermal necrolysis, call for a dermatology consultation immediately, and transfer the patient to a burn unit or intensive care unit (ICU)—do not procrastinate, and do not give systemic steroids. Common drugs involved include allopurinol, sulfonamides, and anticonvulsants. With *toxic shock syndrome* (see page 182) and *necrotizing fasciitis* (see page 192), the patient is more ill or complains of more local pain than you would expect from objective signs. Obtain a dermatology or infectious disease consultation immediately.

BEDSIDE

Quick-Look Test

Does the patient look well (comfortable), sick (uncomfortable or distressed), or critical (about to die)?

Patients with upper airway obstruction due to angioedema and those with anaphylactic reactions look apprehensive and usually have SOB and are sitting upright in bed.

Airway and Vital Signs

What is the respiratory rate?

Tachypnea, particularly if associated with audible stridor or wheezing, is an ominous sign. Inspiratory stridor suggests impending upper airway obstruction—notify your resident and an anesthetist immediately.

What is the blood pressure?

Hypotension suggests impending or established anaphylactic shock, and the patient requires immediate treatment. If anaphylaxis is suspected, insert a large-bore IV line (size 16 if possible) if this has not already been done, and run in NS as fast as possible.

What is the temperature?

Skin rashes are often more prominent when the patient is febrile.

Selective Physical Examination

Is there evidence of an impending anaphylactic reaction?

HEENT	Tongue, pharyngeal, or facial edema (angioedema)
Resp	Wheezing (anaphylaxis)
	If evidence of an impending anaphylactic reaction exists, refer to page 287 for immediate treatment.
Skin	If an urticarial rash due to angioedema or anaphylaxis has been ruled out, provide an accurate description of the rash to establish the diagnosis or perhaps to help someone else diagnose it if it disappears or changes by morning

Where is the rash located?

Is it generalized, acral (hands, feet), or localized? Remember to examine the buttocks, a common site for the onset of drug eruptions.

What color is the rash?

It may be red, pink, brown, or white.

What does the primary lesion look like? (Fig. 25–1)

- *Macule*—flat (noticeable from the surrounding skin because of the color difference)
- *Patch*—a large macule

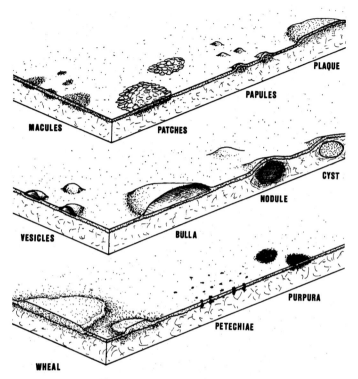

Figure 25–1 Primary skin lesions.

- *Papule*—solid, elevated, size <1 cm
- *Plaque*—solid, elevated, size >1 cm
- *Vesicle*—elevated, well circumscribed, size <1 cm
- *Bulla*—elevated, well circumscribed, size >1 cm
- *Nodule*—deep-seated mass, indistinct borders, size <0.5 cm in both width and depth
- *Cyst*—nodule filled with expressible fluid or semisolid material
- *Wheal (hives)*—well-circumscribed, flat-topped, firm elevation (papule, plaque, or dermal edema) ± central pallor and irregular borders
- *Petechia*—red or purple nonblanchable macule, size <3 mm
- *Purpura*—red or purple nonblanchable macule or papule, size >3 mm

What does the secondary lesion look like? (Fig. 25–2)
- *Scale*—dry, thin plate of thickened keratin layers (white color differentiates it from crust)

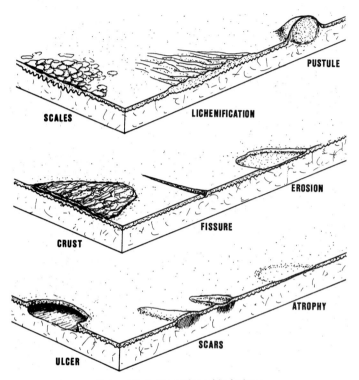

Figure 25–2 Secondary skin lesions.

- *Lichenification*—dry, leathery thickening; shiny surface; accentuated skin markings
- *Pustule*—vesicle containing purulent exudate
- *Crust*—dried, yellow exudate of plasma (result of broken vesicle, bulla, or pustule)
- *Fissure*—linear, epidermal tear
- *Erosion*—wide, epidermal fissure; moist and well circumscribed
- *Ulcer*—erosion into the dermis
- *Scar*—flat, raised, or depressed area of fibrosis
- *Atrophy*—depression secondary to thinning of the skin

What is the configuration of the rash?
- *Annular*—circular
- *Linear*—in lines
- *Grouped*—clusters, such as the vesicular lesions of herpes zoster or herpes simplex

Selective History and Chart Review

How long has the rash been present?

Does it itch?

How has it been treated?

Is this a new or a recurrent problem?

Which drugs was the patient receiving before the rash started?

Management

1. If the rash is associated with urticaria and is thought to be secondary to a drug reaction, the drug should be withheld until the diagnosis is confirmed in the morning.

2. Seemingly minor nonurticarial maculopapular rashes may occasionally be the initial presentation of a more serious reaction, such as toxic epidermal necrolysis. Ideally, if the rash is thought to be a drug reaction, the offending drug should be stopped. If the offending medication is essential to the patient's management overnight, a suitable alternative may be chosen. If no suitable alternative exists, the decision to stop or continue the offending medication must be made with the help of your resident or attending physician.

3. When the skin rash is not a drug eruption and the diagnosis is clear, the standard recommended treatment can be instituted. (Refer to a dermatology text for specific treatment.)

4. Often, house staff have difficulty diagnosing skin rashes with confidence. If you are uncertain, it is often sufficient to describe the lesion accurately and refer the patient to a dermatologist in the morning. Several important exceptions exist:

   a. A *petechial rash* suggests a disorder of platelet number or function; a *purpuric rash* may indicate a coagulation disorder. Activated partial thromboplastin time (aPTT), prothrombin time (PT), and platelet studies should be ordered when appropriate.

   b. *Herpes zoster* in an immunocompromised patient (e.g., one with AIDS) may require urgent treatment because of the risk of systemic dissemination, especially to the central nervous system. If you suspect herpes zoster (initially erythematous macules and papules in a dermatomal distribution progressing to grouped vesicles and hemorrhagic crusts) in an immunocompromised patient, consult your resident or attending physician for possible treatment with IV acyclovir.

   c. Patients with hereditary *deficiency of protein C* may develop skin necrosis, typically 3 to 5 days after beginning warfarin therapy. The skin lesions usually begin as painful red plaques overlying areas of fat. In these cases, warfarin must be stopped immediately, its effect reversed with vitamin K, and heparin substituted as an anticoagulant.

Syncope

Syncope is a brief loss of consciousness due to sudden reduction in cerebral blood flow. Another term, *presyncope*, refers to the situation in which there is sufficient reduction in cerebral blood flow to result in a sensation of impending loss of consciousness, although the patient does not actually pass out. Presyncope and syncope represent degrees of the same disorder and should be addressed as manifestations of the same underlying problem. Your task is to discover the cause of the syncopal attack.

PHONE CALL

Questions

1. **Did the patient actually lose consciousness?**
2. **Is the patient still unconscious?**
3. **What are the vital signs?**
4. **Is the patient diabetic?**
5. **Was the patient recumbent, sitting, or standing when the episode occurred?**
   Syncope while the patient is in the recumbent position is almost always cardiac in origin.
6. **Was any seizure-like activity witnessed?**
7. **What was the admitting diagnosis?**
   An admitting diagnosis of seizure disorder, transient ischemic attack (TIA), or cardiac disease may help direct you to the cause of the syncopal attack.
8. **Has the patient sustained any evidence of injury?**

Orders

If the patient is still *unconscious*, order the following:

1. Intravenous (IV) D5W to keep the vein open (TKVO) immediately, if an IV line is not already in place.
2. Turn the patient on the left side.
   This maneuver prevents the tongue from falling back into the throat and obstructing the upper airway and minimizes the risk of aspiration should vomiting occur.
3. Stat 12-lead electrocardiogram (ECG) and rhythm strip.

Although almost all patients with syncope regain consciousness within a few minutes, you are more likely to be able to document a cardiac dysrhythmia early, while the patient is still symptomatic.

4. If the patient is diabetic, take a stat finger-prick blood glucose (FPBG) reading, then give 50 mL D50W IV.

If the patient has *regained consciousness*, there is no evidence of head or neck injury, and the vital signs are stable, do the following:

1. To return the patient to bed, ask the RN to slowly raise the patient to a sitting position, then a standing position.
2. The patient should be placed back in bed, with instructions to remain there until you are able to assess the problem.
3. Order an ECG and a rhythm strip.
4. Have the vital signs taken every 15 minutes until you arrive at the bedside. Ask the RN to call you back immediately should the vital signs become unstable before you are able to assess the patient.

Inform RN

"I will arrive at the bedside in . . . minutes."

Syncope requires you to see the patient immediately if the patient is still unconscious or if there are abnormalities in the heart rate (HR) or blood pressure (BP). If the patient is alert and conscious with normal vital signs (and if there are other more urgent problems to be assessed), the RN should observe the patient and call you if a problem arises before you are able to get there.

ELEVATOR THOUGHTS

What causes syncope?

1. Cardiac causes
   a. Dysrhythmias
      (1) Tachycardias
         (a) Ventricular tachycardia
         (b) Ventricular fibrillation
      (2) Bradycardias
         (a) Sinus bradycardia
         (b) Second- and third-degree atrioventricular (AV) block
         (c) Sick sinus syndrome (SSS)
   b. Pacemaker syncope
      (1) Pacemaker failure to capture
      (2) Pacemaker syndrome (i.e., uncoordinated AV contractile sequence)

    c. Syncope with exertion
      (1) Aortic stenosis
      (2) Pulmonic stenosis
      (3) Hypertrophic obstructive cardiomyopathy
      (4) Subclavian steal syndrome
2. Neurologic causes
    a. Brain stem TIA or stroke (drop attacks)
    b. Seizure
    c. Subarachnoid hemorrhage (SAH)
    d. Cervical spondylosis
3. Neurally mediated (reflex) syncope
    a. Common faint (vasodepressor reaction)
    b. Situational syncope (e.g., cough, micturition, defecation, sneezing, postprandial)
    c. Carotid sinus syncope
4. Orthostatic hypotension
    a. Drug induced
    b. Volume depletion
    c. Autonomic failure
5. Miscellaneous
    a. Pulmonary embolism
    b. Hyperventilation
    c. Anxiety attacks

MAJOR THREAT TO LIFE

- Aspiration pneumonia or adult respiratory distress syndrome (ARDS)

  Because most patients recover from syncopal attacks within a few minutes, the actual loss of consciousness is not the major problem. Of greater importance is that while the patient is unconscious, the tongue may block the oropharynx or the patient may aspirate oral or gastric contents into the lungs, which may result in the development of *aspiration pneumonia* or *ARDS*. Therefore, in an unconscious patient, your primary goal is to protect the airway until the patient regains consciousness and the cough reflexes are again effective.

- Recurrence of an unrecognized, potentially fatal cardiac dysrhythmia.

  Once the patient has regained consciousness, the major threat to life is the recurrence of an unrecognized, potentially fatal *cardiac dysrhythmia*. This can best be identified and managed by transferring the patient to an intensive care unit/cardiac care unit (ICU/CCU) or other setting with ECG monitors if there is suspicion that a dysrhythmia caused the syncopal episode.

BEDSIDE

Quick-Look Test

Does the patient look well (comfortable), sick (uncomfortable or distressed), or critical (about to die)?

This simple observation helps determine the necessity of immediate intervention. Most patients who have had episodes of syncope and have regained consciousness look perfectly well.

Airway and Vital Signs

If the patient is still unconscious, ensure that the RN has placed him or her on the left side and that the patient's tongue has not fallen into the back of the throat. Most episodes of syncope are short-lived, and by the time you arrive at the bedside, the patient will have regained consciousness. Look for abnormalities in the vital signs, which may help you diagnose the specific cause of syncope.

What is the HR?

Supraventricular or *ventricular tachycardia* should be documented on ECG tracings, and the patient should be treated immediately. (Refer to Chapter 15, page 144, for the treatment of supraventricular tachycardia and Chapter 15, page 147, for the treatment of ventricular tachycardia.)

Any patient with a transient or persistent supraventricular or ventricular tachycardia or its history should be transferred to the ICU/CCU or other setting with ECG monitoring for appropriate management if no other cause of syncope can be found.

What is the BP?

A patient with resting or orthostatic hypotension should be managed as outlined in Chapter 18.

> Remember that a massive internal hemorrhage (such as a gastrointestinal bleed or ruptured aortic aneurysm) can occasionally manifest with a syncopal attack.

Hypertension, if found in association with headache and neck stiffness, may indicate SAH. A brief loss of consciousness is common at the onset of SAH and is often associated with dizziness, vertigo, or vomiting.

What is the temperature?

Patients with syncope are rarely febrile. If fever is present, it is usually due to a concomitant illness unrelated to the syncopal attack. However, especially if the syncopal attack was unwitnessed, be careful to exclude the possibility of a seizure secondary to meningitis, which may manifest as "fever + syncope."

Selective History and Chart Review

Has this ever happened before?

If it has, ask the patient whether a diagnosis was made after the previous attack.

What does the patient or witness recall about the time immediately before the syncope?

- Syncope occurring while in the upright position after an emotional or painful stimulus and preceded by nausea, diaphoresis, pallor, and a *gradual* loss of consciousness is typical of the common faint (vasodepressor syncope).
- Syncope occurring while changing from the supine or sitting position to the standing position suggests orthostatic hypotension.
- An *aura,* though rare, is helpful in pointing to a seizure as the cause of syncope in an unwitnessed attack.
- *Palpitations* preceding an attack may suggest a cardiac dys-rhythmia as the cause of syncope.
- Syncope during or immediately after performance of *Valsalva's maneuver,* such as a bout of coughing, micturition, straining at stool, or sneezing, may occur because of transient reduction of venous return to the right atrium and neurally mediated reflex bradycardia.
- Syncope after *turning the head to one side* (especially if one is wearing a tight collar) or while shaving may represent carotid sinus syncope. This condition is seen most often in elderly men.
- Syncope occurring during *arm exercise* suggests subclavian steal syndrome.
- *Numbness and tingling* in the hands and feet are commonly experienced just before presyncope or syncope due to hyper-ventilation or anxiety.

Is there any history of cardiac disease?

A patient with preexisting cardiac disease may have an increased risk of developing dysrhythmias.

Has the patient ever had a seizure?

An unwitnessed seizure may be perceived as a syncopal attack. Ask whether, during the attack, the patient bit his or her tongue or was incontinent of stool or urine. Either one is suggestive of seizure activity. *Hypoglycemia* should be suspected as a possible cause of seizure or syncope in a diabetic patient receiving oral hypoglycemic agents or insulin.

Has the patient ever had a stroke?

A patient with known cerebrovascular disease is a likely candidate for a brain stem TIA or stroke. However, because atherosclerosis is a diffuse process, a patient with a history of stroke may also have coronary atherosclerosis, which may result in cardiac dysrhythmias.

What does the patient remember on waking from the syncopal attack?

Headache, drowsiness, and mental confusion are common sequelae of seizures but not of cardiac or orthostatic causes of syncope.

What medications is the patient taking?

Check the chart to see what medications the patient is being given.

- Digoxin, beta blockers, and calcium channel blockers may result in bradycardias. Digoxin, if present in toxic amounts, may also precipitate ventricular tachycardia.
- Quinidine, procainamide, disopyramide, sotalol, amiodarone, tricyclic antidepressants, phenothiazines, and some of the "nonsedating" antihistamines may prolong the QT interval, leading to ventricular tachycardia (torsades de pointes) (Fig. 26–1A) or the prolonged QT interval syndrome (see Fig. 26–1B).
- Agents that reduce afterload or preload (angiotensin-converting enzyme [ACE] inhibitors, hydralazine, prazosin,

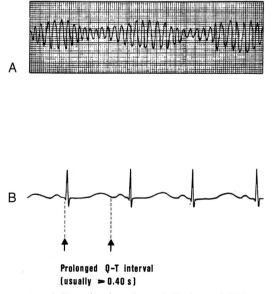

Prolonged Q-T interval
(usually ≥ 0.40 s)

Figure 26–1 A, Torsades de pointes. B, Prolonged QT interval.

nitroglycerin) may cause syncope, especially in elderly or volume-depleted patients.

- Phenothiazines, tricyclic antidepressants, alcohol, and cocaine lower the seizure threshold and may result in a seizure.
- Oral hypoglycemic agents and insulin may cause hypoglycemic seizures or syncope. Many factors can contribute to erratic glucose levels in hospitalized diabetic patients, including coexisting illnesses, changing activity levels, poor appetite, and medication interactions.

Selective Physical Examination

The physical examination is directed toward finding a cause for the syncope. However, a search for evidence of injuries sustained if the patient fell during the syncopal attack is equally important.

Vitals	Repeat now; at this time, take the BP in both arms A difference >20 mm Hg may indicate subclavian steal syndrome.
HEENT	Funduscopy—look for subhyaloid hemorrhages (SAH); blood diffuses between the retinal fiber layer and the internal limiting membrane, forming a pocket of blood with sharp borders and often a fluid level Tongue or cheek laceration (seizure disorder) Neck stiffness (meningitis leading to a seizure, SAH) Supraclavicular or subclavicular bruit (subclavian steal syndrome)
Resp	Crackles, wheezes (aspiration during the syncopal episode)
CVS	Pacemaker (pacemaker syncope) Flat JVP (volume depletion) Atrial fibrillation (vertebrobasilar embolism) Systolic murmur (aortic stenosis, pulmonic stenosis, hypertrophic obstructive cardiomyopathy)
GU	Urinary incontinence (seizure disorder)
Rectal	Fecal incontinence (seizure disorder)
MSS	Palpate bones for evidence of fractures sustained if the patient fell
Neuro	A complete neurologic examination must be done, looking for evidence of residual localizing signs that may indicate a TIA, completed stroke, SAH, space-occupying intracranial lesion, or Todd's paralysis; vertebrobasilar TIAs or strokes are frequently accompanied by other evidence of brain stem dysfunction (i.e., cranial nerve abnormalities) such as diplopia, nystagmus, facial paralysis, vertigo, dysphagia, and dysarthria

Management

Often, an immediate cause for syncope cannot be found. Because treatment of the various causes of syncope is so different, one must have *documented proof* of the cause of a syncopal episode before proceeding to definitive treatment. Investigations may take several days to complete. Your job, once you have assessed a patient with syncope, is to decide from the history, physical findings, and laboratory data what the most likely cause of syncope is and to arrange for further investigation, if necessary.

Cardiac Causes

If a cardiac cause of syncope is suspected, whether related to a dysrhythmia, a valvular problem, or a pacemaker, the patient should be transferred to the CCU or to an intermediate care unit where continuous ECG monitoring is available. If there are no ECG-monitored beds available and if there is no suspicion of ischemia-induced dysrhythmia, 24-hour Holter monitoring should be arranged for the patient first thing in the morning.

Always consider a silent myocardial infarction (MI) with subsequent transient AV block, ventricular tachycardia, or ventricular fibrillation as the cause for syncope of cardiac origin.

Treatment of specific dysrhythmias, if still present when you are assessing the patient, is discussed in Chapter 15:

1. Tachycardias
   a. Ventricular tachycardia (page 147)
   b. Supraventricular tachycardia (page 144)
2. Bradycardias
   a. Sinus bradycardia (page 154)
   b. AV blocks (page 155)
   c. Atrial fibrillation with slow ventricular response (page 155)

Pacemaker syncope requires a cardiology consultation for reprogramming of the pacing rate, output, or mode or for an upgrade to AV sequential pacing.

If *aortic stenosis, pulmonic stenosis,* or *hypertrophic obstructive cardiomyopathy* is thought to be responsible for exertional syncope, arrange for an echocardiogram in the morning to document the suspected cardiac lesion, and ask for a cardiology consultation.

Neurologic Causes

Suspected *brain stem TIA* or *stroke* should be evaluated by a computed tomography (CT) scan of the head. Anticoagulation or platelet inhibitors should be started only after consultation with a neurologist.

If a *seizure* is suspected, you must first document the cause of the seizure, as outlined in Chapter 23, page 252.

If *SAH* is suspected, arrange for an urgent noncontrast CT scan of the head, looking for evidence of aneurysm or blood in the subarachnoid space. A normal CT scan does not, however, exclude SAH, and a lumbar puncture may be required to look for xanthochromic cerebrospinal fluid. If such a lesion is identified, a neurosurgeon should be consulted for further investigation and management.

Neurally Mediated (Reflex) Syncope

Most vasodepressor attacks can be managed without transfer to the ICU/CCU, as outlined in Chapter 18, page 177.

The definitive diagnosis of *carotid sinus syncope* requires potentially dangerous carotid sinus pressure, which must be done while the ECG is being monitored for cardiac dysrhythmias. Although the patient does not require ICU/CCU admission overnight, arrangements should be made in the morning to evaluate the cardiac rhythm during carotid sinus massage.

Orthostatic Hypotension

Syncope due to *volume depletion* can be managed with IV fluid replacement, as outlined in Chapter 18, page 180.

Drug-induced orthostatic hypotension and *autonomic failure* are complex treatment problems. As long as the patient's volume status is normal, they can be addressed in the morning through consultation with a neurologist or clinical pharmacologist.

Until the underlying problem responsible for orthostatic hypotension is corrected, instruct patients that if they must be out of bed during the night, they should ask the RN for assistance and should move slowly from the supine to sitting position and then move slowly again from the sitting to standing position.

Miscellaneous

Syncope due to *hyperventilation* or *anxiety states* can be alleviated by instructing the patient to breathe into a paper bag when he or she begins to feel anxious or presyncopal. This step corrects hypocapnia and thereby prevents a syncopal attack.

REMEMBER

1. In an elderly patient, the main hazard of a syncopal attack is not necessarily an underlying disease but rather a fracture or other injury sustained during a fall.
2. Except for the Stokes-Adams attack (third-degree AV block), true syncope rarely occurs when a patient is in the recumbent position.

Transfusion Reactions

Blood transfusions are given around the clock in hospitals. Reactions to blood products may vary from severe to mild. An organized approach will help you sort out both the nature of the reaction and what to do about it.

PHONE CALL

Questions

1. **What symptoms does the patient have?**
   Fever, chills, chest pain, back pain, diaphoresis, and shortness of breath (SOB) all can be manifestations of a transfusion reaction.
2. **What are the vital signs?**
3. **Which blood product is being transfused, and how long ago was it started?**
4. **What was the reason for admission?**

Orders

1. Stop the transfusion immediately if the patient has any of the following symptoms:
   a. Sudden onset of hypotension
   b. Chest or back pain, tachypnea
   c. Any symptom (even fever, chills, or urticaria) occurring within minutes of the start of the transfusion
   d. Fever in a patient who has never before received a blood transfusion or who has never been pregnant; this symptom may represent an acute hemolytic reaction

   An acute hemolytic transfusion reaction can appear with any of the aforementioned symptoms. Such reactions, though rare, are associated with an extremely high mortality rate, which is proportionate to the volume of blood infused. In previously pregnant or previously transfused patients, fever may be a nonhemolytic febrile reaction.

2. If the blood transfusion has been stopped, keep the intravenous (IV) line open with normal saline (NS).

Inform RN

"I will arrive at the bedside in . . . minutes."
Any suspected hemolytic or anaphylactic transfusion reaction requires you to see the patient immediately.

ELEVATOR THOUGHTS

What causes transfusion reactions?

1. Immune hemolysis.
    a. Acute hemolytic reaction. Errors in either identification of the patient or labeling of the blood can result in mismatched red blood cells (RBCs) (ABO incompatibility), leading to an *acute hemolytic reaction*. Such errors are exceedingly rare and usually occur in emergency situations (e.g., in the postanesthetic, operating, or emergency room), when the usual procedures for patient identification and blood labeling are breached.
    b. Delayed hemolyitc reaction. *Delayed hemolytic reactions* develop as a consequence of prior exposure to foreign red cell antigens (i.e., pregnancy or previous transfusion). Re-exposure to these antigens results in an anamnestic rise in alloantibodies that were not detectable at the time of the original crossmatch. Hemolysis occurs 3 to 14 days after transfusion and may be accompanied by fever, jaundice, and increasing anemia.
2. Nonimmune hemolysis. Nonimmune hemolysis may occur if the blood has been overheated or has undergone trauma. Trauma to blood products occurs either by excessive hand squeezing or pumping of the infusion bag during the rapid administration of blood in an emergency, or by delivery through a needle that is too small.
3. Anaphylaxis (immunoglobulin G [IgG] response to immunoglobulin A [IgA] antibodies). Anaphylaxis may result from transmission of IgA antibodies from the donor's blood into a presensitized IgA-deficient patient.
    a. Congenital IgA deficiency is a common (1 in 1000), asymptomatic disorder. The first transfusion that an IgA-deficient patient receives will contain IgA antibodies, which are recognized by the patient's immune system as foreign antigens. Thus, the IgA-deficient patient becomes sensitized and develops anti-IgA antibodies, which may result in anaphylaxis or urticaria with subsequent transfusions.
    b. There are two known IgA *allotypes* (an allotype is simply a genetic variation in the structure of the immunoglobulin).

Anaphylactic reactions are more common in patients who lack both allotypes of IgA, but they have been reported in patients who lack only one allotype. Individuals with IgA molecules of one allotype may develop antibodies against the other allotype, with subsequent transfusion reactions manifesting as urticaria or, occasionally, anaphylaxis.

4. Urticaria. Transmission of the following antigens from the donor's blood can cause urticaria:
   a. Food allergens, such as shrimp (IgE response)
   b. Other plasma protein allergens
   c. IgA antibodies into an IgA-deficient patient (i.e., deficient in one of the two allotypes); this is a rare cause of urticaria

5. Fever
   a. Nonhemolytic febrile reaction. This is the most common cause of febrile transfusion reactions and does not require stopping the transfusion. It is usually seen in multiparous or multitransfused patients and is due to a white blood cell (WBC) antigen-antibody reaction.
   b. Early sign of acute hemolytic transfusion reaction, particularly in patients who have not had prior transfusions or pregnancies.
   c. Pulmonary leukoagglutinin reaction. The donor's blood (usually from a multiparous woman) contains antibodies to the patient's WBCs, causing the agglutinated WBCs to lodge in the pulmonary capillaries, resulting in noncardiogenic pulmonary edema.
   d. Microbial contamination (very rare). Although many infectious agents can be transmitted via blood transfusions (causing, e.g., non-A, non-B hepatitis, malaria, syphilis, cytomegalovirus, infectious mononucleosis, rubella, Rocky Mountain spotted fever), they do not result in reactions during infusion of the blood product.
   e. Blood banks in Canada screen for human immunodeficiency virus (HIV)-1, HIV-2, human T-cell lymphocytic virus type 1 (HTLV-1), hepatitis B virus (HBV), and hepatitis C virus (HCV) before blood is released for transfusion.

6. Pulmonary edema
   a. Congestive heart failure (CHF). Volume overload may be induced in a patient with a history of CHF because blood transfusions expand the intravascular volume.
   b. Pulmonary leukoagglutinin reaction (see 5c above).

MAJOR THREAT TO LIFE

- Anaphylaxis
- Acute hemolytic reaction

Both of these reactions are rare, but when they do occur, they can be fatal. *Anaphylaxis* may cause death either by severe laryngospasm or bronchospasm or by profound peripheral vasodilatation and cardiovascular collapse. An *acute hemolytic reaction* is a medical emergency because of the possible development of renal failure, acute disseminated intravascular coagulation (DIC), or both.

BEDSIDE

Quick-Look Test

Does the patient look well (comfortable), sick (uncomfortable or distressed), or critical (about to die)?

A patient with impending anaphylaxis may look sick (agitated, restless, or short of breath). A patient with pulmonary edema secondary to a transfusion reaction may look critical, with severe SOB.

Airway and Vital Signs

What is the respiratory rate?

Tachypnea may be a manifestation of CHF or, particularly if associated with audible wheezing, may indicate impending anaphylaxis.

What is the blood pressure?

Hypotension is an ominous sign—ensure that the transfusion has been stopped. Hypotension is seen in acute hemolytic reactions and in anaphylactic reactions. However, if the transfusion is being given for volume depletion, such as in acute blood loss, hypotension may represent continued loss of intravascular volume from uncontrolled bleeding.

Have the patient's tag and wristband been checked?

Compare the identification tag on the blood with the patient's wristband.

Selective Physical Examination

HEENT	Flushed face (hemolytic reaction or anaphylaxis)
	Facial or pharyngeal edema (anaphylaxis)
Resp	Wheezes (anaphylaxis)
Neuro	Decreased level of consciousness (anaphylaxis or hemolytic reaction)
Skin	Heat along the vein being used for the transfusion (hemolytic reaction)
	Oozing from IV sites may be the only sign of hemolysis in an unconscious or anesthetized patient; DIC is a late manifestation of an acute hemolytic transfusion reaction
Urine	Check the urine color: free Hb turns urine red or brown and is indicative of a hemolytic reaction

If there is evidence of anaphylaxis or hemolysis, *stop the transfusion* and immediately begin emergency treatment (see later).

Selective History

Has the patient developed any symptoms since the initial telephone call?
- Fever or chills (nonhemolytic febrile reaction)
- Headache, chest pain, back pain, or diaphoresis (hemolytic reaction)
- SOB (volume overload or pulmonary leukoagglutinin reaction)—a leukoagglutinin reaction in an elderly patient is often misdiagnosed as cardiogenic pulmonary edema

Has the patient had previous transfusion reactions?
Chills and fever are most common in a patient who has received multiple transfusions or who has had several pregnancies.

Management

Anaphylaxis

1. Ensure that the transfusion has been stopped.
2. Epinephrine is the most important drug for any anaphylactic reaction.

   Through its alpha-adrenergic action, epinephrine reverses peripheral vasodilatation, and through its beta-adrenergic action, it reduces bronchoconstriction and increases the force of cardiac contraction. In addition, it suppresses histamine and leukotriene release.

   Two strengths of epinephrine are available for injection. *Make sure that you are using the right strength.*

   For profound anaphylactic shock that is immediately life threatening, use the IV route. Give *epinephrine* 1:10,000, 20 µg (0.2 mL)/min, up to a total dose of 300 µg (3 mL) in 15 minutes. Repeat every 15 minutes if indicated.

   For less severe situations, epinephrine can be given IM. *Note the different concentration.* Give *epinephrine* 1:1000, 500 µg (0.5 mL) IM; repeat after 5 minutes in the absence of improvement or if deterioration occurs. Several doses may be necessary.
3. *Hydrocortisone* 500 mg by slow IV or by IM injection, followed by 100 mg IV or IM every 6 hours to help avert late sequelae.

   | This is particularly important in asthmatics who have previously been treated with corticosteroids.
4. *Salbutamol* 2.5 mg/3 mL NS by nebulizer.

   | This is an adjunctive measure if bronchospasm is a major feature.
5. *Diphenhydramine* 50 to 75 mg by slow IV or by IM injection.

   | The benefits of antihistamines in anaphylactic shock are controversial.
6. Intubation if necessary.

Acute Hemolytic Reaction

1. Ensure that the transfusion has been stopped.
2. Replace all IV tubing.
3. NS 500 mL IV as fast as possible. Try to maintain the urine output >100 mL/hr with IV fluids and diuretics.
4. *Furosemide* 40 mg IV by slow, direct injection at a rate no faster than 4 mg/min or *mannitol* 25 g IV over 5 minutes (to promote diuresis).
5. Draw 20 mL of the patient's blood and send for the following:
   a. Repeat crossmatch
   b. Coombs' test, free hemoglobin (Hb)
   c. Complete blood cell count (CBC), RBC morphology
   d. Platelets, prothrombin time (PT), activated partial thromboplastin time (aPTT), fibrin degradation products (FDP)
   e. Urea, creatinine levels
   f. Unclotted blood for a stat spin—hemolysis is demonstrated when the plasma remains pink despite spinning for 5 minutes (i.e., hemoglobinemia)
6. Obtain a urine sample for free Hb. In addition, urine can be tested with dipsticks. If there is hemoglobinuria, the dipstick results will be positive for Hb and negative for RBCs.
7. Send the donor's blood back to the blood bank for the following:
   a. Repeat crossmatch
   b. Coombs' test
8. If oliguria develops despite adequate IV fluids and appropriate diuretics, *acute renal failure* should be suspected. (For management of acute renal failure, see Chapter 9, pages 77 to 79.)

Urticaria

1. Do not stop the transfusion.
   | Hives alone are rarely serious, but hives with hypotension is considered an anaphylactic reaction until proved otherwise.
2. *Diphenhydramine* 50 mg PO or IV (not IM).
3. Before future transfusions, the patient should be premedicated with *diphenhydramine* 50 mg PO or IV (not IM). If this fails to prevent urticarial reactions, washed RBCs should be given.

Fever

1. Do not stop the transfusion unless a hemolytic reaction is suspected. Fever developing within minutes of the start of a blood transfusion is likely a symptom of a hemolytic reaction.
2. Often, no treatment is required. If the fever is high and the patient is distressed, however, an antipyretic drug, such as *acetaminophen* 650 mg PO, is usually effective.
3. If the patient has documented fever with two consecutive blood transfusions, premedication with an antipyretic before

subsequent transfusions is indicated. If this step fails to prevent fever, washed RBCs can be given.

Pulmonary Edema

1. Stop the transfusion or slow the rate of transfusion, unless the patient urgently needs blood.
2. *Furosemide* 40 mg IV. If the patient is already receiving a diuretic or if there is renal insufficiency, a higher dose of furosemide may be required.
3. For the management of CHF, refer to Chapter 24, page 271. Volume overload, with subsequent pulmonary edema, should be anticipated in a patient with a history of CHF. This problem may be prevented by administering a diuretic (e.g., *furosemide* 40 mg IV) during the transfusion.

Laboratory-Related Problems: The Common Calls

Acid-Base Disorders

Most cases of acidemia or alkalemia are first discovered by measurement of arterial pH.

ACIDEMIA (pH ≤7.35)

First decide whether the acidemia is a respiratory acidemia (i.e., due to hypoventilation) or a metabolic acidemia (i.e., due to acid gain or HCO_3 loss).

Respiratory Acidemia

- pH ≤7.35
- P_{CO_2} ↑
- HCO_3 normal or ↑

Metabolic Acidemia

- pH ≤7.35
- P_{CO_2} normal or ↓
- HCO_3 ↓

The normal response to respiratory acidemia is an increase in HCO_3. An immediate increase in HCO_3 occurs because the increase in P_{CO_2} results in the generation of HCO_3, according to the law of mass action:

$$CO_2 + H_2O \rightleftharpoons H + HCO_3$$

Later, renal tubular preservation of HCO_3 occurs to buffer the change in pH. The expected increase in HCO_3 in *acute respiratory acidemia* is 0.1 (ΔP_{CO_2}). The expected increase in HCO_3 in *chronic respiratory acidemia* is 0.4 (ΔP_{CO_2}). When the HCO_3 is less than expected, a mixed respiratory and metabolic acidemia should be suspected. An HCO_3 greater than expected suggests a combined respiratory acidemia and metabolic alkalemia.

The normal respiratory response to metabolic acidemia is hyperventilation, with a decrease in P_{CO_2}. The expected decrease in P_{CO_2} in uncomplicated metabolic acidemia is 1 to 1.5 (ΔHCO_3). When the P_{CO_2} is higher than expected, a mixed metabolic and respiratory acidemia should be suspected. When the P_{CO_2} is lower than expected, a combined metabolic acidemia and respiratory alkalemia should be suspected.

Respiratory Acidemia

- pH ≤7.35
- P_{CO_2} ↑
- HCO_3 normal or ↑

Causes

1. Central nervous system (CNS) depression
   a. Drugs (e.g., morphine)
   b. Lesions of the respiratory center
2. Neuromuscular disorders
   a. Drugs (e.g., succinylcholine)
   b. Muscular disease
   c. Hypokalemia, hypophosphatemia
   d. Neuropathies
3. Respiratory disorders
   a. Acute airway obstruction
   b. Severe parenchymal lung disease
   c. Pleural effusion
   d. Pneumothorax
   e. Thoracic cage limitation

Manifestations

Respiratory acidemia occurs when there is a failure (either acute or chronic) in ventilation. The manifestations of respiratory acidemia are often overshadowed by those due to the accompanying hypoxia. Symptoms and signs directly attributable to CO_2 retention are uncommon with P_{CO_2} <70 mm Hg but include the following:

- Bradypnea
- Drowsiness
- Confusion
- Papilledema
- Asterixis

Management

Mild. pH 7.30 to 7.35. Patients with mild respiratory acidemia can be observed while reversible causes are searched for and corrected. Repeat arterial blood gases (ABGs) should be obtained, depending on the patient's clinical condition and course. The exception here is a patient with an acute asthmatic attack, in whom even a normal or certainly an elevated P_{CO_2} is a warning sign of impending respiratory failure.

Moderate. pH 7.20 to 7.29. A patient with moderate respiratory acidemia is in the gray zone. Any further decrease in pH would put the patient at risk for life-threatening ventricular dysrhythmias. If a readily reversible cause can be found, the patient can be carefully monitored while treatment measures are instituted. Such a patient should not be left alone until it is determined that he or she is improving. Sequential determinations of pH should be guided by the patient's clinical condition and course.

Severe. pH ≤7.19. This patient is at high risk for cessation of respiration, life-threatening ventricular dysrhythmias, or both. Call your resident for help now. The patient will likely require transfer to the intensive care unit (ICU) for monitoring, intubation, and mechanical ventilation while reversible causes are searched for.

Metabolic Acidemia

- pH ≤7.35
- PCO_2 normal or ↓
- HCO_3 ↓

Causes

The metabolic acidemias are conveniently divided into *normal anion gap* and *high anion gap* varieties. The normal anion gap $(Na + K) - (Cl + HCO_3) = 10$ to 12 mmol/L. Most of the normal anion gap is accounted for by negatively charged plasma proteins. Remember that for every decline in serum albumin of 10 g/L, you must add 4 to the calculated anion gap. Failure to correct for hypoalbuminemia may lead to the overlooking of serious acidemias of the high anion gap type.

Normal Anion Gap Acidemia

1. Loss of HCO_3
   a. Diarrhea, ileus, fistula
   b. High-output ileostomy
   c. Renal tubular acidosis
   d. Carbonic anhydrase inhibitors
2. Addition of H^+
   a. NH_4Cl
   b. HCl

High Anion Gap Acidemia

1. Lactic acidemia
2. Ketoacidosis (type 1 diabetes, alcohol, starvation)
3. Renal failure
4. Drugs (aspirin, ethylene glycol, methyl alcohol, toluene, paraldehyde)
5. High-flux dialysis acetate buffer

The change in anion gap should equal the change in HCO_3. Any deviation from this reveals a mixed acid-base disorder. Always remember to *calculate the osmolar gap* (see Chapter 34, pages 369 to 370) in high anion gap acidemias to determine whether ingestions have contributed to the abnormalities.

Occasionally, the pH may be normal, but the presence of a wide anion gap may be a clue to underlying metabolic acidemia.

Manifestations

The signs and symptoms of metabolic acidemia are nonspecific and include the following:
- Hyperventilation (in an effort to blow off CO_2)
- Fatigue
- Confusion → stupor → coma
- Decreased cardiac contractility
- Peripheral vasodilatation → hypotension

Management

Mild. pH 7.30 to 7.35.

Moderate. pH 7.20 to 7.29.

Severe. pH ≤7.19.

For all causes of metabolic acidemia, management involves reversal of the underlying cause. In most cases of mild or moderate metabolic acidemia, the acid-base disorder can be treated effectively by reversing the underlying condition. However, in some conditions (e.g., chronic renal failure), the condition is not easily reversed. In this situation, mild or moderate metabolic acidemia does not require treatment. Severe metabolic acidemia from chronic renal failure can be treated with PO or IV $NaHCO_3$, being careful not to precipitate volume overload.

For other causes of metabolic acidemia, it is occasionally necessary to raise the blood pH by administering $NaHCO_3$, but this is usually reserved for severe metabolic acidemias only. Some important precautions should be considered:

1. The amount of $NaHCO_3$ given depends on the pH and how effective and rapid the therapy for reversing the underlying cause is going to be. For instance, metabolic acidemia with a pH of 6.9 is a medical emergency and may require an initial dose of 150 mmol of IV $NaHCO_3$ while other resuscitation measures are instituted. Metabolic acidemia with a pH of 7.10 in a patient with diabetic ketoacidosis may require only 50 mmol of IV $NaHCO_3$ while insulin and fluids are administered. An estimate of the amount of bicarbonate required can be made by calculating the extracellular buffer deficit, as follows:

$$\text{Buffer deficit} = (\text{normal serum } HCO_3 - \text{measured serum } HCO_3)(\text{body weight in kg})(0.4),$$

where 0.4 is a correction factor representing the proportion of body weight composed of extracellular fluid (0.2) and the buffering provided by intracellular components. The initial dose of HCO_3 should be approximately half of the calculated buffer deficit. Full correction should not be attempted within the first 24 hours because of the risk of delayed compensation and alkalemia with tetany, seizures, and ventricular dysrhythmias.

The HCO_3 should be diluted (50 to 150 mmol/L is achieved by adding one to three 50-mmol vials to 1 L of 5% dextrose in water [D5W]) and given slowly, because direct infusion of undiluted $NaHCO_3$ can result in fatal ventricular dysrhythmias.

2. In the presence of cardiac arrest, metabolic acidemia can be treated with HCO_3, but only after alveolar ventilation is ensured, because there is a risk of further depression of respiration from a shift in intracellular pH in the respiratory control center in the CNS. When ventilation is ensured, an initial dose of 1 mmol/kg body weight of HCO_3 can be given by rapid IV injection, with repeated doses of 0.5 mmol/kg body weight every 10 minutes during continued cardiac arrest.

Remember that IV $NaHCO_3$ is a significant sodium load and may put a patient in congestive heart failure (CHF). Do not substitute one problem for another.

ALKALEMIA (pH ≥7.45)

First decide whether the patient has a respiratory or a metabolic alkalemia.

Respiratory Alkalemia

- pH ≥7.45
- P_{CO_2} ↓
- HCO_3 ↓

Metabolic Alkalemia

- pH ≥7.45
- P_{CO_2} normal or ↑
- HCO_3 ↑

The normal response to respiratory alkalemia is a decrease in HCO_3. An immediate decrease in HCO_3 occurs because the decrease in P_{CO_2} results in a reduction of HCO_3, according to the law of mass action:

$$CO_2 + H_2O \rightleftharpoons H + HCO_3$$

Later, renal tubular loss of HCO_3 occurs to buffer the change in pH. The expected decrease in HCO_3 in acute respiratory alkalemia is 0.2 (ΔP_{CO_2}). The expected decrease in HCO_3 in chronic respiratory alkalemia is 0.4 (ΔP_{CO_2}). When the HCO_3 is greater than expected, a combined respiratory and metabolic alkalemia should be suspected. When the HCO_3 is less than expected, a combined respiratory alkalemia and metabolic acidemia should be suspected.

The normal response to metabolic alkalemia is hypoventilation, with an increase in the P_{CO_2}. The expected increase in uncomplicated metabolic alkalemia is 0.6 (ΔHCO_3). When the P_{CO_2} is greater than expected, a combined metabolic alkalemia and respiratory acidemia should be suspected. When the P_{CO_2} is less than expected, a combined metabolic and respiratory alkalemia should be suspected.

Respiratory Alkalemia

- pH ≥7.45
- P_{CO_2} ↓
- HCO_3 ↓

Causes

1. Physiologic conditions (pregnancy, high altitude)
2. CNS disorders (anxiety, pain, fever, tumor)
3. Drugs (aspirin, nicotine, progesterone)
4. Pulmonary disorders (CHF, pulmonary embolism, asthma, pneumonia)
5. Miscellaneous (hepatic failure, hyperthyroidism)

Manifestations

- Confusion
- Numbness, tingling, paresthesias (perioral, hands, feet)
- Lightheadedness
- Tetany in severe cases

Management

Mild. pH 7.45 to 7.55.

Moderate. pH 7.56 to 7.69.

Severe. pH ≥7.70.

Mild respiratory alkalemia is commonly seen in physiologic conditions (pregnancy, high altitude) and in these cases requires no treatment. Any of the other causes listed may result in mild respiratory alkalemia, and many patients can be treated symptomatically (e.g., a febrile patient can be treated with antipyretics, a patient in pain can be treated with analgesics, and an anxious patient can be treated with reassurance or sedation). In addition to these measures, more pronounced degrees of respiratory alkalemia due to anxiety can be treated by rebreathing into a paper bag. The only effective treatment for the other causes listed is eliminating the underlying condition.

Metabolic Alkalemia

- pH ≥7.45
- P_{CO_2} normal or ↑
- HCO_3 ↑

Causes

1. With extracellular volume depletion and low urinary chloride (usually <10 mEq/L)
   a. Gastrointestinal (GI) losses
      (1) Vomiting
      (2) GI drainage (nasogastric suction)
      (3) Chloride-wasting diarrhea
      (4) Villous adenoma
   b. Renal losses
      (1) Diuretic therapy
      (2) Posthypercapnia
      (3) Nonreabsorbable anions
      (4) Penicillin, carbenicillin, ticarcillin
      (5) Bartter's syndrome
2. With extracellular volume expansion and the presence of urinary chloride (usually >20 mEq/L)
   a. Mineralocorticoid excess
      (1) Endogenous
         (a) Hyperaldosteronism
         (b) Cushing's syndrome
      (2) Exogenous
         (a) Glucocorticoids
         (b) Mineralocorticoids
         (c) Carbenoxolone
         (d) Licorice excess
   b. Alkali ingestion
   c. Poststarvation feeding

Manifestations

There are no specific signs or symptoms of metabolic alkalemia. Severe alkalemia may result in the following:

- Apathy
- Confusion or stupor

Management

Mild. pH 7.45 to 7.55.

Moderate. pH 7.56 to 7.69.

Severe. pH ≥7.70.

Beyond correcting the underlying cause, mild or moderate metabolic alkalemia rarely requires specific treatment. *Metabolic alkalemia associated with extracellular fluid volume depletion* usually responds to an infusion of normal saline, which enhances renal HCO_3 excretion.

Note that associated electrolyte abnormalities (particularly hypokalemia) may be more threatening to the patient's well-being than the metabolic alkalemia is. Attention to concomitant electrolyte disorders is very important.

In *diuretic-induced alkalemia,* administration of KCl may improve the alkalemia.

If the patient is *volume overloaded* and has a metabolic alkalemia, *acetazolamide* 250 to 500 mg PO or IV every 8 hours enhances the renal HCO_3 excretion and may be helpful.

In *Bartter's syndrome,* the alkalemia may respond to prostaglandin synthetase inhibitors, such as indomethacin.

It is very unusual to require an acidifying agent, such as NH_4Cl or dilute HCl, even for severe metabolic alkalemia. Such agents should be given only under the direct guidance of your resident and the patient's attending physician.

Anemia

Serum hemoglobin (Hb) is one of the most common laboratory determinations made in hospitalized patients. Remember that Hb is a *concentration*, and its value can be modified by both a change in its *content* and a change in its *diluent* (plasma). For instance, a patient's Hb may be elevated (i.e., in the "normal" range) despite a sudden loss of intravascular volume, as is seen in an acute hemorrhage. Because of the possibility of transfusion-related illnesses, one must avoid the reflex administration of red blood cell (RBC) transfusions to correct a low Hb level. *Remember to treat the patient, not the laboratory value.*

Causes

1. Blood loss
   a. Acute
      (1) Gastrointestinal (GI) hemorrhage
      (2) Trauma
      (3) Concealed hemorrhage
         (a) Ruptured aortic aneurysm
         (b) Ruptured ectopic pregnancy
         (c) Retroperitoneal hematoma
         (d) Postsurgical bleeding
   b. Chronic
      (1) GI bleeding
      (2) Uterine bleeding
2. Inadequate production of RBCs
   a. Anemia of chronic disease (chronic inflammation, uremia, endocrine failure, liver disease)
   b. Iron deficiency
   c. Megaloblastic anemias (vitamin B_{12} and folate deficiency, drugs, inherited)
   d. Sideroblastic anemias (drugs, alcohol, malignancy, rheumatoid arthritis, inherited)
   e. Acquired disorders of marrow stem cells (aplastic anemia, myelodysplastic syndromes, chemotherapy, drugs)
3. Hemolysis
   a. Extrinsic factors (immune hemolysis, splenomegaly, mechanical trauma, infection, microangiopathic hemolytic anemia)

   b. Membrane defects (e.g., hereditary spherocytosis, paroxysmal nocturnal hemoglobinuria)

   c. Internal RBC defects (e.g., thalassemia, sickle cell disease)

   d. Acute or delayed RBC transfusion reactions

Manifestations

The manifestations of anemia depend on the underlying medical conditions, the severity of the anemia, and the rapidity with which it develops. The body's reaction to an acute reduction in RBC mass is usually manifested by (compensatory) alterations in the cardiovascular and respiratory systems.

Acute anemias due to hemorrhage result in symptoms and signs of intravascular volume depletion, including the following:

- Pallor, diaphoresis, tachypnea
- Cold, clammy extremities
- Hypotension, tachycardia
- Shock

Anemias that develop slowly over weeks or months are not usually accompanied by signs of intravascular volume depletion. In these cases, symptoms and signs are often not so obvious and may vary, depending on the presence of disease in other organ systems.

Common Symptoms

- Fatigue, lethargy
- Dyspnea
- Palpitations
- Worsening of symptoms in patients with angina pectoris or claudication, or presentation with a transient ischemic attack (TIA)
- GI disturbances (due to shunting of blood from the splanchnic bed)—anorexia, nausea, bowel irregularity
- Abnormal menstrual patterns

Signs

- Pallor
- Tachypnea
- Tachycardia, wide pulse pressure, hyperdynamic precordium
- Jaundice or splenomegaly (in hemolytic anemias)

Management

Assess the Severity

The severity of the situation should be determined according to the level of Hb, the patient's volume status, the rapidity with which the anemia developed, and the likelihood that the underlying process will continue unabated.

Treatment of a Patient Who Is in Shock or Volume Depleted

An acute anemia due to blood loss (and thus intravascular volume depletion) results in compensatory tachycardia and tachypnea. If full hemodynamic compensation is inadequate, hypotension or shock will result. In your assessment of the patient's volume status, do not forget to check for postural changes (see Chapter 3, pages 10 to 11), which may be the earliest manifestation of acute blood loss.

1. Notify your resident.
2. Ensure that at least one—preferably, two—large-bore (size 16 if possible) intravenous (IV) line is in place.
3. If there is evidence of active bleeding, ensure that there is blood on hold. If not, order stat crossmatch for 2, 4, or 6 units of packed RBCs, depending on your estimate of blood loss.
4. **Replenish intravascular volume by giving IV fluids.** The best immediate choice is a crystalloid (normal saline [NS] or Ringer's lactate), which stays in the intravascular space at least temporarily. Albumin or banked plasma can be given, but it is expensive, carries a risk of virus transmission, and is not always available. When a new, severe anemia is associated with intravascular volume depletion, the assumption is that blood has been lost from the intravascular space—so, ideally, blood should be replaced. If there is no blood on hold for the patient, a stat crossmatch usually takes 50 minutes. If blood is on hold, it should be available at the bedside in 30 minutes. In an emergency, O-negative blood may be given, although this practice is usually reserved for acute trauma victims. If the patient refuses blood or blood products, refer to Chapter 13, page 113.

   > Transfusion-related infections can be minimized by transfusing only when necessary. *Rule of thumb:* Maintain the Hb level at 90 to 100 g/L.

5. **Order the appropriate IV rate,** which depends on the patient's volume status. Shock requires IV fluid wide open through at least two large-bore IV sites. Elevating the IV bag, squeezing the IV bag, or using IV pressure cuffs may help speed the rate of delivery of the solution. *Mild or moderate volume depletion* can be treated with 500 to 1000 mL of NS given as rapidly as possible, with serial determinations of volume status and assessment of cardiac status. If blood is not at the bedside within 30 minutes, delegate someone to find out the reason for the delay.

   Note: Aggressive volume replacement in a patient with a history of congestive heart failure may result in pulmonary edema. Do not overshoot the mark.

6. **Determine the site of hemorrhage.**
   a. Look for obvious signs of external bleeding—from IV sites, skin lesions, hematemesis, menstrual bleeding.

b. Examine for signs of occult blood loss.
    (1) Perform a rectal examination to look for melena.
    (2) Occult blood loss should be suspected if there is swelling at biopsy or surgical sites (e.g., flank swelling after renal biopsy, ascites after liver biopsy) or if there are flank or periumbilical ecchymoses (possible hemoperitoneum).
    (3) If the patient is woman in her childbearing years, a ruptured ectopic pregnancy must be considered. If indicated, a pelvic examination should be performed by an experienced physician.
    (4) If a ruptured thoracic or abdominal aortic aneurysm is likely, immediate surgical referral is necessary.
7. Review the chart for exacerbating factors that may contribute to ongoing hemorrhage (e.g., administration of aspirin, heparin, warfarin, or thrombolytic agents or presence of coagulopathies) and for recent pertinent laboratory values (activated partial thromboplastin time [aPTT], prothrombin time [PT], platelets).
8. Request surgical consultation when appropriate.

Treatment of a Patient Who Is Normovolemic

Patients can tolerate even severe anemia (Hb <70 g/L) if it develops slowly. Mild chronic anemias (Hb 100 to 120 g/L) in the context of normal intravascular volume often do not alter the vital signs. If the patient is normovolemic, transfusion therapy is seldom warranted on an urgent basis. If you have excluded the presence of active hemorrhage, the anemia must be due to (1) chronic blood loss, (2) inadequate production of RBCs, or (3) hemolysis.

1. An unexpected Hb of <100 g/L merits a repeat measurement to exclude laboratory error while other assessments are taking place. An asymptomatic patient with mild anemia (Hb 100 to 120 g/L) and normal vital signs usually can wait if other problems of higher priority exist. One must always keep in mind, however, that if active bleeding is responsible for the anemia, a stable patient may become unstable very quickly.
2. **What is the patient's usual Hb?** Look in the current or old chart to determine whether the anemia is a new finding. If the current Hb is more than 10 or 20 g/L lower than previous values, assume that the underlying cause of anemia has worsened or a second factor has developed (e.g., a patient with a chronic disease, such as systemic lupus erythematosus, may normally have an Hb of 90 g/L; a new value of 75 g/L may represent further marrow suppression, hemolysis, or new onset of bleeding).
3. If the patient is comfortable and has a normal cardiovascular examination and your examination reveals no suspicion of active bleeding, further investigation can take place in the morning. Several baseline studies are helpful in pointing you

Oval macrocyte
of megaloblastic
anemia

 Target cell of
liver disease

Sickle cell
of sickle
cell anemia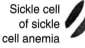

 Normal RBC

Microcytic
hypochromic
cell of iron
deficiency

Burr cells
of uremia

Spherocytes
seen in hemolysis

Helmet cells
of traumatic
hemolysis

Figure 29–1 Blood smear demonstrating helpful diagnostic features associated with specific anemias.

in the right direction to diagnose the cause of the anemia:

a. **Measurement of RBC volume.** The mean corpuscular volume (MCV) is useful in classifying the anemias due to decreased RBC production (microcytic, normocytic, macrocytic).

b. **Examination of the blood smear** by an individual experienced in hematology often provides valuable clues for diagnosing specific anemias (Fig. 29–1).

c. A **reticulocyte count** provides a measure of marrow erythropoiesis. An elevated reticulocyte count suggests hemolysis, recent hemorrhage, or a recently treated chronic anemia (e.g., vitamin B_{12} deficiency). An inappropriately low reticulocyte count suggests a failure to produce RBCs (e.g., untreated iron, vitamin B_{12}, or folate deficiency or anemia of chronic disease).

Calcium Disorders

HYPERCALCEMIA

Causes

1. Increased intake or absorption
   a. Vitamin D or A intoxication
   b. Excessive calcium supplementation
   c. Milk-alkali syndrome (excessive antacid ingestion)
   d. Sarcoidosis and other granulomatous diseases
2. Increased production or mobilization from bone
   a. Primary hyperparathyroidism*
   b. Neoplasm.* There are four mechanisms for hypercalcemia of malignancy:
      (1) Bony metastasis (prostate, thyroid, kidney, breast, lung)
      (2) Parathyroid hormone (PTH)–like substance elaborated by tumor cells (lung, kidney, ovary, colon)
      (3) Prostaglandin E_2, which increases bony resorption (multiple myeloma)
      (4) Osteoclast-activating factor (multiple myeloma, lymphoproliferative disorders)
   c. Severe secondary hyperparathyroidism associated with renal failure
   d. Paget's disease
   e. Immobilization
   f. Hyperthyroidism
   g. Adrenal insufficiency
   h. Acromegaly
   i. Sarcoidosis. In addition to sarcoidosis increasing absorption from the gastrointestinal (GI) tract, there is an increased conversion of 25(OH) vitamin D to the active form, $1,25(OH)_2$ vitamin D.
   j. Chronic lithium use
3. Decreased excretion
   a. Thiazide diuretics
   b. Familial hypocalciuric hypercalcemia

---

*Primary hyperparathyroidism and tumors account for 90% of cases of hypercalcemia.

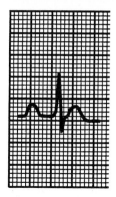

Figure 30–1 Hypercalcemia (short QT interval, prolonged PR interval).

Manifestations

The manifestations of hypercalcemia are numerous and nonspecific, often referred to as "bones, stones, and groans."

HEENT	Corneal calcification (band keratopathy)
CVS	Short QT interval, prolonged PR interval (Fig. 30–1), dysrhythmias, digoxin sensitivity, hypertension
GI	Anorexia, nausea, vomiting, constipation, abdominal pain, pancreatitis ("groans")
GU	Polyuria, polydipsia, nephrolithiasis ("stones")
Neuro	Restlessness, delirium, dementia, psychosis, lethargy, coma
MSS	Muscle weakness, hyporeflexia, bone pain, fractures ("bones")
Misc	Hyperchlorhydric metabolic acidosis

Management

How severe is the situation?

The severity of the situation should be determined according to the serum calcium concentration, the rate of progression, and the presence or absence of symptoms. It is important to recognize that most laboratories measure total serum calcium (ionized plus albumin bound), but the primary determinant of the physiologic effect is the ionized component.

If the patient is hypoalbuminemic, a correction factor can be used to estimate the total calcium concentration. For every 10 g/L of hypoalbuminemia, add 0.2 mmol/L to the serum calcium value—for example, if the measured serum calcium value is 2.6 mmol/L (the upper limit of normal) but the serum albumin value is low at 30 g/L (with an anticipated normal concentration of 40 g/L), the correct serum calcium value is 0.2 + 2.6 = 2.8 mmol/L (mild elevation).

How high is the serum calcium level?
- Normal range = 2.2 to 2.6 mmol/L
- Mild elevation = 2.6 to 2.9 mmol/L
- Moderate elevation = 2.9 to 3.2 mmol/L
- Severe elevation = >3.2 mmol/L

Is there a progressive cause that is likely to result in further increases?
     If the situation is progressive, the patient requires immediate treatment.

Is the patient symptomatic?
     Any symptomatic patient requires immediate treatment.

Treatment of Severe Hypercalcemia

Severe hypercalcemia (>3.2 mmol/L) requires immediate treatment because of the danger of a fatal cardiac dysrhythmia.
1. *Correct volume depletion and expand extracellular volume.* Give normal saline (NS) 500 mL IV as fast as possible. Further NS boluses can be given, depending on the volume status. Titrate the NS maintenance rate to keep the patient slightly volume expanded. If the patient has a history of congestive heart failure (CHF), this volume expansion should be undertaken in the intensive care unit/cardiac care unit (ICU/CCU) to allow close monitoring of the volume status. A reduction in the serum calcium level is expected because of hemodilution and because increased urinary sodium excretion is accompanied by increased calcium excretion.
2. *Establish diuresis >2500 mL/day.* If this cannot be achieved by volume expansion alone, *furosemide* 20 to 40 mg IV every 2 to 4 hours may be given. Care must be taken not to induce volume depletion with the administration of furosemide. The patient may require 4 to 10 L of NS per day to maintain the volume-expanded state. Furosemide inhibits the tubular reabsorption of calcium, thus increasing calcium excretion by the kidneys. Do not use thiazides to establish diuresis, because they elevate the serum calcium level.
3. *Dialysis.* Occasionally, when the serum calcium level is extremely high (e.g., >4.5 mmol/L) and a saline diuresis cannot be achieved, hemodialysis or peritoneal dialysis may be required.
4. *If hypercalcemia is secondary to neoplasm,* in addition to the administration of NS and furosemide (as previously discussed), one of the following medications may be of value:
   a. Corticosteroids: *prednisone* 40 to 100 mg PO daily or *hydrocortisone* 200 to 500 mg IV daily in divided doses.
      > Steroids antagonize the peripheral action of vitamin D (decreased absorption, decreased mobilization from bone, and decreased renal tubular reabsorption of calcium).

   b. *Plicamycin* 25 µg/kg in 1 L of 5% dextrose in water (D5W) or NS IV over 4 to 6 hours.

> Plicamycin inhibits bone resorption. The onset of action is 48 hours.

   c. Bisphosphonates inhibit bone resorption and are effective agents in the control of cancer-associated hypercalcemia. *Etidronate disodium may be given in a dose of* 7.5 mg/kg IV daily for 3 days. Each daily dose should be diluted in 250 mL NS or D5W and given IV over a period of at least 2 hours. Alternatively, give *pamidronate* 60 to 90 mg in 1 L NS or D5W IV over 24 hours.

   d. *Indomethacin* 50 mg PO every 8 hours.

> Indomethacin inhibits the synthesis of prostaglandin E_2, which is produced by some solid tumors (e.g., of the breast).

   e. Synthetic salmon calcitonin may temporarily lower the serum calcium concentration but should not be initiated at night before first skin-testing the patient for allergy (see package insert).

Treatment of Moderate Hypercalcemia or Symptomatic Mild Hypercalcemia

Moderate hypercalcemia (2.9 to 3.2 mmol/L) or symptomatic mild hypercalcemia (2.6 to 2.9 mmol/L) should be managed as follows:

1. *Correct volume depletion and expand extracellular fluid volume* with NS 500 mL IV given over 1 to 2 hours. More NS can be given at a rate to keep the patient slightly volume expanded.
2. *Establish diuresis >2500 mL/day* if volume expansion alone is unsuccessful in lowering the serum calcium.
3. Oral phosphate 0.5 to 3 g/day, depending on GI tolerance (flatulence, diarrhea), may be given to patients with low or normal serum phosphate levels.

Treatment of Asymptomatic Mild Hypercalcemia

Asymptomatic mild hypercalcemia (2.6 to 2.9 mmol/L) does not require immediate treatment. The appropriate investigations can be ordered in the morning.

HYPOCALCEMIA

Causes

1. Decreased intake or absorption
   a. Malabsorption
   b. Intestinal bypass surgery
   c. Short bowel syndrome
   d. Vitamin D deficiency

2. Decreased production or mobilization from bone
   a. Hypoparathyroidism (after subtotal thyroidectomy or parathyroidectomy)
   b. Pseudohypoparathyroidism (PTH resistance)
   c. Vitamin D deficiency [decreased production of 25(OH) vitamin D or 1,25(OH)$_2$ vitamin D]
   d. Acute hyperphosphatemia (tumor lysis, acute renal failure, rhabdomyolysis)
   e. Acute pancreatitis
   f. Hypomagnesemia
   g. Alkalosis (hyperventilation, vomiting, fistula)
   h. Neoplasm
      (1) Paradoxical hypocalcemia associated with osteoblastic metastasis (lung, breast, prostate)
      (2) Medullary carcinoma of the thyroid (calcitonin-producing tumor)
      (3) Rapid tumor lysis with phosphate release
3. Increased excretion
   a. Chronic renal failure
   b. Drugs (aminoglycosides, loop diuretics)

Manifestations

The earliest symptoms are paresthesias of the lips, fingers, and toes.

HEENT	Papilledema, diplopia
CVS	Prolonged QT interval without U waves (Fig. 30–2)
GI	Abdominal cramps
Neuro	Confusion, irritability, depression
	Hyperactive tendon reflexes
	Carpopedal spasm, laryngospasm (stridor), tetany
	Generalized tonic-clonic seizures
	Paresthesias of lips, fingers, toes

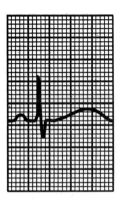

Figure 30–2 Hypocalcemia (long QT interval).

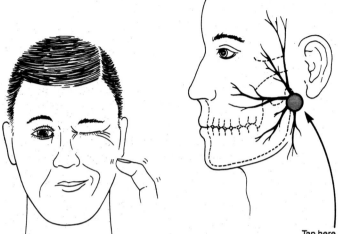

Tap here

Figure 30–3 Chvostek's sign. Facial muscle spasm elicited by tapping the facial nerve immediately anterior to the earlobe and below the zygomatic arch.

Special tests	*Chvostek's sign* (Fig. 30–3): facial muscle spasm elicited by tapping the facial nerve immediately anterior to the earlobe and below the zygomatic arch (this is a normal finding in 10% of the population)
	Trousseau's sign (Fig. 30–4): carpal spasm elicited by occluding the arterial blood flow to the forearm for 3 to 5 minutes

Management

How severe is the situation?

The severity of the situation should be determined based on the serum calcium and phosphate concentrations and the presence or absence of symptoms. If the serum albumin is not within the normal range, a correction factor can be used to estimate the total serum calcium (ionized plus albumin bound). See page 327 for a discussion of this correction factor.

How low is the serum calcium level?

- Normal range = 2.2 to 2.6 mmol/L
- Mild depletion = 1.9 to 2.2 mmol/L
- Moderate depletion = 1.5 to 1.9 mmol/L
- Severe depletion = <1.5 mmol/L

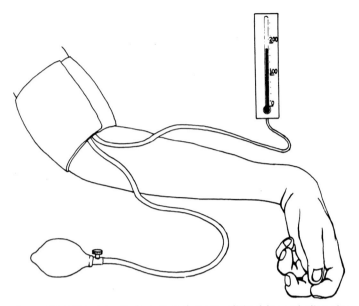

Figure 30–4 Trousseau's sign. Carpal spasm elicited by occluding the arterial blood flow to the forearm for 3 to 5 minutes.

What is the serum phosphate concentration?

If the serum phosphate concentration is markedly elevated (>6 mmol/L) in severe hypocalcemia, correction of hyperphosphatemia must be accomplished with IV glucose and insulin before calcium is given, to avoid metastatic calcification.

Is the patient symptomatic?

Hypocalcemic patients who are asymptomatic do not require urgent correction with IV calcium.

Is the patient receiving digoxin?

Caution is required if the patient is receiving digoxin, because calcium potentiates its action. Ideally, if IV calcium administration is required, the patient should have continuous electrocardiographic monitoring.

Treatment of Severe Symptomatic Hypocalcemia

Severe symptomatic hypocalcemia (<1.5 mmol/L) requires immediate treatment because of the danger of respiratory failure from laryngospasm.

1. Provided the patient's PO_4 is normal or low, give 10 to 20 mL (93 mg elemental calcium/10 mL) of 10% solution of *calcium*

gluconate IV in 100 mL D5W over 30 minutes. If the patient has evidence of tetany or laryngeal stridor, the same dose should be given over 2 minutes as a direct injection, that is, calcium gluconate 10% solution 10 to 20 mL IV over 2 minutes. Oral calcium can be started immediately: 1 to 2 g of *elemental calcium* PO three times a day. If the corrected serum calcium value is <1.9 mmol/L 6 hours after initiating this treatment, a calcium infusion is required. Add 10 mL (93 mg elemental calcium) of a 10% calcium gluconate solution to 500 mL D5W and infuse over 6 hours. If the serum calcium value is not within the normal range after 6 hours of this infusion, 5 mL (46.5 mg elemental calcium) of calcium gluconate can be added to the initial infusion dose every 6 hours until a satisfactory serum calcium level is achieved. A postparathyroidectomy patient may require 100 to 150 mg of elemental calcium per hour. Once a satisfactory response has been achieved with IV calcium gluconate, oral replacement may begin in doses of 0.5 to 2 g elemental calcium three times a day.

2. If the patient is hyperphosphatemic (PO_4 >6 mmol/L), correction with glucose and insulin is required before the administration of IV calcium. Consult the nephrology services immediately.

Treatment of Mild and Moderate Asymptomatic Hypocalcemia

Mild and moderate asymptomatic hypocalcemia does not require urgent IV calcium replacement. Oral calcium replacement with *elemental calcium* 1000 to 1500 mg/day can be started to achieve a corrected serum calcium level in the 2.2 to 2.6 mmol/L range. Long-term treatment with oral calcium or vitamin D depends on the cause, which can be evaluated in the morning.

Coagulation Disorders

While on call, you will be confronted with abnormal results of tests of hemostasis. These must always be interpreted in the clinical context in which the measurements were made. Bleeding is the most common clinical manifestation of a coagulation disorder, and the type of bleeding can alert you to the probable type of disorder present.

Patients with *vessel* or *platelet abnormalities* may have petechiae, purpura, or easy bruising. The bleeding characteristically occurs superficially (e.g., oozing from mucous membranes or intravenous sites). The bleeding of scurvy is seen only rarely in North America and is usually manifested by perifollicular hemorrhages, although gingival bleeding and intramuscular hematomas also may occur.

Bleeding due to *coagulation factor deficiencies* may occur spontaneously and in deeper organ sites (e.g., visceral hemorrhages and hemarthroses), and it tends to be delayed and prolonged. Bleeding associated with *thrombolytic agents* is usually manifested by continuous oozing from intravenous sites.

TESTS TO ASSESS HEMOSTASIS

Three tests are commonly used to assess hemostasis—prothrombin time (PT), activated partial thromboplastin time (aPTT), and platelet count. A fourth test, bleeding time, is used infrequently because it is rarely helpful in making a specific diagnosis and it carries the risk of accidental exposure to hepatitis and human immunodeficiency virus (HIV). Laboratory features of the common coagulation disorders are listed in Table 31-1.

Prothrombin Time

The one-stage PT tests the *extrinsic coagulation system* (Fig. 31-1). It is affected by deficiencies in factors I, II, V, VII, and X. However, antagonists of the extrinsic system, including unfractionated heparin, activated antithrombin III, and fibrin degradation products, can prolong the PT.

TABLE 31–1 Laboratory Features of Common Coagulation Disorders

Disorder	Diagnostic Laboratory Test				
	aPTT	PT	Platelets	Bleeding Time	Other
Vessel Abnormalities					
Vasculitis	Normal	Normal	Normal	Normal or ↑	C3, C4 C1Q binding
Increased vascular fragility	Normal	Normal	Normal	↑	
Hereditary connective tissue disorders	Normal	Normal	Normal	↑	
Paraproteinemias	Normal	Normal	Normal	↑	
Coagulation Factor Abnormalities					
Unfractionated heparin	↑	↑ or Normal	Normal or ↓	Normal or ↑	
Low-molecular-weight heparin	Normal	Normal	Normal	Normal or ↑	
Warfarin	Normal or ↑	↑	Normal	Normal	

Continued

TABLE 31–1 Laboratory Features of Common Coagulation Disorders—cont'd

	Diagnostic Laboratory Test				
Disorder	aPTT	PT	Platelets	Bleeding Time	Other
Vitamin K deficiency	↑	↑	Normal	Normal	
DIC	↑	↑	↓	Normal or ↑*	↑ Fibrin degradation products; ↓ fibrinogen
Factor VIII deficiency	↑	Normal	Normal	Normal	↓ Factor VIII assay
Factor IX deficiency	↑	Normal	Normal	Normal	Normal factor IX assay
Von Willebrand's disease	Normal or ↑	Normal	Normal	Normal or ↑	Normal or ↓ factor VIII assay; ↓ factor VIII antigen ↓ Ristocetin cofactor
Liver disease	↑	↑	Normal or ↓	Normal or ↑	
Platelet Disorders					
Thrombocytopenia	Normal	Normal	↓	Normal or ↑*	
Impaired platelet function	Normal	Normal	Normal	↑	

*Depends on degree of thrombocytopenia.
aPTT, activated partial thromboplastin time; DIC, disseminated intravascular coagulation; PT, prothrombin time.

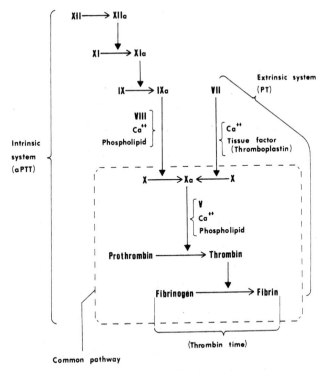

Figure 31–1 The coagulation cascade.

Disorders Associated with Prothrombin Time Prolongation

- Coagulation factor abnormalities
- Oral anticoagulants
- Vitamin K deficiency
- Liver disease
- Disseminated intravascular coagulation (DIC)
- Unfractionated heparin (variable)

Activated Partial Thromboplastin Time

The aPTT is a test of the *intrinsic coagulation system* (see Fig. 31–1). It is most sensitive to deficiencies and abnormalities in the sequence of procoagulant activities that occur before factor X activation.

Disorders Associated with Activated Partial Thromboplastin Time Prolongation

- Circulating anticoagulant
- Unfractionated heparin
- Factor VIII, factor IX deficiency
- Von Willebrand's disease (variable)
- DIC
- Vitamin K deficiency
- Oral anticoagulants (variable)

A frequent benign cause of aPTT prolongation in the hospital is the presence of an acquired anticoagulant, such as the lupus erythematosus anticoagulant. This situation can be differentiated from a factor deficiency by demonstrating failure to normalize the aPTT when a sample of the plasma of a patient with an acquired anticoagulant is mixed with normal plasma 50:50.

Note that low-molecular-weight heparin (LMWH) does not prolong the PT or aPTT. It exerts its anticoagulant effect by binding to antithrombin III, resulting in anti–factor Xa and IIa activity.

Platelet Count

The platelet count is a reflection of the production and destruction (sequestration) of platelets.

Disorders Associated with Low Platelet Count

Decreased Marrow Production

- Marrow replacement by tumor, granuloma (e.g., tuberculosis, sarcoid), fibrous tissue
- Storage disease (e.g., Gaucher's disease)
- Marrow injury by drugs (e.g., sulfonamides, chloramphenicol)
- Defective maturation (e.g., vitamin B_{12} or folate deficiency)

Increased Peripheral Destruction

IMMUNE MEDIATED
- Drugs (e.g., quinine, quinidine, heparin)
- Connective tissue disorders (e.g., systemic lupus erythematosus [SLE])
- Lymphoproliferative disorders (e.g., chronic lymphocytic leukemia)
- HIV infection
- Idiopathic
- Post-transfusion purpura

NON–IMMUNE MEDIATED
- Consumption (e.g., DIC, thrombotic thrombocytopenic purpura [TTP], prosthetic valves)
- Dilutional (e.g., massive transfusion)

- For instance, any cause of splenomegaly

Factitious Thrombocytopenia

Some patients have platelets that are susceptible to clumping when exposed to edetate disodium (EDTA), a preservative used in the lavender-topped blood collection tubes. This platelet clumping results in a falsely low platelet count when the blood specimen is read by an autoanalyzer. To diagnose factitious thrombocytopenia, verify platelet clumping by direct examination of the blood smear. An accurate platelet count can be obtained in these patients by collecting a blood sample in a sodium citrate (blue-topped) tube.

VESSEL OR PLATELET FUNCTION ABNORMALITIES

If the patient has a normal PT, aPTT, and platelet count and is not receiving LMWH, bleeding can still occur. This may be a result of *vessel abnormalities* or *abnormal platelet function.*

Vessel Abnormalities (Vascular Factor)

Hereditary Disorders

- Hereditary hemorrhagic telangiectasia
- Ehlers-Danlos syndrome
- Marfan's syndrome
- Pseudoxanthoma elasticum
- Osteogenesis imperfecta

Acquired Disorders

VASCULITIS
- Schönlein-Henoch purpura
- SLE
- Polyarteritis nodosa
- Rheumatoid arthritis
- Cryoglobulinemia

INCREASED VASCULAR FRAGILITY
- Senile purpura
- Cushing's syndrome
- Scurvy

Impaired Platelet Function

Hereditary Disorders

- Von Willebrand's disease
- Bernard-Soulier disease
- Glanzmann's thrombasthenia

Acquired Disorders

- Drugs (e.g., aspirin; clopidogrel; ticlopidine; glycoprotein IIb/IIIa inhibitors; nonsteroidal anti-inflammatory drugs [NSAIDs]; antibiotics such as high-dose penicillin, cephalosporins, nitrofurantoin)
- Uremia
- Paraproteins (e.g., amyloidosis, multiple myeloma, Waldenström's macroglobulinemia)
- Myeloproliferative and lymphoproliferative disease (e.g., chronic granulocytic leukemia, essential thrombocytosis)
- Post–cardiopulmonary bypass

BLEEDING IN COAGULATION DISORDERS

Manifestations

Bleeding in a patient with a coagulation disorder is of concern for two reasons:

1. Progressive loss of intravascular volume, if uncorrected, may lead to hypovolemic shock, with inadequate perfusion of vital organs.
2. Hemorrhage into specific organ sites may produce local tissue or organ injury (e.g., intracerebral hemorrhage, epidural hemorrhage with spinal cord compression, hemarthrosis).

TTP characteristically occurs with a combination of hemolytic anemia, thrombocytopenia, fever, neurologic disorders, and renal dysfunction. The *hemolytic uremic syndrome* has a presentation similar to that of TTP, but without the neurologic manifestations. These two syndromes can be distinguished from *DIC*, in which prolonged aPTT and PT, reduced fibrinogen level, and elevated fibrin degradation products are seen. DIC most often occurs in the context of infection (e.g., gram-negative sepsis), obstetric catastrophe, malignancy (e.g., prostate cancer), and tissue damage or shock.

Management

Vessel Abnormalities

Treatment of bleeding due to vessel abnormalities usually consists of treatment of the underlying disorder.

1. Serious bleeding due to *hereditary disorders of connective tissue* and to hereditary hemorrhagic telangiectasia most often requires local mechanical or surgical measures at the site of hemorrhage to control blood loss. In some patients with hereditary hemorrhagic telangiectasia, bleeding may be controlled with aminocaproic acid.[1]

2. In the *vasculitides*, control of bleeding is best achieved by the use of corticosteroids, other immunosuppressive agents, or both.
3. There is no good treatment for the increased vascular fragility that results in senile purpura. Purpura due to *Cushing's syndrome* is preventable with normalization of plasma cortisol levels. However, in a patient receiving therapeutic corticosteroids, the underlying indication for therapy often prevents a significant reduction in steroid levels. Hemorrhages associated with *scurvy* do not recur after adequate dietary supplementation of ascorbic acid.

Coagulation Factor Abnormalities

Treatment of coagulation factor abnormalities is dependent on the specific factor deficiency or deficiencies.

1. *Specific factor deficiencies* should always be treated in consultation with a hematologist. Factor VIII deficiency (hemophilia A) can be treated with fresh frozen plasma or cryoprecipitate, but factor VIII concentrate is the treatment of choice. Nonblood products may also be of benefit, such as desmopressin acetate (DDAVP) injection or aminocaproic acid. Factor IX deficiency (hemophilia B) may be treated with fresh frozen plasma or prothrombin complex concentrate, but factor IX concentrate is the treatment of choice.
2. Active bleeding in patients with *liver disease* and an elevated PT, aPTT, or international normalized ratio (INR) should be managed with fresh frozen plasma. Because many patients with liver disease are also vitamin K deficient, it is worthwhile to administer *vitamin K* 10 mg SC, IM, or PO daily for 3 days. Intravenous vitamin K occasionally causes an anaphylactic reaction. Factor IX concentrates carry a risk of thrombosis and are contraindicated in liver disease.
3. *Vitamin K deficiency* can be treated in an identical manner to that outlined later for the correction of warfarin coagulopathy. Ideally, however, one should identify and treat the underlying cause of vitamin K deficiency.
4. The treatment of *DIC* is both complicated and controversial. All medical authorities agree, however, that definitive management involves treating the underlying cause. Additionally, a patient with DIC often requires coagulation factor and platelet support in the form of fresh frozen plasma, cryoprecipitate, and platelet transfusions. The role of heparin in the treatment of DIC is controversial and should not be used without hematologic consultation.
5. Bleeding due to *anticoagulant therapy* can be reversed slowly or rapidly, depending on the clinical status of the patient and the site of bleeding.
   a. *Unfractionated heparin* has a half-life of only 1½ hours, so simply discontinuing a heparin infusion should normalize

the aPTT and correct a heparin-induced coagulopathy involving minor episodes of bleeding. *LMWH*, however, has a longer half-life, and it may be necessary to reverse the heparin effect with protamine sulfate. This may also be necessary in cases of serious bleeding associated with unfractionated heparin. The usual dose is *protamine sulfate 1 mg/100 units* (either fractionated or unfractionated heparin) approximately, IV slowly. The dosage is determined by estimating the amount of circulating heparin; for example, for a patient on a maintenance infusion of unfractionated heparin 1000 units/hr IV, the heparin infusion should be stopped and sufficient protamine should be given to neutralize approximately half of the preceding hour's dose—a total protamine dose of 5 mg. No more than 50 mg per single dose in a 10-minute period should be given. Side effects of protamine include hypotension, bradycardia, flushing, and bleeding.

b. Rapid reversal of *warfarin* effect, as may be required in life-threatening hemorrhages, can be achieved by administering *plasma* (e.g., 2 units at a time), with subsequent redetermination of PT. Although both fresh frozen plasma and banked plasma contain the vitamin K–dependent clotting factors, banked plasma is considerably less expensive and is thus preferred. Prothrombin complex concentrates, if available, may achieve a more rapid or complete reversal of warfarin effect than plasma alone. Severe bleeding (e.g., intracranial hemorrhage) requires urgent hematologic consultation. When prolonged reversal of anticoagulant effect is desired, *vitamin K 10 mg PO, SC, or IM* may be given daily for 3 days. Minor bleeding complications in patients on warfarin may require temporary discontinuation of this drug. Intravenous vitamin K occasionally causes an anaphylactic reaction and should be given with caution.

6. For *bleeding due to thrombolytic agents*, localized oozing at sites of invasive procedures can often be controlled by local pressure dressings or avoided by not doing invasive procedures. More serious hemorrhage requires discontinuation of the thrombolytic agent. Fibrinolytic agents that are not fibrin specific cause systemic fibrinogenolysis, so fresh frozen plasma may be required to replace fibrinogen. Cryoprecipitate can also be used to replace fibrinogen and factor VIII levels. Aminocaproic acid, which is an inhibitor of plasminogen activator, has also been used (20 to 30 g/day) but should not be initiated before hematologic consultation.

Platelet Abnormalities

Treatment of bleeding in a thrombocytopenic patient varies, depending on the presence of either an abnormality in platelet production or an increase in platelet destruction.

1. *Decreased marrow production* of platelets is treated in the long term by identifying and, if possible, correcting the underlying cause (e.g., chemotherapy for tumor, removal of marrow toxins, vitamin B_{12} or folate supplementation when indicated). In the short term, however, a serious bleeding complication should be treated by platelet transfusion (e.g., 6 to 8 units at a time). One unit of platelets can be expected to increase the platelet count by 1000 in a patient with inadequate marrow production of platelets. Check the response to transfusion by ordering a 1-hour post–platelet transfusion count.

2. *Increased peripheral destruction* of platelets is best managed by identifying and correcting the underlying problem. Often, this involves the systemic use of corticosteroids or other immunosuppressive agents. Such patients tend to have less serious bleeding manifestations than do those with inadequate marrow production of platelets, but platelet transfusion may be required for life-threatening bleeding episodes. Significant bleeding in patients with *idiopathic thrombocytopenic purpura* may respond to immune globulin IV followed by platelet transfusions.[2] Platelet transfusion therapy should not be used to treat thrombocytopenia in a patient with *TTP*, because it may actually worsen the condition. The platelet abnormality in TTP is best treated with plasma infusion[3] or, preferably, plasma exchange.[4]

3. *Dilutional thrombocytopenia* due to massive red blood cell (RBC) transfusion and intravenous fluid therapy is treated with platelet transfusion as required. Dilutional thrombocytopenia can usually be prevented by remembering to transfuse 8 units of platelets for every 10 to 12 units of RBCs transfused. (Because massive transfusion may also result in consumption and dilution of coagulation factors in the recipient, plasma should be administered if there is evidence of bleeding and a significantly elevated PT, aPTT, or INR.)

4. *Von Willebrand's disease* may be treated with factor VIII concentrates or cryoprecipitate. DDAVP injection is useful in type I von Willebrand's disease but may exacerbate thrombocytopenia in type II disease.

5. Bleeding disorders resulting from *acquired platelet dysfunction* are best managed by identification and correction of the underlying problem. Temporary treatment of bleeding disorders due to these conditions may involve platelet transfusion or other more specialized measures (e.g., cryoprecipitate, DDAVP injection, plasmapheresis, conjugated estrogens, intensive dialysis in uremia).

References

1. Saba HI, Morelli GA, Logrono LA: Treatment of bleeding in hereditary hemorrhagic telangiectasia with aminocaproic acid. N Engl J Med 1994; 330:1789-1790.

2. Baumann MA, Menitove JE, Aster RH, et al: Urgent treatment of idiopathic thrombocytopenic purpura with single-dose gammaglobulin infusion followed by platelet transfusion. Ann Intern Med 1986;104: 808-809.

3. Byrnes JJ, Khurana M: Treatment of thrombotic thrombocytopenic purpura with plasma. N Engl J Med 1997;297:1386-1389.

4. Rock GA, Shumak KH, Buskard NA, et al: Comparison of plasma exchange with plasma infusion in the treatment of thrombotic thrombocytopenic purpura: Canadian Apheresis Study Group. N Engl J Med 1991; 325:393-397.

Glucose Disorders

The management of glucose disorders has become increasingly complex because of the proliferation of insulin types and the popular use of new insulin delivery devices. For this reason, it is important to be familiar with the insulin brands commonly used in your institution and to have an understanding of the various insulin delivery devices. The common insulins available in the United States and their manufacturers are listed in Table 32–1. International name equivalents are listed in Table 32–2. Premixed insulin is also commercially available in some countries (Table 32–3). Comparative duration of action of insulins is listed in the On-Call Formulary, page 466.

Bovine, porcine, and human insulins are available, and each has different antigenicities. Bovine insulin is the most immunogenic, and human insulin is the least. Human insulin is derived from DNA recombinant techniques using either baker's yeast (Novolin ge insulins) or *Escherichia coli* bacteria (Humulin insulins). Human insulins are associated with fewer adverse reactions (e.g., insulin allergy, antibody-mediated insulin resistance, lipoatrophy) and should be considered, especially when treatment is intermittent. If the patient is already receiving bovine or porcine insulin without complications, it is fine to adjust the dosage of the same preparation the patient is receiving.

Insulin may be given intravenously (usually reserved for emergencies) or subcutaneously. The subcutaneous route may involve direct injection, a pen device, or a continuous infusion system (the "insulin pump"). Insulin pens are available through a variety of manufacturers and often use particular types of insulin or pre-mixtures. Usually the patient is familiar with the use and limitations of his or her pen. If simple adjustments cannot be made and you need to change a patient's insulin dosage, it is best to use direct injection with a needle and syringe, or consult your resident or a diabetes education nurse. The insulin pump is a more complex method of continuous insulin delivery. Principles of insulin use with the insulin pump are described in Box 32–1. Unless you are familiar with this device, it is best to contact your resident or attending physician before making changes in the patient's insulin regimen.

TABLE 32–1 **Insulins Available in the United States**

Insulin	Manufacturer
Rapid-Acting Analogs	
Humalog (insulin lispro)	Lilly
NovoLog (insulin aspart)	Novo Nordisk
Short-Acting Insulin	
Humulin R (regular)	Lilly
Novolin R (regular)	Novo Nordisk
Velosulin BR (regular buffered)	Novo Nordisk
Intermediate-Acting Insulin	
Humulin L (lente)	Lilly
Humulin N (NPH)	Lilly
Novolin N (NPH)	Novo Nordisk
Lente Iletin II (pork)	Lilly
NPH Iletin II (pork)	Lilly
Long-Acting Insulin	
Humulin-U (ultralente)	Lilly
Long-Acting Analog	
Lantus (insulin glargine)	Aventis
Combinations	
Humulin 50/50 (50% NPH, 50% regular)	Lilly
Humulin 70/30 (70% NPH, 30% regular)	Lilly
Humalog 75/25 (75% insulin protamine suspension [NPH], 25% insulin lispro)	Lilly
Novolin 70/30 (70% NPH, 30% regular)	Novo Nordisk

HYPERGLYCEMIA

Causes

Patients with Documented Diabetes Mellitus

- Poorly controlled type 1 or type 2 diabetes mellitus
- Stress (surgery, infection, severe illness)
- Drugs (corticosteroids, thiazides, beta blockers, phenytoin, nicotinic acid, opiates)
- Total parenteral nutrition (TPN) administration
- Pancreatic injury (pancreatitis, trauma, surgery)
- Insulin delivery problems in patients using an insulin pump (e.g., programming errors, pump or alarm malfunctions, reservoir problems, infusion set or injection site problems)

TABLE 32–2 **International Name Equivalents for Insulin Products**

Canada/ Bermuda	United States	Japan	Other Countries
Novolin ge Toronto	Novolin R	Novolin R HM ge	Actrapid HM ge
Novolin ge Toronto Penfill	Novolin R Penfill	Penfill R HM ge	Actrapid HM ge Penfill
Novolin ge NPH	Novolin N	Novolin N HM ge	Protophane HM ge
Novolin ge NPH Penfill	Novolin N Penfill	Penfill N HM ge	Protophane HM ge Penfill
Novolin ge 30/70 Penfill	Novolin 70/30	Novolin 30R HM ge	Actraphane HM ge
Novolin ge 30/70 Penfill	Novolin 70/30 Penfill	Penfill 30R HM ge	Actraphane HM ge Penfill
Novolin Pen	NovoPen	NovoPen	NovoPen
Novolin Pen 3	NovoPen 3	NovoPen 3	NovoPen 3
N/A	NovoPen 1.5	NovoPen 1.5	Available in selected countries

N/A, not available.

Patients without Previously Documented Diabetes Mellitus

- New onset of diabetes mellitus
- Stress (surgery, infection, severe illness)
- Drugs (corticosteroids, thiazides, beta blockers, phenytoin, nicotinic acid, opiates)
- TPN administration
- Pancreatic injury (pancreatitis, trauma, surgery)

TABLE 32–3 **Premixed Insulins Available for Pen-Device Injection**

Insulin	Manufacturer
Novolin 10/90 (10% regular, 90% NPH)	Novo Nordisk
Novolin 20/80 (20% regular, 80% NPH)	Novo Nordisk
Novolin 30/70 (30% regular, 70% NPH)	Novo Nordisk
Novolin 40/60 (40% regular, 60% NPH)	Novo Nordisk
Novolin 50/50 (50% regular, 50% NPH)	Novo Nordisk

These insulins are available in 3- and 1.5-mL cartridges that are used in the Novolin Pen, which is available in some countries.

BOX 32–1 **The Insulin Pump**

An insulin pump is a small mechanical device that delivers insulin subcutaneously via an infusion set. The pump is worn outside the body in a pouch or on a belt. The infusion set is a long, thin plastic tube connected to a flexible plastic cannula that is inserted into the skin at the infusion site, usually in the subcutaneous abdominal tissue. The infusion set remains in place for 2 to 4 days and is then replaced, using a new location each time.

When a patient with an insulin pump is admitted to the hospital, the pump should remain on the patient at all times, unless other arrangements are made for insulin replacement. These patients have been trained in insulin pump therapy and, in most situations, can aid in maintaining glycemic control with the pump, together with the diabetes education nurse and the attending physician. If the patient is unconscious, in most cases the pump can be removed, and insulin can be administered by alternative methods.

The insulin pump is not an artificial pancreas. It is a computer-controlled unit that delivers insulin in precise amounts at prepro-grammed times. It uses only Humalog or NovoLog (NovoRapid) insulin. The pump is not "automatic." The patient has to decide how much insulin will be given, based on blood glucose results and the amount of food that will be consumed.

The device contains a small reservoir of insulin (up to 3 mL), a small battery-powered pump, and a computer to control its operation. The pump is set to deliver insulin in two ways:

1. Basal rate—a small, continuous flow of insulin automatically delivered every 15 minutes. The basal rate is programmed by the operator and may vary at different times of the day.
2. Bolus dose—designed to cover the food eaten during a meal or to correct elevated blood glucose levels. Bolus doses can be programmed at any time, which gives the patient greater flexibility with regard to when and what he or she eats.

Acute Manifestations

Mild Hyperglycemia: Fasting Blood Glucose 6.1 to 11.0 mmol/L

- May be asymptomatic
- Polyuria, polydipsia, thirst

Moderate Hyperglycemia: Fasting Blood Glucose 11.1 to 22.5 mmol/L

- Volume depletion (tachycardia, decreased jugular venous pressure [JVP], ± hypotension)
- Polyuria, polydipsia, thirst
- May be asymptomatic

Severe Hyperglycemia: Fasting Blood Glucose >22.5 mmol/L

TYPE 1 DIABETES MELLITUS

- Musty odor on breath (ketone breath)
- Kussmaul's breathing (deep, pauseless respirations seen when pH is <7.2)
- Volume depletion (tachycardia, decreased JVP, ± hypotension)
- Anorexia, nausea, vomiting, abdominal pain (may mimic a surgical abdomen)
- Ileus, gastric dilatation
- Hyporeflexia, hypotonia, delirium, coma

TYPE 2 DIABETES MELLITUS

- Polyuria, polydipsia
- Volume depletion
- Confusion, coma

Management

Assess the Severity

The severity of the situation should be determined based on the blood glucose level (Table 32–4) and the patient's symptoms.

Treatment of Mild, Asymptomatic Hyperglycemia

Regardless of whether a patient is taking oral hypoglycemics or an insulin preparation, mild, asymptomatic hyperglycemia does not require urgent treatment. If the patient is not known to be diabetic, it may be useful to take the initial steps to determine whether the patient has diabetes, impaired fasting glucose, or impaired glucose tolerance. Order the following:
1. Fasting blood glucose in the morning.
   A fasting blood glucose of >7.0 mmol/L on more than one occasion confirms the diagnosis of diabetes mellitus. Make sure that the patient is not receiving glucose-containing IV solutions, which would make these results invalid. In addition, the diagnosis of diabetes mellitus cannot be made in the setting of stress (e.g., infection, surgery, severe illness).

TABLE 32–4 **Blood Glucose Levels**

	Fasting or AC Blood Glucose (mmol/L)	2-Hour PC Blood Glucose (mmol/L)
Normal range	3.5–6.0	<11.0
Mild hyperglycemia	6.1–11.0	11.1–16.5
Moderate hyperglycemia	11.1–22.5	16.6–27.5
Severe hyperglycemia	>22.5	>27.5

AC, before meals; PC, after meals.

Any one of the following criteria[1] is diagnostic for diabetes mellitus:
a. Fasting blood glucose >7.0 mmol/L × 2 (venous plasma)
b. Random blood glucose >11.1 mmol/L × 2 (venous plasma)
c. A glucose tolerance test (GTT) with a 2-hour PC blood glucose ≥11.1 mmol/L (venous plasma)

2. Finger-prick blood glucose (FPBG) readings before meals and at bedtime. If the readings are >25 or <2.8 mmol/L, a stat blood glucose sample should be drawn and a physician informed.

Treatment of Moderate Hyperglycemia

Moderate hyperglycemia may require an adjustment in the insulin being given. Whenever possible, adjustments in a patient's insulin regimen should be made using the same insulins and the same delivery device that the patient is already using. Examine the diabetic record for the past 3 days.

A sample adjustment in insulin dosage is given in Table 32–5. The FPBG readings are in millimoles per liter, and the SC insulin dose given is indicated in parentheses (e.g., 20/10 indicates that 20 units of neutral protamine Hagedorn [NPH] and 10 units of regular insulin have been given).

You have been called at night because of a FPBG reading of 25 mmol/L. Order the following:
1. Stat random blood glucose to confirm the FPBG.
2. *Regular insulin* 5 to 10 units SC now.

> It is not your job to devise a schedule that will achieve perfect blood glucose control for the rest of the patient's hospital stay. Short-term control of blood glucose levels has not been shown to decrease complications in diabetic patients. When the blood glucose level is elevated at night, your aim is to prevent the development of ketoacidosis in a patient with type 1 diabetes mellitus or the development of the hyperosmolar state in a patient with type 2 diabetes mellitus without producing symptomatic hypoglycemia with your treatment.

TABLE 32–5 **Sample Insulin Dosage Adjustment**

Date	Before Breakfast (NPH/Regular)	Before Lunch (NPH/Regular)	Before Supper (NPH/Regular)	QHS (NPH/Regular)
August 1	16.7* (20/10)†	13.9 (0/0)	16.7 (10/10)	18.1 (0/0)
August 2	13.9 (20/10)	16.7 (0/4)	8.3 (10/10)	19.4 (0/0)
August 3	16.7 (20/10)	15.2 (0/0)	13.1 (10/10)	25.0 (0/0)

NPH, neutral protamine Hagedorn; QHS, at bedtime.
*Finger-prick blood glucose reading given in mmol/L.
†Indicates 20 units of NPH and 10 units of regular insulin.

3. An 0300 FPBG reading. Determining the reason for poor control of blood glucose before breakfast may aid in the ongoing adjustment of the patient's insulin.

> Hypoglycemia documented at 3 AM would suggest that pre-breakfast hyperglycemia is due to hyperglycemic rebound (the Somogyi effect), which is correctly managed by reducing the before-supper NPH insulin dose. Hyperglycemia documented at 3 AM would suggest that pre-breakfast hyperglycemia is due to inadequate insulin coverage overnight. This is correctly managed by increasing the before-supper NPH insulin dose.

Treatment of Severe Hyperglycemia

Severe hyperglycemia requires urgent treatment. In most cases, this involves temporarily stopping the patient's previous diabetic medications and giving intravenous hydration and insulin.

1. **Diabetic ketoacidosis (DKA).** This complication may be seen in a patient with poorly controlled type 1 diabetes mellitus. It is due to an absolute insulin deficit, resulting in impaired resynthesis of long-chain fatty acids from acetate, with subsequent conversion to the acidic ketone bodies (ketosis).

   a. *Correct volume depletion.* Give 500 to 1000 mL NS IV over the first hour, with subsequent IV rates guided by reassessment of volume status.

   > Patients with DKA often have a 3- to 5-L volume deficit. It is therefore not unusual to require NS at rates of 500 mL/hr for an additional 2 to 8 hours to restore euvolemia. If the patient has a history of congestive heart failure (CHF), weighs <50 kg, or is 80 years or older, NS should be given cautiously to avoid iatrogenic CHF.

   b. *Begin an insulin infusion.* Give a single dose of 5 to 10 units of IV regular insulin by direct slow injection, followed by an infusion rate based on close monitoring of blood glucose. Start the insulin infusion at 0.1 U/kg per hour in NS.

   > Regular insulin can bind to the plastic IV tubing. To ensure accurate insulin delivery, 30 to 50 mL of the infusion solution should be run through the IV tubing and discarded before connecting the tubing to the patient.

   Discontinue the standing order for SC insulin or oral hypoglycemics before beginning the insulin infusion.

   c. *Monitor blood glucose hourly* by FPBG measurements. When the blood glucose has fallen to 14 mmol/L, continue the insulin infusion but switch the delivery solution from NS to D5W. Continue the insulin infusion until the blood glucose remains stable at 8 to 10 mmol/L. As the blood glucose falls, the rate of insulin infusion should be slowed (e.g., 0.025 to 0.05 U/kg per hour).

> The rate of fall of blood glucose should be approximately 2 mmol/L per hour; more aggressive treatment of hyperglycemia may result in severe hypokalemia and cerebral edema.

d. When the glucose has stabilized at 8 to 10 mmol/L, *restart SC insulin*, remembering that the insulin infusion must be continued for 1 to 2 hours after the injection of SC insulin, or ketogenesis will be reactivated. Continue to monitor the bedside glucose every 4 hours, adding supplemental regular insulin to keep blood glucose between 8 and 10 mmol/L.

e. Monitor blood glucose, serum electrolytes, and arterial blood gases (ABGs).

> Hyperglycemic patients can have metabolic acidemia and hypokalemia. As NS and insulin are administered, the acidemia is corrected, and the potassium shifts into the cells from the extracellular fluid. This can result in a worsening of hypokalemia.

Order baseline ABGs, electrolytes, urea, creatinine, and glucose levels. Repeat the ABGs and potassium level in 2 hours and thereafter as required. When hypokalemia is first noted, add KCl to the IV NS, provided the patient is passing urine and has normal urea and creatinine levels. If the patient is in renal failure, use caution when adding potassium to the IV, to avoid iatrogenic hyperkalemia.

f. *Search for the precipitating cause.* Common precipitating factors include the following:
   (1) Infection
   (2) Inadequate insulin dosage
   (3) Dietary indiscretion
   (4) Pancreatitis

2. **Hyperosmolar, hyperglycemic, nonketotic state.** This condition may be seen in a patient with poorly controlled type 2 diabetes mellitus. It is a syndrome of profound volume depletion resulting from a sustained hyperglycemic diuresis without compensatory fluid intake. Typically, the patient is 50 to 70 years old. Many have no prior histories of diabetes mellitus. The precipitating event is often stroke, infection, pancreatitis, or drugs. The blood glucose level is often very high (>55 mmol/L), but significant ketosis is absent.

a. *Correct volume depletion and water deficit.* The objective of fluid therapy in the nonketotic hyperosmolar state is to both correct the volume deficit and resolve the hyperosmolarity. This can be achieved by giving NS 500 to 1000 mL IV over 1 to 2 hours, with further IV rates guided by reassessment of volume status. Once the volume deficit is corrected using NS, remaining water deficits—as indicated by persistent hypernatremia or hyperglycemia—are best corrected using hypotonic IV solutions, such as ½ NS.

b. *Begin an insulin infusion.* See the previous discussion of the treatment of DKA. Rehydration alone often produces a substantial fall in blood glucose through renal excretion. As a result, patients with the hyperosmolar, hyperglycemic, nonketotic state generally require less insulin than does a patient with type 1 diabetes and ketoacidosis.

c. *Monitor blood glucose level and serum electrolytes.* Order baseline electrolytes, urea, creatinine, and glucose levels. Repeat the blood glucose level and electrolytes in 2 hours and thereafter as required.

d. *Search for the precipitating cause.*
   (1) Infection
   (2) Inadequate fluid intake
   (3) Other acute illnesses (myocardial infarction, stroke)

HYPOGLYCEMIA

Causes

Patients with Documented Diabetes Mellitus

- Excess insulin or oral hypoglycemic administration
- Decreased caloric intake
- Missed meals or missed snacks
- Increased exercise

Patients without Documented Diabetes Mellitus

- Surreptitious intake of insulin or oral hypoglycemics
- Insulinoma
- Supervised 72-hour fasting for the investigation of hypoglycemia
- Drugs (ethanol, pentamidine, disopyramide, monoamine oxidase [MAO] inhibitors)
- Hepatic failure
- Adrenal insufficiency

Manifestations

Adrenergic Response (Catecholamine Release Due to Rapid Decrease in Glucose Level)

- Diaphoresis
- Palpitations
- Tremulousness
- Tachycardia
- Hunger
- Acral and perioral numbness
- Anxiety
- Combativeness

- Confusion
- Coma

Central Nervous System Response (Slow Response May Develop over 1 to 3 Hours)

- Headache
- Diplopia
- Bizarre behavior
- Focal neurologic deficits
- Confusion
- Seizures
- Coma

The adrenergic response does not always precede the central nervous system response, and some patients may progress directly from confusion or inability to speak to seizure or coma.

Management

Assess the Severity

Any symptomatic patient with suspected hypoglycemia requires treatment. Symptoms may be precipitated by either a rapid fall in blood glucose level or an absolute low level of blood glucose.

1. *Draw 1 mL of blood* to be sent for blood glucose testing to confirm the diagnosis. If the cause of hypoglycemia is not clear, draw 10 mL and ask the laboratory to save an aliquot for later insulin and C peptide measurement. **Do not wait to receive the blood glucose results before beginning treatment.**

   Insulin produced endogenously includes the C peptide fragment; commercial preparations of insulin do not. Thus, a high insulin level associated with a high C peptide level and hypoglycemia suggests endogenous production of excess insulin (e.g., insulinoma), whereas a high insulin level associated with a low C peptide level and hypoglycemia suggests surreptitious or therapeutic administration of exogenous insulin.

2. In a cooperative, awake patient, oral glucose in the form of sweetened fruit juice can be given. If the patient is unable to take oral fluids or is unconscious, D50W 50 mL IV should be given by direct slow injection. If there is no IV access and the patient is unable to take oral fluids (e.g., unconscious), *glucagon* 1 mg SC or IM should be given. After glucagon administration, vomiting may develop, so a patient who is not fully conscious should be monitored carefully to prevent aspiration.

3. If ongoing hypoglycemia is anticipated, or if the patient's symptoms were severe (e.g., seizure, coma), begin a maintenance IV of D5W or D10W at a rate of 100 mL/hr. Ask the RN to reassess the patient in 1 hour. In addition, remeasure the

blood glucose level in 2 to 4 hours to ensure that a hypoglycemic relapse has not occurred. Hypoglycemia due to oral hypoglycemics may require repeated doses of D50W because of the slow metabolism and excretion of these drugs.

Reference

1. Report of the Expert Committee on the Diagnosis and Classification of Diabetes Mellitus. Diabetes Care 1997;20:1183-1197.

Potassium Disorders

HYPERKALEMIA

Causes

Excessive Intake

- K^+ supplements (oral or intravenous)
- Salt substitutes
- High-dose IV therapy with K^+ salts of penicillin
- Blood transfusions

Decreased Excretion

- Renal failure (acute or chronic)
- Drugs
- K^+-sparing diuretics (spironolactone, triamterene, amiloride)
- Angiotensin-converting enzyme (ACE) inhibitors
- Nonsteroidal anti-inflammatory drugs (NSAIDs)
- Trimethoprim-sulfamethoxazole
- Pentamidine
- Cyclosporine
- Addison's disease, hypoaldosteronism
- Distal tubular dysfunction (i.e., type IV renal tubular acidosis [RTA])

Shift from Intracellular to Extracellular Fluid

- Acidemia (especially nonanion gap)
- Insulin deficiency
- Tissue destruction (hemolysis, crush injuries, rhabdomyolysis, extensive burns, tumor lysis)
- Drugs (succinylcholine, digoxin, arginine, beta blockers)
- Hyperkalemic periodic paralysis

Factitious

- Prolonged tourniquet placement for venipuncture
- Blood sample hemolysis
- Leukocytosis
- Thrombocytosis

Manifestations

Cardiac

- Fatal ventricular dysrhythmias

    The progressive electrocardiogram (ECG) changes seen in hyperkalemia are peaked T waves → depressed ST segments → decreased amplitude of R waves → prolonged PR interval → small or absent P waves → wide QRS complexes → biphasic sine wave pattern (Fig. 33–1). Dysrhythmias associated with hyperkalemia include bradycardias, complete heart block, ventricular fibrillation, and asystole.

Neuromuscular

- Weakness, often beginning in the lower extremities
- Paresthesias
- Depressed tendon reflexes

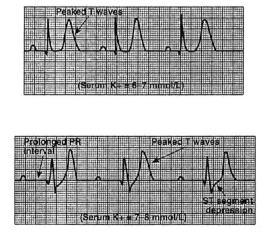

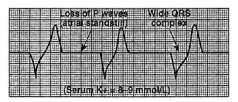

Figure 33–1 Progressive electrocardiographic manifestations of hyperkalemia.

Management

Electrocardiogram

Fatal ventricular dysrhythmias can occur at any time during treatment; hence, continuous ECG monitoring is required if the K^+ level is >6.5 mmol/L.

Assess the Severity

The severity of the situation should be determined based on the serum K^+ concentration, the ECG findings, and whether the underlying cause is immediately remediable.

IF SEVERE
- Serum K^+ >8.0 mmol/L
- ECG findings more advanced than peaked T waves alone
- Cause not immediately remediable

1. Notify your resident.
2. Place the patient on continuous ECG monitoring.
3. Correct contributing factors (acidemia, hypovolemia).
4. Give one or more of the following:
   a. *Calcium gluconate* 5 to 10 mL of a 10% solution IV over 2 minutes. This temporarily antagonizes the cardiac and neuromuscular effects of hyperkalemia. The onset of calcium gluconate is immediate, and its effect lasts 1 hour. It does not, however, reduce the serum concentration of K^+. *Caution:* The administration of calcium to a patient on digoxin may precipitate ventricular dysrhythmias due to the combined effects of digoxin and calcium.
   b. *Fifty percent dextrose in water* (D50W) 50 mL IV, followed by *regular insulin* 5 to 10 units IV. This shifts K^+ from the extracellular fluid (ECF) to the intracellular fluid (ICF). Its effect is immediate and lasts 1 to 2 hours. If the patient is already hyperglycemic, the D50W should be omitted. Subsequent serum glucose levels should be obtained to determine whether additional doses of insulin are required and to ensure that hypoglycemia does not occur.
   c. *Sodium bicarbonate* 1 ampule (44.6 mmol) IV. This shifts K^+ from the ECF to the ICF. Its effect is immediate and lasts 1 to 2 hours.
   d. *Glucose-insulin-HCO_3* cocktail—D10W 1000 mL with 3 ampules of $NaHCO_3$ and 20 units of regular insulin at 75 mL/hr—until more definitive measures are taken.
   e. *Sodium polystyrene sulfonate* (Kayexalate) 15 to 30 g (4 to 8 teaspoonfuls) in 50 to 100 mL of 20% sorbitol PO every 3 to 4 hours or 50 g in 200 mL D20W PR by retention enema for 30 to 60 minutes every 4 hours. This is the only drug treatment that actually removes K^+ from the total

body pool. Watch carefully for evidence of volume overload, because this resin works by exchanging Na^+ for K^+.

   f. *Beta-2-adrenergic agonists* can temporarily reduce serum K^+ by stimulating cyclic AMP and shifting K^+ from the ECF to the ICF. *Salbutamol 10 to 20 mg by nebulizer* may be transiently effective in lowering serum K^+ in patients on hemodialysis.[1]

5. *Hemodialysis* should be considered on an urgent basis if the aforementioned measures have failed or if the patient is in acute or chronic oliguric renal failure.

6. Monitor the serum K^+ concentration every 1 to 2 hours until it is <6.5 mmol/L.

IF MODERATE

- Serum K^+ between 6.5 and 8.0 mmol/L
- ECG findings show peaked T waves only
- Cause is not progressive

1. Place the patient on continuous ECG monitoring.
2. Correct contributing factors (acidemia, hypovolemia).
3. Give one or more of the following in the dosages previously outlined:
   a. $NaHCO_3$
   b. Glucose and insulin
   c. Sodium polystyrene sulfonate
4. Monitor the serum K^+ concentration every 1 to 2 hours until it is <6.5 mmol/L.

IF MILD

- Serum K^+ <6.5 mmol/L
- ECG findings show peaked T waves only
- Cause is not progressive

1. Correct contributing factors (acidemia, hypovolemia).
2. Remeasure the serum K^+ concentration 4 to 6 hours later, depending on the cause.

HYPOKALEMIA

Causes

Renal Losses (Urine K^+ >20 mmol/Day)

- Diuretics, osmotic diuresis
- Antibiotics (carbenicillin, ticarcillin, nafcillin, amphotericin, aminoglycosides)
- RTA (classic type I)
- Hyperaldosteronism
- Glucocorticoid excess
- Magnesium deficiency
- Chronic metabolic alkalosis

- Bartter's syndrome
- Fanconi's syndrome
- Ureterosigmoidostomy
- Vomiting, nasogastric (NG) suction (hydrogen ions are lost with vomiting and NG suction, inducing alkalosis that results in renal K^+ wasting)

Extrarenal Losses (Urine K^+ <20 mmol/Day)

- Diarrhea
- Intestinal fistula

Inadequate Intake

- Over 1 to 2 weeks

Shift from Extracellular to Intracellular Space

- Acute alkalosis
- Drugs
- Insulin therapy
- Vitamin B_{12} therapy
- Salbutamol
- Lithium
- Hypokalemic periodic paralysis
- Hypothermia

Manifestations

Cardiac

- Premature atrial contractions (PACs)
- Premature ventricular contractions (PVCs)
- Digoxin toxicity
- ECG changes (Fig. 33–2)
    - T wave flattening
    - U waves
    - ST segment depression

Neuromuscular

- Weakness
- Depressed deep tendon reflexes

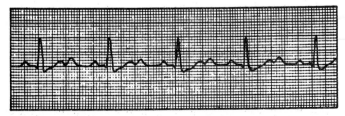

Figure 33–2 Electrocardiographic manifestations of hypokalemia.

- Paresthesias
- Ileus

Miscellaneous

- Nephrogenic diabetes insipidus
- Metabolic alkalosis
- Worsening of hepatic encephalopathy

Management

If possible, correct the underlying cause.

Assess the Severity

The severity of the situation should be determined based on the serum K^+ concentration, the ECG findings, and the clinical setting in which hypokalemia is occurring.

IF SEVERE

- Serum K^+ <3.0 mmol/L with PVCs in the setting of myocardial ischemia or with digoxin toxicity

1. Notify your resident.
2. Place the patient on continuous ECG monitoring.
3. IV replacement therapy may be required: 10 mmol KCl in 100 mL normal saline (NS) IV over 1 hour. Repeat once or twice as necessary.

   > KCl in small volumes should be given through central IV lines, because these high concentrations of K^+ are sclerosing to peripheral veins.

   Further replacement can be achieved with maintenance therapy containing up to 40 to 60 mmol KCl/L of IV fluid at a maximum rate of 20 mmol/hr. K^+ can also be given by administering the liquid salt by NG tube or by oral supplementation.
4. Recheck serum K^+ concentration after each 20 to 30 mmol KCl IV has been given.

IF MODERATE

- Serum K^+ ≤3.0 mmol/L with PACs but no (or infrequent) PVCs and no digoxin toxicity

1. Notify your resident.
2. Oral K^+ supplementation is usually adequate: Slow-K = 8 mmol KCl per tablet, Kay Ciel Elixir = 20 mmol/15 mL, and K-Lyte = 25 mmol/packet.
3. In this situation, IV replacement therapy should be reserved for patients with marked hypokalemia or for those who are unable to take oral supplements (see previous recommendations).
4. Recheck serum K^+ concentration in the morning or sooner if clinically indicated.

IF MILD

- Serum K$^+$ between 3.1 and 3.5 mmol/L, no (or infrequent) PVCs, and patient asymptomatic

1. Oral supplementation is usually adequate (see previous recommendations).
2. Recheck serum K$^+$ concentration in the morning or sooner if clinically indicated.

REMEMBER

1. Serious hyperkalemia can occur as a result of K$^+$ supplementation. Hence, serum K$^+$ levels should be closely monitored during treatment. Be particularly cautious in patients with renal impairment.
2. Hypokalemia and hypocalcemia may coexist. Correction of hypokalemia without accompanying correction of hypocalcemia may increase the risk of ventricular dysrhythmias.
3. Hypokalemia and hypomagnesemia may coexist. Correction of hypokalemia may be unsuccessful unless hypomagnesemia is corrected simultaneously.

Reference

1. Allon M, Dunlay R, Copkney C: Nebulized albuterol for acute hyperkalemia in patients on hemodialysis. Ann Intern Med 1989;110:426-429.

Sodium Disorders

HYPERNATREMIA

Causes

1. Inadequate intake of water
   a. Coma
   b. Hypothalamic dysfunction
2. Excessive water losses
   a. Renal losses
      (1) Diabetes insipidus (nephrogenic or pituitary)
      (2) Osmotic diuresis (hyperglycemia, mannitol administration, urea)
   b. Extrarenal losses
      (1) Gastrointestinal (GI) losses (vomiting, nasogastric [NG] suction, diarrhea)
      (2) Insensible losses (burns, febrile illness, tachypnea)
3. Excessive sodium gain
   a. Iatrogenic (excessive sodium administration)
   b. Primary hyperaldosteronism

Manifestations

Hypernatremia most often results from extracellular fluid (ECF) volume depletion due to hypotonic fluid loss (e.g., vomiting, diarrhea, sweating, osmotic diuresis). Symptoms are dependent on the absolute increase in serum osmolality, as well as the rate at which it develops. The manifestations of hypernatremia are due to acute brain cell shrinkage from an outward shift of intracellular water, which occurs as a result of increased ECF osmolality. They range from confusion and muscle irritability to seizures, respiratory paralysis, and death.

Management

Assess the Severity

The severity of the situation should be determined based on the symptomatic state of the patient, the serum sodium concentration, the serum osmolality, and the ECF volume.

1. Osmolality can be measured in the laboratory. However, sufficient information may be available to permit its calculation

based on the major osmotically active substances in the ECF, as follows:

$$\text{Osmolality (mmol/kg)} = 2 \text{ Na (mmol/L)} + \text{urea (mmol/L)} + \text{glucose (mmol/L)}$$

The normal range is 281 to 297 mmol/kg.

2. Most patients with hypernatremia have an accompanying extracellular volume deficit that can compromise perfusion of vital organs. Assess the volume status of the patient (see Chapter 3).

3. Most patients with hypernatremia have relatively few symptoms and are not at immediate risk of dying.

Correct the Cause

The cause of hypernatremia is usually evident from the history and physical findings and should be corrected, if possible.

Correct Volume and Water Deficits

The choice of fluid is dependent on the severity of the extracellular volume deficit.

1. In patients who are volume depleted, hypernatremia can be corrected by giving intravenous (IV) normal saline (NS) until the patient is hemodynamically stable and then changing to ½ NS or 5% dextrose in water (D5W) to correct the remaining water deficit.

2. In patients who are not volume depleted, ½ NS or D5W can be used to correct the water deficit.

One can estimate the volume of water required, remembering that the deficit is in *total body water* (TBW), which is approximately 60% of body weight:

$$\text{Water deficit} = \frac{[\text{serum Na (observed)} - \text{serum Na (normal)}] \times 0.6 \text{ weight (kg)}}{\text{Serum Na (normal)}}$$

Example: A 65-year-old man is admitted to the hospital after being found in his apartment 2 days after falling and fracturing his hip. He is moderately volume depleted and has a serum sodium value of 156 mmol/L. His weight is 70 kg. Calculate the volume of water required to correct the serum sodium as follows:

$$\text{Free water deficit} = \frac{[156 \text{ mmol/L} - 140 \text{ mmol/L}] \times 0.6(70 \text{ L})}{140 \text{ mmol/L}} = 4.8L$$

Remember to correct the osmolality abnormality at a rate similar to that at which it developed. Biologic systems are more responsive to rates of change than to absolute amounts of change. It is safest to correct half the deficit and then reevaluate. Corrections in serum sodium greater than 1 to 2 mmol/L can lead to brain swelling, resulting in the development of confusion, seizures, or coma.

3. In an occasional patient with hypernatremia who is volume overloaded, the hypernatremia can be corrected by initiating a diuresis using *furosemide* 20 to 40 mg IV and repeating at intervals of 2 to 4 hours as necessary. Once the extracellular volume has returned to normal, if the serum sodium level is still elevated, diuresis should be continued, with urinary volume losses replaced with D5W until the serum sodium level is again in the normal range.

HYPONATREMIA

Causes

Hyponatremia with Decreased Extracellular Fluid Volume

1. Renal loss of sodium
   a. Diuretic excess
   b. Sodium-losing nephropathies
   c. Diuretic phase of acute tubular necrosis
   d. Bartter's syndrome
   e. Hypoaldosteronism
2. Extrarenal losses of sodium
   a. Vomiting, NG suction
   b. Diarrhea
   c. Sweating
   d. Burns
   e. Pancreatitis

Hyponatremia with Excess Extracellular Fluid Volume and Edema

1. Renal failure
2. Nephrotic syndrome
3. Congestive heart failure (CHF)
4. Cirrhosis of the liver

Hyponatremia with Normal Extracellular Fluid Volume

1. Syndrome of inappropriate antidiuretic hormone (SIADH)
   a. Tumors
      (1) Small cell carcinoma of the lung
      (2) Pancreatic carcinoma
      (3) Duodenal adenocarcinoma
      (4) Lymphosarcoma

  b. Central nervous system (CNS) disorders
      (1) Brain tumor
      (2) Brain trauma
      (3) Meningitis
      (4) Encephalitis
      (5) Subarachnoid hemorrhage
      (6) Guillain-Barré syndrome
  c. Pulmonary disorders
      (1) Tuberculosis
      (2) Pneumonia
  d. Drugs
      (1) Hypoglycemic agents (chlorpropamide, tolbutamide)
      (2) Neuroleptics (haloperidol, trifluoperazine, fluphenazine, and others)
      (3) Antidepressants (amitriptyline, desipramine, tranylcypromine)
      (4) Antineoplastic drugs (cyclophosphamide, vincristine)
      (5) Narcotics
      (6) Clofibrate
      (7) Carbamazepine
      (8) Nicotine
  e. The postoperative state (particularly in premenopausal women)
2. Primary polydipsia (water intoxication)
3. Pseudohyponatremia
  a. Hyponatremia with normal serum osmolality
      (1) Hyperlipidemia
      (2) Hyperproteinemia
  b. Hyponatremia with increased serum osmolality
      (1) Excess urea
      (2) Hyperglycemia
      (3) Mannitol
      (4) Ethanol
      (5) Methanol
      (6) Ethylene glycol
      (7) Isopropyl alcohol
4. Endocrine disorders
  a. Hypothyroidism
  b. Addison's disease

Manifestations

Manifestations of hyponatremia depend on the absolute decrease in serum osmolality, the rate of development of hyponatremia, and the volume status of the patient. When associated with a decreased serum osmolality, hyponatremia may cause the following:

- Confusion
- Lethargy
- Weakness

- Nausea and vomiting
- Seizures
- Coma

When hyponatremia develops gradually, a patient may tolerate a serum sodium concentration of less than 110 mmol/L with only moderate confusion or lethargy. However, when the serum sodium concentration decreases rapidly from 140 to 115 mmol/L, a patient may experience a seizure.

Management

Assess the Severity

The severity of the situation should be determined based on the symptomatic state of the patient, the serum sodium concentration, the serum osmolality, and the ECF.

Remember that when attempting to correct disorders manifested by hyponatremia, brain cells try to maintain their volume in dilutional states by losing solutes (e.g., potassium). If the serum sodium level is corrected too rapidly (i.e., to levels >120 to 125 mmol/L), the serum may become hypertonic relative to brain cells, resulting in an outward shift of water, with resultant CNS damage due to acute brain shrinkage.

Correct the Cause (if Possible)

Urinary electrolyte determination may be helpful in identifying the primary cause of hyponatremia when there is more than one possibility. The renal response to salt and water loss differs, depending on the cause of hyponatremia. When extrarenal losses of sodium and water occur through the skin (e.g., sweating, burns) or due to third space losses (e.g., pancreatitis), the renal response is to conserve sodium (urine sodium <20 mmol/L) and to conserve water through secretion of antidiuretic hormone (ADH) (high urine osmolality). However, if volume loss is due to vomiting or NG suction, primarily HCl is lost from gastric secretions. The kidneys generate and excrete $NaHCO_3$ to maintain the acid-base balance, resulting in urine with a normal (>20 mmol/L) sodium but a low (<20 mmol/L) chloride. If volume loss is due to diarrhea, primarily $NaHCO_3$ is lost in the stools. The kidneys generate and excrete NH_4Cl to maintain the acid-base balance, resulting in urine that is low in sodium but not in chloride.

Hyponatremia with ECF excess and edema may be accompanied by a low (<20 mmol/L) urinary sodium (e.g., nephrotic syndrome, CHF, cirrhosis of the liver) or a normal urinary sodium (renal failure).

Assess and Correct the Volume Status (see Chapter 3)

1. If the patient is volume depleted, correct the ECF volume using NS. Aim for a jugular venous pressure (JVP) of 2 to 3 cm H_2O above the sternal angle. In this case, the amount of

sodium required to improve the serum sodium concentration can be calculated using the following formula:

$$\text{mmol Na} = [\text{serum Na (desired)} - \text{serum Na (observed)}] \times \text{TBW},$$

where TBW = $0.6 \times$ weight (in kg).

> Remember that biologic systems are more responsive to rates of change than to absolute amounts of change. Make corrections at a rate similar to that at which the abnormality developed. It is safest to correct half the deficit and then reassess the situation.

Example: If you want to raise the serum sodium level from 120 to 135 mmol/L in a 70-kg man, the amount of sodium required is calculated as follows:

$$
\begin{aligned}
\text{mmol Na} &= (135 \text{ mmol/L} - 120 \text{ mmol/L}) (0.6 \times 70 \text{ L}) \\
&= (15 \text{ mmol/L}) (42 \text{ L}) \\
&= 630
\end{aligned}
$$

Because 1 L of NS contains 154 mmol of sodium, approximately 4 L of NS are required to raise the patient's serum level to 135 mmol/L.

2. If the patient has *extracellular volume excess and edema*, treat the volume excess and hyponatremia with water restriction and diuretics. Because most of these states are accompanied by secondary hyperaldosteronism, spironolactone is a reasonable choice of diuretic, as long as the patient is not hyperkalemic. Remember that the diuretic effect of this drug may be delayed for 3 to 4 days. The dose of *spironolactone* ranges from 25 to 200 mg daily in adults and can be given once daily or in divided doses. In this situation, strict intake-output charts can be useful. To raise the serum sodium, the daily water intake should be less than the daily urine output.

3. If the patient has a normal ECF volume, SIADH, primary polydipsia, pseudohyponatremia, or an endocrine disorder should be considered.

SIADH

The diagnosis of SIADH requires that stringent criteria be met:

1. Hyponatremia with serum hypo-osmolality
2. Urine that is less than maximally dilute when compared with serum osmolality (i.e., a simultaneous urine osmolality that is greater than the serum osmolality)
3. Inappropriately large amounts of urine sodium (>20 mmol/L)
4. Normal renal function
5. Normal thyroid function
6. Normal adrenal function
7. Patient not on diuretics

Management

SIADH should be treated as follows:

1. Correction of the underlying cause or contributory factors (e.g., drugs), if present.
2. Water restriction, usually to less than insensible losses (e.g., 500 to 1000 mL/day).
3. In addition to the first two measures, patients with severe symptomatic hyponatremia (serum sodium <115 mmol/L) may benefit from furosemide-induced diuresis, with hourly replacement of urinary sodium and potassium losses using NS. Very rarely, 3% saline is required.

   Too rapid correction of hyponatremia can result in central pontine myelinolysis and other undesirable side effects. Correct the serum sodium level slowly. Once the serum sodium level is >120 to 125 mmol/L, many of the symptoms of hyponatremia begin to lessen.
4. *Demeclocycline* 300 to 600 mg PO twice a day is occasionally useful in patients with chronic symptomatic SIADH in whom water restriction has been unsuccessful.

Primary Polydipsia

"Water intoxication" should be suspected in a patient with a psychiatric disorder, particularly when excessive drinking and polyuria interfere with sleep or are noticed by the ward staff. The hyponatremia is often exacerbated by the effects of neuroleptic or antidepressant medications the patient is taking. Immediate treatment involves fluid restriction, but this is only temporarily effective if not coupled with psychiatric assessment. *Demeclocycline* 300 to 600 mg PO twice a day may reduce the severity of hyponatremic episodes in patients with this disorder.

Pseudohyponatremia

The diagnosis of pseudohyponatremia can be made by

1. Demonstrating a normal serum osmolality in the presence of hyperlipidemia or hyperproteinemia.
2. Demonstrating a significant (>10 mmol/kg) osmolar gap, indicating the presence of additional osmotically active solutes, which can falsely lower the serum sodium level. This can be done by first having the laboratory *measure* serum osmolality. You should then *calculate* serum osmolality using the following formula:

$$\text{Serum osmolality (mmol/kg)} = 2\,\text{Na (mmol/L)} + \text{glucose (mmol/L)} + \text{urea (mmol/L)}$$

If the *measured* serum osmolality is more than 10 mmol/kg greater than the *calculated* serum osmolality, the hyponatremia is at least partially due to the presence of osmotically active solutes, such as excess lipids or plasma proteins.

Management

Treatment of pseudohyponatremia is restricted to correction of the underlying cause.

In cases of hyperglycemia, the true serum sodium concentration can be estimated by the following formula:

$$\frac{(\text{Observed glucose} - \text{normal glucose})(1.4)}{\text{Normal glucose}} + \text{serum Na (observed)}$$

The factor 1.4 is an arithmetic approximation to account for the shift of water that follows glucose into the extracellular compartment, thereby diluting sodium.

Example: A 35-year-old woman in diabetic ketoacidosis is admitted with the following laboratory results:

- Glucose = 83 mmol/L
- Sodium = 127 mmol/L
- Urea = 25 mmol/L
- Creatinine = 274 mmol/L

The true serum sodium, where normal glucose is taken as 5 mmol/L,

$$= \frac{(83 \text{ mmol/L} - 5 \text{ mmol/L})(1.4)}{5} + 127 \text{ mmol/L}$$

$$= 22 \text{ mmol/L} + 127 \text{ mmol/L}$$

$$= 149 \text{ mmol/L}$$

Endocrine Disorders

Hypothyroidism and *Addison's disease* can be diagnosed by their typical clinical features in association with confirmatory laboratory studies. Hyponatremia in either of these conditions responds to treatment of the underlying endocrine disorder.

Appendix

Adult Emergency Cardiac Care Algorithms

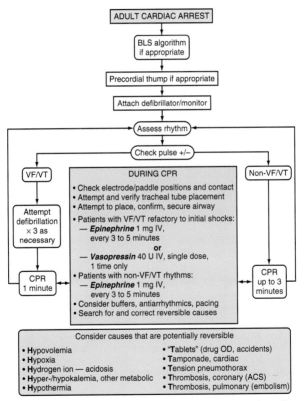

Figure A–1 ILCOR universal/international adult advanced cardiovascular life support algorithm. ACS, acute coronary syndrome; BLS, basic life suport; CPR, cardiopulmonary resuscitation; IV, intravenous; OD, overdose; VF/VT, ventricular fibrillation/ventricular tachycardia. (Redrawn with permission from ACLS Provider Manual, © 2002, Copyright American Heart Association.)

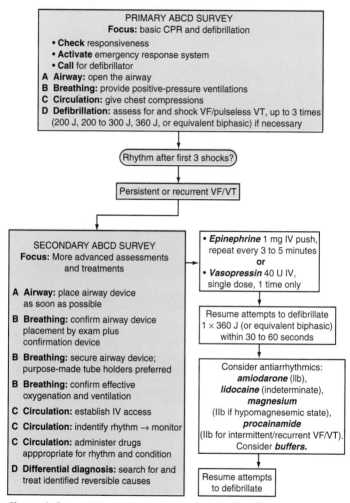

Figure A–2 Algorithm for ventricular fibrillation/pulseless ventricular tachycardia (VF/VT). CPR, cardiopulmonary resuscitation; IV, intravenous. (Redrawn with permission from ACLS Provider Manual, © 2002, Copyright American Heart Association.)

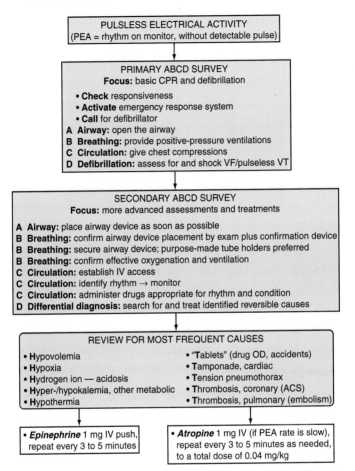

Figure A–3 Algorithm for pulseless electrical activity (PEA). ACS, acute coronary syndrome; CPR, cardiopulmonary resuscitation; OD, overdose; VF, ventricular fibrillation; VT, ventricular tachycadia. (Redrawn with permission from ACLS Provider Manual, © 2002, Copyright American Heart Association.)

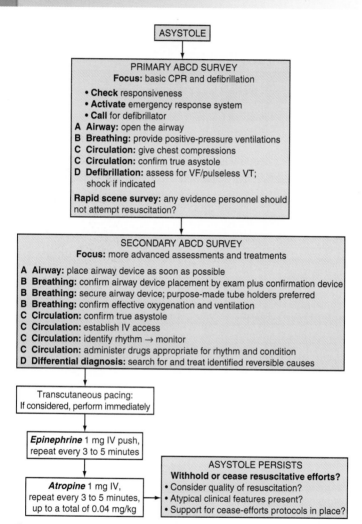

Figure A–4 Algorithm for asystole: the silent heart. CPR, cardio-pulmonary resuscitation; IV, intravenous; VF, ventricular fibrillation; VT, ventricular tachycardia. (Redrawn with permission from ACLS Provider Manual, © 2002, Copyright American Heart Association.)

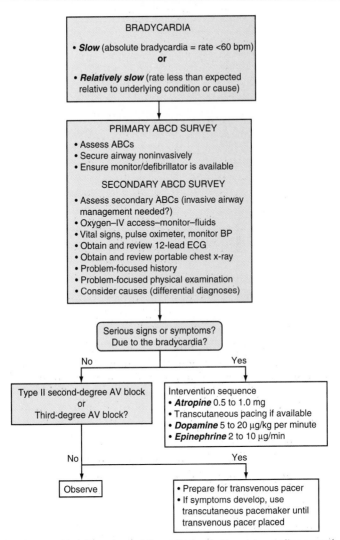

Figure A–5 Algorithm for bradycardia (patient not in cardiac arrest). AV, atrioventricular; BP, blood pressure; bpm, beats per minute; ECG, electrocardiogram; IV, intravenous. (Redrawn with permission from ACLS Provider Manual, © 2002, Copyright American Heart Association.)

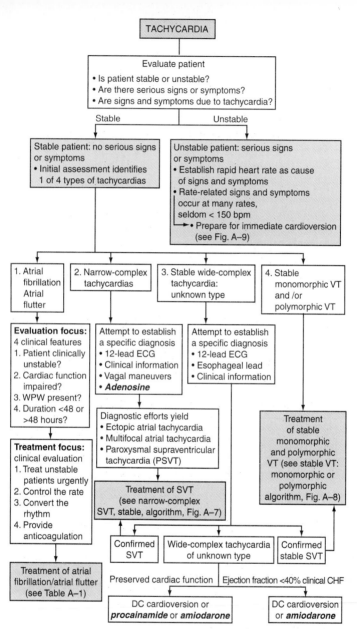

Figure A–6 Overview algorithm: the tachycardias. bpm, beats per minute; CHF, congestive heart failure; DC, direct current; ECG, electrocardiogram; SVT, supraventricular tachycardia; VT, ventricular tachycardia; WPW, Wolff-Parkinson-White syndrome. (Redrawn with permission from ACLS Provider Manual, © 2002, Copyright American Heart Association.)

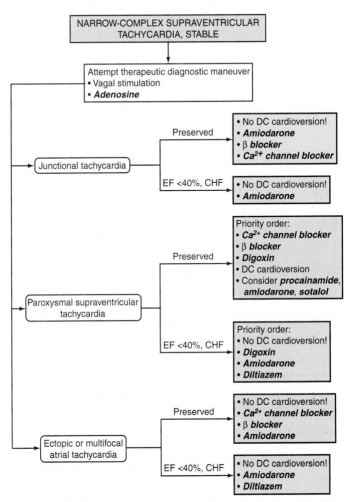

Figure A–7 Algorithm for narrow-complex tachycardia. CHF, congestive heart failure; DC, direct current; EF, ejection fraction. (Redrawn with permission from ACLS Provider Manual, © 2002, Copyright American Heart Association.)

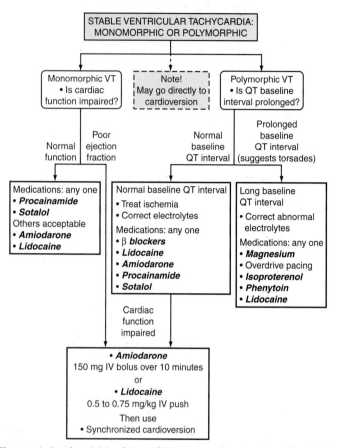

Figure A–8 Algorithm for stable ventricular tachycardia (VT)—monomorphic and polymorphic. IV, intravenous. (Redrawn with permission from ACLS Provider Manual, © 2002, Copyright American Heart Association.)

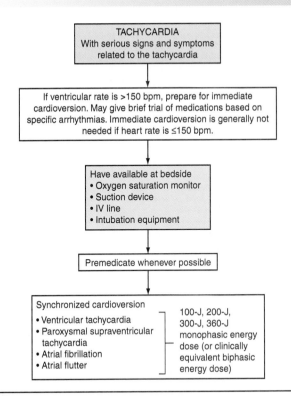

Figure A–9 Algorithm for electrical cardioversion. bpm, beats per minute; IV, intravenous; VF, ventricular fibrillation. (Redrawn with permission from ACLS Provider Manual, © 2002, Copyright American Heart Association.)

TABLE A-1 Tachycardia: Atrial Fibrillation and Flutter

	1. Control Rate		2. Convert Rhythm	
	Heart Function Preserved	Impaired Heart EF <40% or CHF	Duration <48 Hours	Duration >48 Hours or Unknown

Normal cardiac function	**Note:** *If AF >48 hr duration, use agents to convert rhythm with extreme caution in patients not receiving adequate anticoagulation because of possible embolic complications*
	
	Use only 1 of the following agents*
	• Calcium channel blockers (class I)
	• Beta blockers (class I)
		N/A	**Consider** DC cardioversion
			
			Use only 1 of the following agents*
			• Amiodarone (class IIa)
			• Ibutilide (class IIa)
			• Flecainide (class IIa)
			• Propafenone (class IIa)
			• Procainamide (class IIa)
				No DC cardioversion!
				Note: *Conversion of AF to NSR with drugs or shock may cause embolization of atrial thrombi unless patient has adequate anticoagulation*
				Use antiarrhythmic agents with extreme caution if AF >48 hr duration (see note above)
				
				or
				
				Delayed cardioversion
				• Anticoagulation × 3 wk at proper levels
				• Cardioversion, *then*
				• Anticoagulation × 4 wk more
				
				or
				
				Early cardioversion
				• Begin IV heparin at once
				• TEE to exclude atrial clot
				   then
				• Cardioversion within 24 hr
				   then
				• Anticoagulation × 4 wk more

Impaired heart (EF <40% or CHF)	N/A	*Note: If AF >48 hr duration, use agents to convert rhythm with extreme caution in patients not receiving adequate anticoagulation because of possible embolic complications* DC cardioversion *or* Primary antiarrhythmic agents	*Note: If AF >48 hr duration, use agents to convert rhythm with extreme caution in patients not receiving adequate anticoagulation because of possible embolic complications* *Use only 1 of the following agents** • Digoxin (class IIb) • Diltiazem (class IIb) • Amiodarone (class IIb)	Consider DC cardioversion **or** amiodarone (class IIb)	Anticoagulation, as described above, followed by DC cardioversion
WPW		*Note: If AF >48 hr duration, use agents to convert rhythm with extreme caution in patients not receiving adequate anticoagulation because of possible embolic complications* DC cardioversion *or* Amiodarone (class IIb)	DC cardioversion *or* **Primary anti-arrhythmic agents** *Use only 1 of the following agents** • Amiodarone (class IIb) • Flecainide (class IIb) • Procainamide (class IIb)	Anticoagulation, as described above, followed by DC cardioversion

*Occasionally two of the named antiarrhythmic agents may be used, but use of these agents in combination may have proarrhythmic potential. The classes listed represent the Class of Recommendation rather than the Vaughn-Williams classification of antiarrhythmics.

Continued

TABLE A–1 Tachycardia: Atrial Fibrillation and Flutter—cont'd

	1. Control Rate		2. Convert Rhythm	
	Heart Function Preserved	Impaired Heart EF <40% or CHF	Duration <48 Hours	Duration >48 Hours or Unknown
	*Use only 1 of the following agents** • Amiodarone (class IIb) • Flecainide (class IIb) • Procainamide (class IIb) • Propafenone (class IIb) • Sotalol (class IIb) *Class III (can be harmful)* • Adenosine • Beta blockers • Calcium blockers • Digoxin		• Propafenone (class IIb) • Sotalol (class IIb) *Class III (can be harmful)* • Adenosine • Beta blockers • Calcium blockers • Digoxin	

AF, atrial fibrillation; CHF, congestive heart failure; DC, direct current; EF, ejection fraction; IV, intravenous; N/A, not applicable; NSR, normal sinus rhythm; TEE, transesophageal echocardiogram; WPW, Wolff-Parkinson-White syndrome.
*Occasionally two of the named antiarrhythmic agents may be used, but use of these agents in combination may have proarrhythmic potential. The classes listed represent the Class of Recommendation rather than the Vaughn-Williams classification of antiarrhythmics.
Reproduced with permission, ACLS Provider Manual, 2002, Copyright American Heart Association.

Appendix

Advanced Cardiovascular Life Support Drugs and Electrical Therapy

TABLE B–1 Advanced Cardiovascular Life Support Drugs and Electrical Therapy

Drug/Therapy	Adult Dosage	Indications/Precautions
ACE Inhibitors	**Approach**	**Indications**
	ACE inhibitor therapy should start with low-dose oral administration (with possible IV doses for some preparations) and increase steadily to achieve a full dose within 24–28 hr	ACE inhibitors reduce mortality and improve LV dysfunction in post-AMI patients. They help prevent adverse LV remodeling, delay progression of heart failure, and decrease sudden death and recurrent MI.
Enalapril	• PO: Start with a single dose of 2.5 mg; titrate to 20 mg PO BID • IV (enalaprilat): 1.25 mg IV initial dose over 5 min, then 1.25–5.0 mg IV q 6 hr.	They are of greatest benefit in patients with the following conditions: • Suspected MI and ST segment elevation in 2 or more anterior precordial leads • Hypertension • Clinical heart failure without hypotension in patients not responding to digitalis or diuretics • Clinical signs of AMI with LV dysfunction • LV ejection fraction <40%
Captopril	• Start with a single dose of 6.25 mg PO • Advance to 25 mg TID and then to 50 mg TID as tolerated	**Precautions/Contraindications for all ACE inhibitors** • ***Contraindicated*** in pregnancy (may cause fetal injury or death) • Contraindicated in angioedema • Hypersensitivity to ACE inhibitors • Reduce dose in renal failure (creatinine >3 mg/dL); avoid in bilateral renal artery stenosis
Lisinopril	• 5 mg within 24 hr of onset of symptoms, then • 5 mg given after 24 hr, then • 10 mg given after 48 hr, then • 10 mg once daily for 6 wk	

Continued

TABLE B-1 Advanced Cardiovascular Life Support Drugs and Electrical Therapy—cont'd

Drug/Therapy	Adult Dosage	Indications/Precautions
Ramipril	Start with a single dose of 2.5 mg PO; titrate to 5 mg PO BID as tolerated	**Indications/Precautions** • Avoid hypotension, especially following initial dose and in relative volume depletion • Generally not started in ED but within first 24 hr after fibrinolytic therapy has been completed and blood pressure has been stabilized
Adenosine	**IV Rapid Push** • Place patient in mild reverse Trendelenburg's position before administration of drug • Initial bolus of 6 mg given *rapidly* over 1–3 sec followed by NS bolus of 20 mL; then elevate the extremity • Repeat dose of 12 mg in 1–2 min if needed • A third dose of 12 mg may be given in 1–2 min if needed **Injection Technique** • Record rhythm strip during administration • Draw up adenosine dose and flush in 2 separate syringes • Attach both syringes to the IV injection port closest to patient • Clamp IV tubing above injection port • Push IV adenosine *as quickly as possible* (1–3 sec) • While maintaining pressure on adenosine plunger, push NS flush *as rapidly as possible* after adenosine • Unclamp IV tubing	**Indications** • First drug for most forms of narrow-complex PSVT; effective in terminating those due to reentry involving AV node or sinus node • Does *not* convert atrial fibrillation, atrial flutter, or VT **Precautions** • Transient side effects include flushing, chest pain or tightness, brief periods of asystole or bradycardia, ventricular ectopy • Less effective in patients taking theophyllines; avoid in patients receiving dipyridamole • If administered for wide-complex tachycardia/VT, may cause deterioration (including hypotension) • Transient periods of sinus bradycardia and ventricular ectopy are common after termination of SVT • Contraindication: poison/drug-induced tachycardia

Amiodarone

Cardiac Arrest

300 mg IV push; consider repeating 150 mg IV push in 3–5 min (maximum cumulative dose: 2.2 g IV/24 hr)

Wide Complex Tachycardia (Stable)

Maximum cumulative dose: 2.2 g IV/24 hr
May be administered as follows:

- *Rapid infusion:* 150 mg IV over first 10 min (15 mg/min); may repeat rapid infusion (150 mg IV) q 10 min as needed
- *Slow infusion:* 360 mg IV over 6 hr (1 mg/min)
- *Maintenance infusion:* 540 mg IV over 18 hr (0.5 mg/min)

Indications

Used in a wide variety of atrial and ventricular tachyarrhythmias and for rate control of rapid atrial arrhythmias in patients with impaired LV function when digoxin has proved ineffective

Recommended for

- Treatment of shock-refractory VF/pulseless VT
- Treatment of polymorphic VT and wide-complex tachycardia of uncertain origin
- Control of hemodynamically stable VT when cardioversion is unsuccessful; particularly useful in the presence of LV dysfunction
- Use as adjunct to electrical cardioversion of SVT, PSVT
- Acceptable for termination of ectopic or multifocal atrial tachycardia with preserved LV function
- May be used for rate control in treatment of atrial fibrillation or flutter when other therapies are ineffective

Precautions

- May produce vasodilatation and hypotension
- May have negative inotropic effects
- When multiple doses are administered, cumulative doses >2.2 g/24 hr are associated with significant hypotension in clinical trials
- May prolong QT interval; do not routinely administer with other drugs that prolong QT interval (e.g., procainamide)

Continued

387

TABLE B–1 Advanced Cardiovascular Life Support Drugs and Electrical Therapy—cont'd

Drug/Therapy	Adult Dosage	Indications/Precautions
		• Use with caution if renal failure is present • Terminal elimination is extremely long (half-life up to 40 days)
Amrinone	**IV Loading Dose and Infusion** • 0.75 mg/kg, given over 10–15 min • Follow with infusion of 5–15 μg/kg/min titrated to clinical effec • Optimal use requires hemodynamic monitoring	**Indications** Severe CHF refractory to diuretics, vasodilators, and conventional inotropic agents **Precautions** • Do not mix with dextrose solutions or other drugs • May cause tachyarrhythmias, hypotension, or thrombocytopenia • Can increase myocardial ischemia
Aspirin • 160- or 325-mg tablets • Chewable tablets more effective in some trials	• 160–325-mg tablet taken as soon as possible (chewing is preferable to swallowing) and then daily • May use rectal suppository for patients who cannot take PO • Give within minutes of arrival • Higher doses (1000 mg) interfere with prostacyclin production and may limit positive benefits	**Indications** • Administer to all patients with ACS, particularly reperfusion candidates, unless hypersensitive to aspirin • Blocks formation of thromboxane A₂, which causes platelets to aggregate, arteries to constrict; this reduces overall AMI mortality, reinfarction, nonfatal stroke • Any person with symptoms ("pressure," "heavy weight," "squeezing," "crushing") suggestive of ischemic pain

Atropine Sulfate

Can be given via tracheal tube

Asystole or Pulseless Electrical Activity

- 1 mg IV push
- Repeat every 3–5 min (if asystole persists) to a maximum dose of 0.03–0.04 mg/kg

Bradycardia

- 0.5–1 mg IV every 3–5 min as needed, not to exceed total dose of 0.04 mg/kg
- Use shorter dosing interval (3 min) and higher doses (0.04 mg/kg) in severe clinical conditions

Tracheal Administration

- 2–3 mg diluted in 10 mL NS

Precautions

- Relatively contraindicated in patients with active ulcer disease or asthma
- Contraindicated in patients with known hypersensitivity to aspirin

Indications

- First drug for symptomatic sinus bradycardia (class I)
- May be beneficial in presence of AV block at the nodal level (class IIa) or ventricular asystole; **will not be effective when infranodal (Mobitz type II) block is suspected (class IIb)**
- Second drug (after epinephrine or vasopressin) for asystole or bradycardic pulseless electrical activity (class IIb)

Precautions

- Use with caution in presence of myocardial ischemia and hypoxia; increases myocardial oxygen demand
- Avoid in hypothermic bradycardia
- Will not be effective for infranodal (type II) AV block and new third-degree block with wide QRS complexes (in these patients, may cause paradoxical slowing; be prepared to pace or give catecholamines)

Beta Blockers

Metoprolol

- Initial IV dose: 5 mg slow IV at 5-min intervals to a total of 15 mg

Indications

- Administer to all patients with suspected MI and unstable angina in the absence of complications; these are effective antianginal agents and can reduce incidence of VF

TABLE B-1 Advanced Cardiovascular Life Support Drugs and Electrical Therapy—cont'd

Drug/Therapy	Adult Dosage	Indications/Precautions
Atenolol	• Oral regimen to follow IV dose: 50 mg BID for 24 hr, then increase to 100 mg BID • 5 mg slow IV (over 5 min) • Wait 10 min, then give second dose of 5 mg slow IV (over 5 min) • In 10 min, if tolerated well, may start 50 mg PO; then give 50 mg PO BID	• Useful as an adjunctive agent with fibrinolytic therapy; may reduce nonfatal reinfarction and recurrent ischemia • To convert to normal sinus rhythm or to slow ventricular response (or both) in supraventricular tachyarrhythmias (PSVT, atrial fibrillation, or atrial flutter); beta blockers are second-line agents after adenosine, diltiazem, or digitalis derivative • To reduce myocardial ischemia and damage in AMI patients with elevated HR, BP, or both • For emergency antihypertensive therapy for hemorrhagic and acute ischemic stroke
Propranolol	• Total dose: 0.1 mg/kg by slow IV push, divided into 3 equal doses at 2- to 3-min intervals, do not exceed 1 mg/min • Repeat after 2 min if necessary	**Precautions** Concurrent IV administration with IV calcium channel blocking agents such as verapamil or diltiazem can cause severe hypotension
Esmolol	• 0.5 mg/kg over 1 min, followed by continuous infusion at 0.05 mg/kg/min • Titrate to effect; esmolol has a short half-life (2–9 min)	• Avoid in bronchospastic diseases, cardiac failure, or severe abnormalities in cardiac conduction • Monitor cardiac and pulmonary status during administration • May cause myocardial depression
Labetalol	• 10 mg labetalol IV push over 1–2 min • May repeat or double labetalol every 10 min to a maximum dose of 150 mg, or give initial dose as a bolus, then start labetalol infusion at 2–8 µg/min	• Contraindicated in presence of HR <60 beats/min, systolic BP <100 mm Hg, severe LV failure, hypoperfusion, or second-or third-degree AV block

Calcium Chloride

100 mg/mL in 10 mL vial (total = 1 g; a 10% solution)

IV Slow Push

- 8–16 mg/kg (usually 5 to 10 mL) IV for hyperkalemia and calcium channel blocker overdose; may be repeated as needed
- 2–4 mg/kg (usually 2 mL) IV for prophylaxis before IV calcium channel blockers.

Indications

- Known or suspected hyperkalemia (e.g., renal failure)
- Hypocalcemia (e.g., after multiple blood transfusions)
- As an antidote for toxic effects (hypotension and arrhythmias) from calcium channel blocker overdose or beta-adrenergic blocker overdose
- May be used prophylactically before IV calcium channel blockers to prevent hypotension

Precautions

- Do not use routinely in cardiac arrest
- Do not mix with sodium bicarbonate

Cardioversion (Synchronized)

Administered via remote defibrillation electrodes or hand-held paddles from a defibrillator/monitor

Place defibrillator/monitor in synchronized (sync) mode

Technique

- Premedicate whenever possible
- Engage sync mode before each attempt
- Look for sync markers on the R wave
- "Clear" the patient before each shock
- Deliver monophasic shocks in the following sequence: 100 J, 200 J, 300J, 360 J.* Use this sequence for each of the following:
  —VT[†]
  —PSVT[‡]
  —Atrial flutter[‡]
  —Atrial fibrillation

Indications

- All tachycardias (rate >150 beats/min) with serious signs and symptoms related to tachycardia
- May give brief trial of medications based on specific arrhythmias

Precautions

- In critical conditions, go to immediate unsynchronized shocks
- Urgent cardioversion is generally not needed if heart rate is ≤150 beats/min

*Biphasic waveforms using lower energy are acceptable if documented to be clinically equivalent or superior to reports of monophasic shock success.
[†]Treat polymorphic VT (irregular form and rate) with same currents used for VF:200 J, 200 to 300 J, 360 J.
[‡]PSVT and atrial flutter often respond to lower energy levels; start with 50 J.

Continued

Drug/Therapy	Adult Dosage	Indications/Precautions
Sync mode delivers energy just after the R wave	• Press "charge" button, "clear" the patient, and press both "shock" buttons simultaneously	• Reactivation of sync mode is required after each attempted cardioversion (defibrillators/cardioverters default to unsynchronized mode) • Prepare to defibrillate immediately if cardioversion causes VF • Synchronized cardioversion cannot be performed unless the patient is connected to monitor leads; lead select switch must be on lead I, II, or III and not on "paddles" • Contraindication: poison/drug induced tachycardia
Defibrillation Attempt	Adult Monophasic Defibrillation Energy Levels*	Indications
Use conventional monitor/defibrillator	• 200 J, first shock • 200–300 J, second shock • 360 J, third shock • If these shocks fail to convert VF/VT, continue at 360 J for future shocks • If VF recurs, shock again at the last successful energy level	First intervention for VF or pulseless VT (class I) Precautions
Use automated or shock advisory defibrillator		• Always "clear" the patient before discharging a defibrillation shock • Do not delay defibrillation for VF/VT • Asystole should not be routinely shocked • Treat VF/VT in hypothermic cardiac arrest with up to 3 shocks; repeat shocks for VF/VT only after core temperature rises above 30°C
Administer shocks via remoteadhesive electrodes or		

*Biphasic devices shock at lower energy levels (approximately 150 J). In some clinical settings, initial and repeated shocks at these lower energy levels are acceptable.

hand-held
paddles

- If patient in VF/VT has an automatic implantable cardioverter defibrillator (AICD), perform external defibrillation per BLS guidelines; if AICD is delivering shocks, wait 30–60 sec for completion of cycle
- If patient has implanted pacemaker, place paddles and pads several inches from the pacing generator

Digibind (Digoxin-Specific Antibody Therapy)

40-mg vial (each vial binds about 0.6 mg digoxin)

Chronic Intoxication

3–5 vials may be effective

Acute Overdose

- IV dose varies according to amount of digoxin ingested
- Average dose is 10 vials (400 mg); may require up to 20 vials (800 mg)
- See package insert for details

Indications

Digoxin toxicity with the following:
- Life-threatening arrhythmias
- Shock or CHF
- Hyperkalemia (potassium level >5.0 mEq/L)
- Steady-state serum levels >10–15 ng/mL for symptomatic patients

Precautions

Serum digoxin levels rise after digibind therapy and should not be used to guide continuing therapy

Digoxin

0.25 mg/mL or 0.1 mg/mL supplied in 1- or 2-mL ampule (totals = 0.1–0.5 mg)

IV Infusion

- Loading doses of 10–15 µg/kg lean body weight provide therapeutic effect with minimum risk of toxic effects
- Maintenance dose is affected by body size and renal function

Indications

- To slow ventricular response in atrial fibrillation or atrial flutter
- Alternative drug for PSVT

Continued

393

TABLE B-1 Advanced Cardiovascular Life Support Drugs and Electrical Therapy—cont'd

Drug/Therapy	Adult Dosage	Indications/Precautions
		Precautions • Toxic effects are common and are frequently associated with serious arrhythmias • Avoid electrical cardioversion if patient is receiving digoxin unless condition is life threatening; use lower current settings (10–20 J)
Diltiazem	**Acute Rate Control** • 15–20 mg (0.25 mg/kg) IV over 2 min • May repeat in 15 min at 20–25 mg (0.35 mg/kg) over 2 min **Maintenance Infusion** 5–15 mg/hr, titrated to HR	**Indications** • To control ventricular rate in atrial fibrillation and atrial flutter; may terminate reentrant arrhythmias that require AV nodal conduction for their continuation • Use after adenosine to treat refractory PSVT in patients with narrow QRS complex and adequate BP **Precautions** • Do not use calcium channel blockers for wide-QRS tachycardias of uncertain origin or for poison/drug-induced tachycardia • Avoid calcium channel blockers in patients with Wolff-Parkinson-White syndrome plus rapid atrial fibrillation or flutter, in patients with sick sinus syndrome, or in patients with AV block without a pacemaker • Expect BP drop resulting from peripheral vasodilatation (greater drop with verapamil than with diltiazem) • Avoid in patients receiving oral beta blockers • Concurrent IV administration with IV beta blockers can cause severe hypotension

Disopyramide
(IV dose not approved for use in United States)

IV Dose

2 mg/kg over 10 min, followed by continuous infusion of 0.4 mg/kg/hr

Indications

Useful for treatment of a wide variety of arrhythmias; prolongs the effective refractory period, similar to procainamide

Precautions/Contraindications

Must be infused relatively slowly; has potent anticholinergic, negative inotropic, and hypotensive effects that limit its use

Dobutamine
IV infusion: dilute 250 mg (20 mL) in 250 mL NS or D5W

IV Infusion

- Usual infusion rate is 2– 20 μg/kg/min
- Titrate so HR does not increase by >10% of baseline
- Hemodynamic monitoring is recommended for optimal use

Indications

Consider for pump problems (CHF, pulmonary congestion) with systolic BP of 70–100 mm Hg and *no* signs of shock

Precautions

- Avoid with systolic BP <100 mm Hg *and* signs of shock
- May cause tachyarrhythmias, fluctuations in BP, headache, and nausea
- Contraindication: suspected or known poison/drug-induced shock
- Do not mix with sodium bicarbonate

Dofetilide
(Not approved for use in United States)

IV Infusion Dose

Single infusion of 8 μg/kg over 30 min

Indications

Treatment of atrial fibrillation

Precautions/Contraindications

- Adverse effects include QT prolongation, which can be associated with torsades de pointes; this complication is most likely to occur in patients with a history of CHF
- Its use is limited by the need to infuse relatively slowly, which may be impractical under emergent conditions

Continued

TABLE B-1 Advanced Cardiovascular Life Support Drugs and Electrical Therapy—cont'd

Drug/Therapy	Adult Dosage	Indications/Precautions
Dopamine *IV infusion:* Mix 400–800 mg in 250 mL NS, lactated Ringer's solution, or D5W	**Continuous infusions (titrate to patient response)** **Low dose:** 1–5 µg/kg/min **Moderate dose:** 5–10 µg/kg/min ("cardiac doses") **High dose:** 10–20 µg/kg/min ("vasopressor doses")	**Indications** • Second drug for symptomatic bradycardia (after atropine) • Use for hypotension (systolic BP ≤70–100 mm Hg) with signs and symptoms of shock **Precautions** • May use in patients with hypovolemia, but only after volume replacement • Use with caution in cardiogenic shock with accompanying CHF • May cause tachyarrhythmias, excessive vasoconstriction • Taper slowly • Do not mix with sodium bicarbonate
Epinephrine Available in 1:10,000 and 1:1000 concentrations	**Cardiac Arrest** • **IV dose:** 1 mg (10 mL of 1:10,000 solution) administered of 3–5 min during resuscitation; follow each dose with 20 mL IV flush • **Higher dose:** higher doses (up to 0.2 mg/kg) may be used if 1-mg dose fails • **Continuous infusion:** add 30 mg epinephrine (30 mL of 1:1000 solution) to 250 mL NS or D5W; run at 100 mL/hr and titrate to response	**Indications** • **Cardiac arrest:** VF, pulseless VT, asystole, pulseless electrical activity • **Symptomatic bradycardia:** after atropine, dopamine, and transcutaneous pacing • **Severe hypotension** • **Anaphylaxis, severe allergic reactions:** combine with large fluid volumes, corticosteroids, antihistamines

Fibrinolytic Agents

For all agents, use 2 peripheral IV lines, *one line exclusively for fibrinolytic administration*

Alteplase, recombinant *(Activase)*, tissue plasminogen activator (tPA)

50- and 100-mg vials reconstituted with sterile water to 1 mg/mL

• **Tracheal route:** 2–2.5 mg diluted in 10 mL NS

Profound Bradycardia or Hypotension

2–10 μg/min infusion (add 1 mg of 1:1000 to 500 mL NS; infuse at 1–5 mL/min)

Recommended total dose is based on patient's weight. For AMI, the total dose should not exceed 100 mg; for acute ischemic stroke, the total dose should not exceed 90 mg. Note that there are 2 approved dose regimens for AMI patients and a *different* regimen for acute ischemic stroke.

For AMI:

• Accelerated infusion (1.5 hr)
—Give 15-mg IV bolus
—Then 0.75 mg/kg over next 30 min (not to exceed 50 mg)
—Then 0.50 mg/kg over next 60 min (not to exceed 35 mg)

• 3-hour infusion
—Give 60 mg in first hour (initial 6–10 mg is given as a bolus)
—Then 20 mg/hr for 2 additional hr

Precautions

• Raising BP and increasing HR may cause myocardial ischemia, angina, and increased myocardial oxygen demand

• High doses do not improve survival or neurologic outcome and may contribute to postresuscitation myocardial dysfunction

• Higher doses *may* be required to treat poison/drug-induced shock

Indications

For AMI in adults:

• ST elevation (≥1 mm in ≥2 contiguous leads) or new or presumably new LBBB; strongly suspicious for injury (BBB obscuring ST analysis)

• In context of signs and symptoms of AMI

• Time from onset of symptoms <12 hr

For acute ischemic stroke (alteplase is the only fibrinolytic agent approved for acute ischemic stroke):

• Sudden onset of focal neurologic deficits or alterations in consciousness (e.g., language abnormality, motor arm, facial droop)

• Absence of intracerebral or subarachnoid hemorrhage or mass effect on CT scan

• Absence of variable or rapidly improving neurologic deficits

• Alteplase can be started in <3 hr from symptom onset

Continued

TABLE B–1 Advanced Cardiovascular Life Support Drugs and Electrical Therapy—cont'd

Drug/Therapy	Adult Dosage	Indications/Precautions
		Precautions
	For acute ischemic stroke:	*Specific exclusion criteria*
	• Give 0.9 mg/kg (maximum 90 mg) infused over 60 min	• Active internal bleeding (except menses) within 21 days
	• Give 10% of the total dose as an initial IV bolus over 1 min	• History of cerebrovascular, intracranial, or intraspinal event within 3 mo (stroke, arteriovenous malformation, neoplasm, aneurysm, recent trauma, recent surgery)
	• Give the remaining 90% over the next 60 min	
Anistreplase *(Eminase)*; anisoylated plasminogen streptokinase activator complex (APSAC) Reconstitute 30 U in 50 mL sterile water or D5W	30 IU IV over 2–5 min	• Major surgery or serious trauma within 14 days • Aortic dissection • Severe, uncontrolled hypertension • Known bleeding disorders • Prolonged CPR with evidence of thoracic trauma • Lumbar puncture within 7 days • Recent arterial puncture at non compressible site • During the first 24 hr of fibrinolytic therapy for ischemic stroke, do not administer aspirin or heparin
	Reteplase Recombinant	**Adjuvant Therapy for AM**
Reteplase, recombinant *(Retavase)* 10-U vials reconstituted with sterile water to 1 U/mL	• Give first 10-U IV bolus over 2 min • 30 min later, give second 10-U IV bolus over 2 min (give NS flush before and after each bolus)	• 160–325 mg aspirin chewed as soon as possible • Begin heparin immediately and continue for 48 hr if alteplase or reteplase is used

398

Streptokinase
(Streptase)
Reconstitute to 1 mg/mL

1.5 million IU in a 1-hr infusion

Tenecteplase
(TNKase)

Bolus: 30–50 mg

Flecainide

(IV form not approved for use in United States)

IV Dose

Administered at 2 mg/kg body weight at 10 mg/min; *must be infused slowly*

Indications
- Treatment of ventricular arrhythmias
- Treatment of supraventricular arrhythmias in patients without coronary artery disease
- Effective for termination of atrial flutter and fibrillation, ectopic atrial tachycardia, AV nodal reentrant tachycardia, and SVTs associated with an accessory pathway

Precautions/Contraindications
- Should be avoided in patients with impaired LV function because it has significant negative inotropic effects
- *Must be infused slowly*
- Adverse effects include bradycardia, hypotension, and neurologic symptoms such as oral paresthesias and visual blurring

Flumazenil

First Dose

0.2 mg IV over 15 sec

Second Dose

0.3 mg IV over 30 sec; if no adequate response, give third dose

Indications

Reverse respiratory depression and sedative effects from pure benzodiazepine overdose

Precautions
- Effects may not outlast effect of benzodiazepines
- Monitor for recurrent respiratory depression
- Do not use in suspected tricyclic overdose
- Do not use in seizure-prone patients

Continued

399

TABLE B–1 Advanced Cardiovascular Life Support Drugs and Electrical Therapy—cont'd

Drug/Therapy	Adult Dosage	Indications/Precautions
	Third Dose 0.5 mg IV over 30 sec; if no adequate response, repeat once every minute until adequate response or a total of 3 mg is given	• Do not use in unknown drug overdose or mixed drug overdose with drugs known to cause seizures (e.g., tricyclic anti-depressants, cocaine, amphetamines)
Furosemide	**IV Infusion** • 0.5–1 mg/kg given over 1–2 min • If no response, double dose to 2 mg/kg, slowly, over 1–2 min	**Indications** • For adjuvant therapy of acute pulmonary edema in patients with systolic BP >90–100 mm Hg (without signs and symptoms of shock) • Hypertensive emergencies • Increased intracranial pressure **Precautions** Dehydration, hypovolemia, hypotension, hypokalemia, or other electrolyte imbalance may occur
Glucagon Powdered in 1- and 10-mg vials Reconstitute with provided solution	**IV Infusion** 1–5 mg over 2–5 min	**Indications** Adjuvant treatment of toxic effects of calcium channel blocker or beta blocker **Precautions** • Do not mix with saline • May cause vomiting, hyperglycemia
Glycoprotein IIb/IIIa Inhibitors	Check package insert for current indications, doses, and duration of therapy; optimal duration of therapy has not been established	**Indications** These drugs inhibit the integrin glycoprotein IIb/IIIa receptor in the membrane of platelets, inhibiting platelet aggregation; indicated for acute coronary syndromes *without* ST segment elevation

Abciximab
(ReoPro)

- *Acute coronary syndromes with planned PCI within 24 hr:* 0.25 mg/kg IV bolus (10–60 min before procedure), then 0.125 µg/kg/min IV infusion
- *PCI only:* 0.25 mg/kg IV bolus, then 10 µg/kg/min IV infusion

Precautions/Contraindications

Active internal bleeding or bleeding disorder in past 30 days, history of intracranial hemorrhage or other bleeding, surgical procedure or trauma within 1 mo, platelet count <150,000/mm^3, hypersensitivity and concomitant use of another GP IIb/IIIa inhibitor

Indications

FDA-approved for patients with non–Q wave MI or unstable angina with planned PCI within 24 hr

Eptifibatide
(Integrilin)

- *Acute coronary syndromes:* 180 µg/kg IV bolus, then 2 µg/kg/min IV infusion
- *PCI:* 135 µg/kg IV bolus, then begin 0.5 µg/kg/min IV infusion, then repeat bolus in 10 min

Precautions/Contraindications

- Must use with heparin
- Binds irreversibly with platelets; platelet function recovery requires 48 hr (regeneration)
- Readministration may cause hypersensitivity reaction

Indications

Non–Q wave MI, unstable angina managed medically, and unstable angina/non–Q wave MI patients undergoing PCI

Actions/Precautions

Platelet function recovers within 4–8 hr after discontinuation

Tirofiban
(Aggrastat)

Acute coronary syndromes or PCI: 0.4 µg/kg/min IV for 30 min, then 0.1 µg/kg/min IV infusion

Indications

Non–Q wave MI, unstable angina managed medically, and unstable angina/non–Q wave MI patients undergoing PCI

Continued

TABLE B-1 Advanced Cardiovascular Life Support Drugs and Electrical Therapy—cont'd

Drug/Therapy	Adult Dosage	Indications/Precautions

Heparin— Unfractionated (UFH)
 	
Concentrations range from 1000 to 40,000 IU/mL
	IV Infusion
	• Initial bolus 60 IU/kg (maximum bolus, 4000 IU)
	• Continue 12 IU/kg/hr (maximum, 1000 IU/hr for patients >70 kg) (round to the nearest 50 IU)
	• Adjust to maintain aPTT 1.5–2.0 times the control values for 48 hr or until angiography
	• Target range for aPTT after first 24 hr is between 50 and 70 sec (may vary with laboratory)
	• Check aPTT at 6,12,18, and 24 hr
	• Follow institutional heparin protocol
		Actions/Precautions
		Platelet function recovers within 4–8 hr after discontinuation
		
		Indications
		• Adjuvant therapy in AMI
		• Begin heparin with fibrin-specific lytics (e.g., alteplase)
		
		Precautions
		• Same contraindications as for fibrinolytic therapy:active bleeding, recent intracranial, intraspinal, or eye surgery; severe hypertension; bleeding disorders; GI bleeding
		• Doses and laboratory targets appropriate when used with fibrinolytic therapy
		• Heparin reversal: **protamine** 25-mg IV infusion over 10 min or longer (calculate dose as 1 mg protamine per 100 IU of heparin remaining in patient; heparin plasma half-life is 60 min)
		• Do not use if platelet count is or falls below 100,000 or with history of heparin-induced thrombocytopenia; for these patients, consider direct antithrombins:
		  —*Desirudin:* 0.1 mg/kgIV bolus, followed by infusion of 0.1 mg/kg/hr for 72 hr
		  —*Lepirudin:* 0.4 mg/kg IV bolus, followed by infusion of 0.15 mg/kg/hr for 72 hr

Heparin

—Low Molecular Weight (LMWH)

Indications

For use in acute coronary syndromes, specifically patients with non–Q wave MI or unstable angina. These drugs inhibit thrombin generation by factor Xa inhibition and also inhibit thrombin indirectly by formation of a complex with antithrombin III. These drugs are **not** neutralized by heparin-binding proteins.

Precautions

- Hemorrhage may complicate any therapy with LMWH
- Contraindicated in presence of hypersensitivity to heparin or pork products or history of sensitivity to drug
- Use **enoxaparin** with extreme caution, if at all, in patients with heparin-induced thrombocytopenia
- Contraindicated if platelet count <100,000; for these patients, consider direct antithrombins:
  —*Desirudin*: 0.1 mg/kg IV bolus, followed by infusion of 0.1 mg/kg/hr for 72 hr
  —*Lepirudin*: 0.4 mg/kg IV bolus, followed by infusion of 0.15 mg/kg/hr for 72 hr

Dalteparin
(Fragmin)

Subcutaneous Dose

1 mg/kg BID SC for 2–8 days, administered with aspirin

Enoxaparin
(Lovenox)

1 mg/kg BID SC for 2–8 days, administered with aspirin

Nadroparin
(Fraxiparine)
(not available in United States)

Ibutilide

Dose for Adults ≥60 kg

1 mg (10 mL) administered IV (diluted or undiluted) over 10 min; a second dose may be administered at the same rate 10 min later

Indications

Treatment of supraventricular arrhythmias, including atrial fibrillation and atrial flutter. Because it has such a short duration of action, it is most effective for the conversion of atrial fibrillation or flutter of relatively brief duration.

Continued

403

TABLE B–1 Advanced Cardiovascular Life Support Drugs and Electrical Therapy—cont'd

Drug/Therapy	Adult Dosage	Indications/Precautions
	Dose for Adults <60 kg 0.01 mg/kg initial IV dose.	**Precautions/Contraindications** Ventricular arrhythmias develop in approximately 2% to 5% of patients (polymorphic ventricular tachycardia, including torsades de pointes, may be observed). *Monitor ECG continuously for arrhythmias during administration and for 4–6 hr after administration, with defibrillator nearby.* Patients with significantly impaired LV function are at highest risk for arrhythmias.
Isoproterenol *IV infusion:* mix 1 mg in 250 mL NS, lactated Ringer's solution, or D5W	**IV Infusion** • Infuse at 2–10 μg/min • Titrate to adequate HR • In torsades de pointes, titrate to increase HR until VT is suppressed	**Indications** • Use cautiously as *temporizing measure if external pacer is not available* for treatment of symptomatic bradycardia • Refractory torsades de pointes unresponsive to magnesium sulfate • *Temporary control of bradycardia in heart transplant patients (denervated heart unresponsive to atropine)* • Poisoning from beta-adrenergic blockers **Precautions** • Do not use for treatment of cardiac arrest • Increases myocardial oxygen requirements, which may increase myocardial ischemia • Do not give with epinephrine; can cause VF/VT • Do not administer to patients with poison/drug-induced shock (exception: beta-adrenergic blocker poisoning) • Higher doses are class III (harmful) except for beta-adrenergic blocker poisoning

Lidocaine

Can be given via tracheal tube

Cardiac Arrest from VF/VT

- Initial dose: 1–1.5 mg/kg IV
- For refractory VF, may give additional 0.5–0.75 mg/kg IV push, repeat in 5 to 10 min; maximum total dose, 3 mg/kg
- A single dose of 1.5 mg/kg IV in cardiac arrest is acceptable
- Tracheal administration: 2–4 mg/kg

Perfusing Arrhythmia

For stable VT, wide-complex tachycardia of uncertain type, or significant ectopy, use as follows:
- 1–1.5 mg/kg IV push
- Repeat 0.5–0.75 mg/kg in 5–10 min; maximum total dose, 3 mg/kg

Maintenance Infusion

1–4 mg/min (30–50 µg/kg/min)

Magnesium Sulfate

Cardiac Arrest (for Hypomagnesemia or Torsades de Pointes)

1–2 g (2–4 mL of a 50% solution) diluted in 10 mL of D5W IV push

Torsades de Pointes (Not in Cardiac Arrest)

- Loading dose of 1–2 g mixed in 50–100 mL of D5W, over 5–60 min IV
- Follow with 0.5–1 g/hr IV (titrate dose to control the torsades)

Indications

- Cardiac arrest from VF/VT (class IIb)
- Stable VT, wide-complex tachycardias of uncertain type, wide-complex PSVT (class IIb)

Precautions

- *Prophylactic* use in AMI patients is *not* recommended
- Reduce maintenance dose (not loading dose) in presence of impaired liver function or LV dysfunction
- Discontinue infusion immediately if signs of toxicity develop

Indications

- Recommended for use in cardiac arrest only if torsades de pointes of suspected hypomagnesemia is present
- Refractory VF (after lidocaine)
- Torsades de pointes with a pulse
- Life-threatening ventricular arrhythmias due to digitalis toxicity
- Prophylactic administration in hospitalized patients with AMI is not recommended

Continued

TABLE B–1 Advanced Cardiovascular Life Support Drugs and Electrical Therapy—cont'd

Drug/Therapy	Adult Dosage	Indications/Precautions
	Acute Myocardial Infarction (if Indicated) • Loading dose of 1–2 g, mixed in 50–100 mL of D5W, over 5–60 min IV • Follow with 0.5–1 g/hr IV for up to 24 hr	**Precautions** • Occasional fall in BP with rapid administration • Use with caution if renal failure is present
Mannitol Strengths: 5%, 10%, 15%, 20%, and 25%	**IV Infusion** • Administer 0.5–1 g/kg over 5–10 min • Additional doses of 0.25–2 g/kg can be given q 4–6 hr as needed • Use with support of oxygenation and ventilation	**Indications** Increased intracranial pressure in management of neurologic emergencies **Precautions** • Monitor fluid status and serum osmolality (not to exceed 310 mOsm/kg) • Use with caution in renal failure, because fluid overload may result
Morphine Sulfate	**IV Infusion** 2–4 mg IV (over 1–5 min) q 5–30 min	**Indications** • Chest pain with ACS unresponsive to nitrates • Acute cardiogenic pulmonary edema (if BP is adequate) **Precautions** • Administer slowly and titrate to effect • May compromise respiration; therefore, use with caution in the compromised respiratory state of acute pulmonary edema • Causes hypotension in volume-depleted patients • Reverse, if needed, with naloxone (0.4–2 mg IV)

Naloxone Hydrochloride

Available in IV form, sublingual tablets, and aerosol spray

IV Infusion

- 0.4–2 mg q 2 min
- Use higher doses for complete narcotic reversal
- Can administer up to 10 mg over short period (<10 min)
- In suspected opiate-addicted patients titrate dose until ventilations are adequate: begin with 0.2 mg q 2 min x 3 doses, then 1.4 mg IV push

Indications

Respiratory and neurologic depression due to opiate intoxication

Precautions

- May cause opiate withdrawal
- Effects may not outlast effects of narcotics
- Monitor for recurrent respiratory depression
- Rare anaphylactic reactions have been reported

Nitroglycerin

IV Infusion

- IV bolus: 12.5–25 µg
- Infuse at 10–20 µg/min
- Route of choice for emergencies
- Use appropriate IV sets provided by pharmaceutical companies
- Titrate to effect

Sublingual Route

1 tablet (0.3–0.4 mg); repeat every 5 min

Aerosol Spray

Spray for 0.5–1 sec at 5-min intervals (provides 0.4 mg/dose)

Indications

- Initial antianginal for suspected ischemic pain
- For initial 24–48 hr in patients with *AMI and CHF*, large anterior wall infarction, persistent or recurrent ischemia or hypertension
- Continued use (beyond 48 hr) for patients with recurrent angina or persistent pulmonary congestion
- Hypertensive urgency with ACS

Precautions/Contraindications

- With evidence of AMI, limit systolic BP drop to 10% if patient is normotensive, 30% drop if hypertensive, and avoid drop below 90 mm Hg
- Do not mix with other drugs
- Patient should sit or lie down when receiving this medication

Continued

Drug/Therapy	Adult Dosage	Indications/Precautions
		• Do not shake aerosol spray, because this affects metered dose
		• Contraindications
		—Hypotension
		—Severe bradycardia or severe tachycardia
		—RV infarction
		—Viagra within 24 hr
Nitroprusside (Sodium Nitroprusside) Mix 50 or 100 mg in 250 mL D5W only	**IV Infusion** • Begin at 0.10 µg/kg/min and titrate upward every 3–5 min to desired effect (up to 5.0 µg/kg/min) • Use with an infusion pump; use hemodynamic monitoring for optimal safety • Action occurs within 1–2 min • Cover drug reservoir and tubing with opaque material	**Indications** • Hypertensive crisis • To reduce afterload in heart failure and acute pulmonary edema • To reduce afterload in acute mitral or aortic valve regurgitation **Precautions** • Light-sensitive; therefore, wrap drug reservoir in aluminum foil • May cause hypotension, thiocyanate toxicity, and CO_2 retention • May reverse hypoxic pulmonary vasoconstriction in patients with pulmonary disease, exacerbating intrapulmonary shunting, resulting in hypoxemia • Other side effects include headaches, nausea, vomiting, and abdominal cramps

Norepinephrine

Mix 4 mg in 250 mL of D5W or 5% dextrose in NS

Avoid dilution in NS alone

IV Infusion (Only Route)

- 0.5–1 µg/min titrated to improve BP (up to 30 µg/min)
- Do not administer in same IV line as alkaline solutions
- Poison/drug-induced hypotension may require higher doses to achieve adequate perfusion

Indications

- For severe cardiogenic shock and hemodynamically significant hypotension (systolic BP <70 mm Hg) with low total peripheral resistance
- This is an agent of last resort for management of ischemic heart disease and shock

Precautions

- Increases myocardial oxygen requirements because it raises BP and HR
- May induce arrhythmias; use with caution in patients with acute ischemia; monitor cardiac output
- Extravasation causes tissue necrosis
- If extravasation occurs, administer phentolamine 5–10 mg in 10–15 mL saline solution, infiltrated into area

Oxygen

Delivered from portable tanks or installed, wall-mounted sources through delivery devices

Device	Flow Rate	O₂ (%)
Nasal prongs	1–6 L/min	24–44
Venturi mask	4–8 L/min	24–40
Partial rebreather mask		
Bag-mask	15 L/min	Up to 100

Indications

- Any suspected cardiopulmonary emergency, especially (but *not* limited to) complaints of shortness of breath and suspected ischemic chest pain
- **Note:** Pulse oximetry provides a useful method of titrating oxygen administration to maintain physiologic oxygen saturation (see precautions)

Precautions

- Observe closely when using with pulmonary patients known to be dependent on hypoxic respiratory drive (very rare)
- Pulse oximetry inaccurate in low cardiac output states or with vasoconstriction

Continued

TABLE B–1 Advanced Cardiovascular Life Support Drugs and Electrical Therapy—cont'd

Drug/Therapy	Adult Dosage	Indications/Precautions
Procainamide	**Cardiac Arrest** • 20 mg/min IV infusion (maximum total dose; 17 mg/kg) • In refractory VF/VT, 100 mg IV push doses given q 5 min are acceptable **Other Indications** • 20 mg/min IV infusion until one of the following occurs: —Arrhythmia suppression —Hypotension —QRS widens by >50% —Total dose of 17 mg/kg is given **Maintenance Infusion** 1–4 mg/min	**Indications** • Useful for treatment of a wide variety of arrhythmias • May use for treatment of PSVT uncontrolled by adenosine and vagal maneuvers if BP stable • Stable wide-complex tachycardia of unknown origin • Atrial fibrillation with rapid rate in Wolff-Parkinson-White syndrome **Precautions** • If cardiac or renal dysfunction is present, reduce maximum total dose to 12 mg/kg and maintenance infusion to 1–2 mg/min • Proarrhythmic, especially in setting of AMI, hypokalemia, or hypomagnesemia • May induce hypotension in patients with impaired LV function • Use with caution with other drugs that prolong QT interval (e.g., amiodarone, sotalol)
Propafenone *IV form not approved for use in United States*	**IV Dose** 1–2 mg/kg body weight at 10 mg/min *Must be infused slowly*	**Indications** Antiarrhythmic agent used for treatment of ventricular and supraventricular arrhythmias **Precautions/Contraindications** • Significant negative inotropic effects; *must be infused slowly; may increase mortality in patients who have had MI, so should be avoided when coronary artery disease is suspected*

Sodium Bicarbonate

- Increased plasma concentrations can develop if taken with cimetidine; digoxin and warfarin levels increase when these drugs are taken with propafenone
- Reported side effects include bradycardia, hypotension, and GI upset

Indications

Specific indications for bicarbonate use are as follows:
- **Class I** if known preexisting hyperkalemia
- **Class IIa** if known preexisting bicarbonate-responsive acidosis (e.g., diabetic ketoacidosis) or overdose (e.g., tricyclic antidepressant overdose, cocaine, diphenhydramine) to alkalinize urine in aspirin or other overdose
- **Class IIb** if prolonged resuscitation with effective ventilation; upon return of spontaneous circulation after long arrest interval
- **Class III** (not useful or effective) in hypercarbic acidosis (e.g., cardiac arrest and CPR without intubation)

IV Infusion

- 1 mEq/kg IV bolus
- Repeat half this dose q 10 min thereafter
- If rapidly available, use ABG analysis to guide bicarbonate therapy (calculated base deficits or bicarbonate concentration)

Blood Gas Interpretation

An acute change in Paco$_2$ of 1 mm Hg is associated with an increase or decrease in pH of 0.008 U (relative to normal Paco$_2$ of 40 mm Hg and normal pH of 7.4)

Sotalol

IV form not approved for use in United States

Precautions

- Adequate ventilation and CPR, not bicarbonate, are the major "buffer agents" in cardiac arrest
- Not recommended for routine use in cardiac arrest patients

Indications

In the United States, oral form is approved for treatment of ventricular and atrial arrhythmias. Outside the United States, used for treatment of supraventricular and ventricular arrhythmias in patients without structural heart disease

Dose

Administered at 1–1.5 mg/kg body weight, then infused at rate of 10 mg/min
Must be infused slowly

Continued

TABLE B–1 Advanced Cardiovascular Life Support Drugs and Electrical Therapy—cont'd

Drug/Therapy	Adult Dosage	Indications/Precautions
		Precautions/Contraindications
		• Should be avoided in patients with poor perfusion because of significant negative inotropic effects; *must be infused slowly*
		• Adverse effects include bradycardia, hypotension, and arrhythmias (torsades de pointes)
		• Use with caution with other drugs that prolong QT interval (e.g., procainamide, amiodarone)
Thrombolytic Agents (see *Fibrinolytic Agents, page 397*)		
Transcutaneous Pacing	**Technique**	**Indications**
External pace-makers have either *fixed* rates (nondemand or asynchronous mode) or *demand* rates (range, 30–180 beats/min)	• Place pacing electrodes on chest per package instructions	• Class I for hemodynamically unstable bradycardia, (e.g., BP changes, altered mental status, angina, pulmonary edema)
	• Turn the pacer ON	• Class I for pacing readiness in setting of AMI, as follows:
	• Set demand rate to approximately 80 beats/min	— Symptomatic sinus node dysfunction
	• Set current (mA) output as follows:	— Type II second-degree heart block
	—*Bradycardia:* Increase milliamperes from minimum setting until consistent capture is achieved (characterized by a widening QRS and a broad T wave after each pacer spike); then add 2 mA for safety margin	— Third-degree heart block
		— New left, right, or alternating BBB or bifascicular block

Current outputs range from 0 to 200 mA

—*Asystole:* Begin at full output (mA); if capture occurs, slowly decrease output until capture is lost (threshold); then add 2 mA for safety margin

- Class IIa for bradycardia with symptomatic ventricular escape rhythms
- Class IIa for overdrive pacing of tachycardias refractory to drug therapy or electrical cardioversion
- Class IIb for bradyasystolic cardiac arrest. Not routinely recommended, but if used, use early

Precautions

- Contraindicated in severe hypothermia or prolonged bradyasystolic cardiac arrest
- Conscious patients may require analgesia for discomfort
- Avoid using carotid pulse to confirm mechanical capture; electrical stimulation causes muscular jerking that may mimic carotid pulse

Vasopressin

IV, IO, and ET Doses for Cardiac Arrest

40 U IV push x 1

Indications

- May be used as an alternative pressor to epinephrine in the treatment of adult shock-refractory VF (class IIb)
- May be useful for hemodynamic support in vasodilatory shock (e.g., septic shock)

Precautions/Contraindications

- Potent peripheral vasoconstrictor; increased peripheral vascular resistance may provoke cardiac ischemia and angina
- Not recommended for responsive patients with coronary artery disease

Continued

413

TABLE B–1 Advanced Cardiovascular Life Support Drugs and Electrical Therapy—cont'd

Drug/Therapy	Adult Dosage	Indications/Precautions
Verapamil	**IV Infusion** • 2.5–5 mg IV bolus over 2 min • Second dose: 5–10 mg, if needed, in 15–30 min; maximum dose, 20 mg • Alternative: 5-mg bolus q 15 min to total dose of 30 mg • Older patients: administer over 3 min	**Indications** • Alternative drug (after adenosine) to terminate PSVT with narrow QRS complex and adequate BP and *preserved LV function* • May control ventricular response in patients with atrial fibrillation, flutter, or multifocal atrial tachycardia **Precautions** • Give *only* to patients with narrow-complex PSVT or arrhythmias known to be of supraventricular origin; do not use calcium channel blockers for wide-QRS tachycardias of uncertain origin • Avoid calcium channel blockers in patients with Wolff-Parkinson-White syndrome and atrial fibrillation, sick sinus syndrome, or second- or third-degree AV block without pacemaker • Expect BP drop caused by peripheral vasodilation; IV calcium is an antagonist that may restore BP in toxic cases • May decrease myocardial contractility and may exacerbate CHF in patients with LV dysfunction • Concurrent IV administration with IV beta blockers may produce severe hypotension • Use with extreme caution in patients receiving oral beta blockers

Reproduced with permission, ACLS Provider Manual, 2002, Copyright American Heart Association.

TABLE B–2 Emergency Treatment of Hyperkalemia

Therapy	Dose	Onset of Effect	Duration of Effect
Antagonize			
Calcium chloride	5–10 mL IV of 10% solution (500–1000 mg)	1–3 min	30–60 min
Shift into Cells			
Sodium bicarbonate	1 mEq/kg IV bolus	5–10 min	1–2 hr
Insulin plus glucose (use 1 U insulin/2.5 g glucose)	Regular insulin 10 U IV plus 50 mL D$_{50}$ (25 g glucose) IV bolus (1 50-mL prefilled syringe or vial or D$_{50}$)	30 min	4–6 hr
Nebulized albuterol	10–20 mg nebulized over 15 min	15 min	15–90 min
Remove from Body			
Diuresis with furosemide	40–80 mg IV bolus	When diuresis starts, 1–2 hr	When diuresis ends, 4–6 hr
Cation-exchange resin (Kayexalate)	15–50 g PO or PR, plus sorbitol		
Peritoneal dialysis or hemodialysis	Per institution	As soon as started	Until dialysis completed

Reproduced with permission, ACLS Provider Mamual, 2002, Copyright American Heart Association.

TABLE B-3 Sympathomimetic, Inotropic, and Inodilator Drugs

Drug	IV Infusion	Adrenergic		Arrhythmogenic Potential
		Alpha	Beta	
Epinephrine	2–10 μg/min	++	+++	+++
Norepinephrine	0.5–30 μg/min	+++	++	++
Dopamine	1–5 μg/kg/min	+	+*	+
	5–10 μg/kg/min	++	++*	++
	10–20 μg/kg/min	+++	++	+++
Dobutamine	2–20 μg/kg/min	+	+++	++
Isoproterenol	2–10 μg/min	0	+++	+++
Amrinone†	5–15 μg/kg/min (after loading dose)	0	0*	++

*Increases renal and splanchnic blood flow.
†Phosphodiesterase inhibitor.
Reproduced with permission, ACLS Provider Manual, 2002, Copyright American Heart Association.

Appendix

Blood Products

The maximum time over which blood products can be administered is 4 hours for 1 unit, because of the danger of bacterial infection and red blood cell (RBC) hemolysis. For the same reasons, if the flow is interrupted for more than 30 minutes, the unit must be discarded.

Packed Red Blood Cells

- Volume: 300 ± 25 mL
- Maximum administration time: 4 hours
- Rate of infusion: dependent on patient's clinical condition
- Administration: standard blood set for each unit hung, or Y-type set if blood is to be reconstituted
- Indications: active bleeding with loss of ≥15% of total blood volume; anemia that is adversely influencing another medical disorder (e.g., unstable angina); symptomatic chronic anemia unrelated to nutritional deficiency
- Outcome measurement: hemoglobin (Hb) level within 24 hours

Deleukocyted Red Blood Cells

- Volume: 300 ± 25 mL
- Maximum administration time: 4 hours
- Rate of infusion: dependent on patient's clinical condition
- Administration: standard blood set for each unit hung, plus a filter (filter not required if RBCs are washed)
- Indications: clinically significant transfusion reactions; to reduce sensitization to histocompatibility antigens

Frozen Red Blood Cells (Deglycerolized)

- Volume: approximately 200 mL
- Maximum administration time: 4 hours
- Rate of infusion: dependent on patient's clinical condition
- Administration: standard blood set for each unit hung
- Indications: storing of rare blood groups and autotransfusion
- *Note:* use only in special situations

Plasma

- Volume: approximately 200 mL
- Maximum administration time: 4 hours

- Rate of infusion: dependent on patient's clinical condition
- Administration: standard blood set
- Indications: as a source of coagulation factors. *Frozen plasma* is frozen within 24 hours of collection and contains higher levels of labile coagulation factors (V and VIII). Nonlabile factors are well maintained in both frozen and *stored (banked) plasma.* Plasma may be used for the following:
  1. Significant hemorrhage due to a deficiency of coagulation factors
  2. Immediate hemostasis in a patient on warfarin
  3. Abnormal clotting tests and active bleeding in a patient with severe liver disease or massive transfusion (whole blood volume replaced within 24 hours)
  4. Thrombotic thrombocytopenic purpura
  5. Prophylaxis before an invasive procedure associated with a significant bleeding risk
- Outcome measurement: prothrombin time (PT), activated partial thromboplastin time (aPTT), or both within 4 hours of transfusion

Platelets

- Volume: approximately 50 mL
- Rate of infusion: as rapidly as tolerated by patient
- Administration: blood component recipient set
- Indications: to improve hemostasis. Platelet use should be considered in the following situations:
  1. Patients with platelet counts of less than 20 g/L on the basis of decreased platelet production
  2. Patients with consumptive thrombocytopenia (e.g., immune thrombocytopenia; disseminated intravascular coagulation [DIC]) only when there is significant bleeding
  3. Patients with significant platelet dysfunction
- Outcome measurement: platelet count 1 hour after transfusion
- *Note:* Platelet transfusion reactions are common. In patients with a history of reactions, the use of acetaminophen 650 mg PO and diphenhydramine 50 mg IV may prevent reactions. Narcotics (morphine 5 to 10 mg IV) or steroids (hydrocortisone 100 mg IV) also may be helpful. If these measures fail, deleukocyted platelets are recommended.

In patients who are unresponsive to random donor platelets (defined by a <5 g/L increment in platelets 1 hour after transfusion on two successive transfusions), platelets collected from a single donor by apheresis should be considered.

Cryoprecipitate

- Volume: 5 to 10 mL
- Rate of infusion: as rapidly as possible
- Administration: blood component recipient set

- Indications: Cryoprecipitate contains significant amounts of factor VIII (100 units/unit of cryoprecipitate), fibrinogen (250 mg/unit), and von Willebrand's factor. It is therefore useful in the treatment of mild hemophilia A and von Willebrand's disease and in the repletion of fibrinogen (e.g., DIC, dilutional coagulopathy). The dose is dependent on body mass, the indication for use, and the severity of the preexisting deficiency.
- Outcome measurement: factor VIII level and aPTT (hemophilia A); von Willebrand's factor antigen level, bleeding time, or both (von Willebrand's disease); fibrinogen level (DIC, dilutional coagulopathy)— all within 4 hours of transfusion

Factor VIII Concentrate

- Lyophilized, fractionated plasma product
- Specific activity and storage conditions stated on label
- Must be reconstituted before use
- Indications: moderate to severe factor VIII deficiency and low titer of factor VIII inhibitors
- *Note:* Not for use in von Willebrand's disease. Consult a hematologist before administration.

Factor IX Complex

- Lyophilized, fractionated plasma product
- Factor IX content and storage conditions stated on labels
- Must be reconstituted before use
- Indications: factor IX deficiency. Consult a hematologist before administration.

Normal Serum Albumin

- Concentrates of 25% in vials of 100 mL and 5% in vials of 250 and 500 mL
- Sodium content approximately 145 mmol/L
- Indications: hypoproteinemia with peripheral edema (give 25%); volume depletion when IV normal saline (NS) is contraindicated (give 5%); *not indicated* in an asymptomatic hypoproteinemic patient

Blood Tubes

Lavender Top (EDTA)

Complete blood count (CBC) and differential
Sickle cell
Reticulocyte count
Malaria stain
Direct Coombs' test
Adrenocorticotropic hormone (ACTH)
Glucose-6-phosphate dehydrogenase (G-6-PD)

Red/Gray ("Tiger Top")

SMAC (glucose)*
C3, C4, cryoglobulins
Cardiac enzymes
Osmolality
Liver enzymes
Pregnancy test
Drug concentrations (e.g., alcohol, digoxin, gentamicin)
C peptide/insulin
Protein electrophoresis

Red Top

Crossmatch
Rheumatoid arthritis (RA)
Haptoglobin
Antinuclear antibody (ANA)
Tricyclic antidepressants (TCA) concentrations

Green Top

Lactate*
Ammonia*

Blue Top (Citrate)

PT, aPTT
Fibrinogen
Circulating anticoagulants
Coagulation factor assays

Blue Top (for FDPs only)

Fibrin degradation products (FDPs)

---

*These specimens must be delivered to the laboratory immediately or put on ice for transportation.

Appendix

D

Reading Electrocardiograms

Rate

Multiply the number of QRS complexes in a 6-second period (30 large squares) by 10 to obtain the number of beats/min (Fig. D–1).
- Normal = 60 to 100 beats/min
- Tachycardia = >100 beats/min
- Bradycardia = <60 beats/min

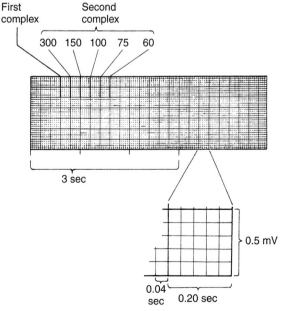

First complex   Second complex

300 150 100 75 60

3 sec

0.5 mV

0.04 sec   0.20 sec

Figure D–1 Rate.

Rhythm

Is the rhythm regular?

Is there a P wave preceding every QRS complex? Is there a QRS complex following every P wave?

1. Yes = sinus rhythm
2. No P waves with irregular rhythm = atrial fibrillation
3. No P waves with regular rhythm = junctional rhythm—look for retrograde P waves in all leads

Axis

See Figure D–2.

P Wave Configuration

Normal P Wave

Look at all leads (Fig. D–3A).

Left Atrial Enlargement

See Figure D–3B.

- Duration: 120 msec (three small squares in lead II); often notched indicates P mitrale
- Amplitude: negative terminal P wave in lead V_1 >1 mm in depth and >40 msec (one small square)

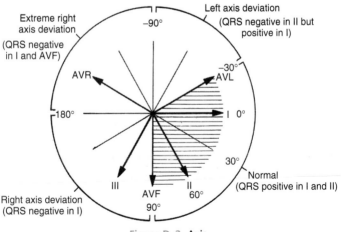

Figure D–2 **Axis.**

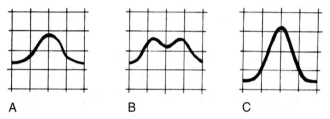

Figure D-3 P wave configuration in lead II. *A*, Normal P wave. *B*, Left atrial enlargement. *C*, Right atrial enlargement.

Right Atrial Enlargement

See Figure D-3C.
- Amplitude: 2.5 mm in lead II, III, or aVF (i.e., tall peaked P wave of P pulmonale); 1.5 mm in the initial positive deflection of the P wave in lead V_1 or V_2

QRS Configuration

Left Ventricular Hypertrophy

1. Increased QRS voltage (S in lead V_1 or V_2 plus R in V_5 >35 mm or R in aVL ≥11 mm)
2. ST segment depression and negative T wave in left lateral leads are common

Right Ventricular Hypertrophy

1. R > S in V_1
2. Right axis deviation (>+90 degrees)
3. ST segment depression and negative T wave in right precordial leads

Conduction Abnormalities

First-Degree Block

- PR interval ≥0.20 second (≥one large square)

Second-Degree Block

- Occasional absence of QRS and T after a P wave of sinus origin
  Type I (Wenckebach's): progressive prolongation of the PR interval before the missed QRS complex (see Fig. 15–18)
  Type II: absence of progressive prolongation of the PR interval before the missed QRS complex (see Fig. 15–19)

Third-Degree Block

- Absence of any relationship between P waves of sinus origin and QRS complexes (see Fig. 15–20)

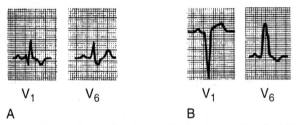

Figure D–4 QRS configuration. *A,* Complete right bundle branch block. *B,* Complete left bundle branch block.

Left Anterior Hemiblock

- Left axis deviation, Q in I and aVL, and a small R in III, in the absence of left ventricular hypertrophy

Left Posterior Hemiblock

- Right axis deviation, a small R in I, and a small Q in III, in the absence of right ventricular hypertrophy

Complete Right Bundle Branch Block

See Figure D–4*A.*

Complete Left Bundle Branch Block

See Figure D–4*B.*

Ventricular Preexcitation

1. PR interval <0.11 second with widened QRS (>0.12 second) due to a delta wave indicates Wolff-Parkinson-White syndrome
2. PR interval <0.11 second with a normal QRS complex indicates Lown-Ganong-Levine syndrome

TABLE D–1 **Myocardial Infarction Patterns**

Type of Infarct	Patterns of Changes (Q Waves, ST Elevation or Depression, T Wave Inversion)*
Inferior	Q in II, III, aVF
Inferoposterior	Q in II, III, aVF, and V_6
	R > S and positive T in V_1
Anteroseptal	V_1 to V_4
Anterolateral to posterolateral	V_1 to V_5; Q in I, aVL, and V_6
Posterior	R > S in V_1, positive T, and Q in V_6

*A significant Q wave is >40 msec wide or more than one third of the QRS height. ST segment or T wave changes in the absence of significant Q waves may represent a non–Q wave infarction.

Appendix

E

Miscellaneous

CALCULATION OF CREATININE CLEARANCE

$$\text{CrCl (mL/sec)} = \frac{(140 - \text{age in years}) \times 1.5}{\text{Serum creatinine (}\mu\text{mol/L)}} \ (\times 0.85 \text{ in females})$$

CALCULATION OF ALVEOLAR-ARTERIAL OXYGEN GRADIENT [$P(A-a)O_2$]

The $P(A - a)O_2$ can be calculated easily from the arterial blood gas (ABG) results. It is useful in confirming the presence of a shunt.

$$P(A - a)O_2 = PAO_2 - PaO_2$$

- PAO_2 = alveolar oxygen tension, calculated as shown subsequently
- PaO_2 = arterial oxygen tension measured by ABG determination

PAO_2 can be calculated by the following formula:

$$PAO_2 = (PB - PH_2O) \ (FIO_2) \ PaCO_2/R$$

- PB = barometric pressure (760 mm Hg at sea level)
- PH_2O = 47 mm Hg
- FIO_2 = fraction of O_2 in inspired gas
- $PaCO_2$ = arterial CO_2 tension measured by ABG determination
- R = respiratory quotient (0.8)

Normal $P(A - a)O_2$ ranges from 12 mm Hg in a young adult to 20 mm Hg at age 70.

In pure ventilatory failure, the $P(A - a)O_2$ remains 12 to 20 mm Hg. In oxygenation failure, it increases.

INTERNATIONAL NORMALIZED RATIO

The international normalized ratio (INR) was developed to improve the consistency of oral anticoagulant therapy. It is calculated using the mean normal prothrombin time (PT) for a laboratory's system, not the PT of "normal control material." The relation between PT and INR is as follows:

$$INR = (PT_{patient}/PT_{mean})^{ISI},$$

where $PT_{patient}$ is the patient's PT, PT_{mean} is the mean of the normal PT range (measured by the laboratory), and ISI is the International

Sensitivity Index, which is a measure of the responsiveness of the thromboplastin used to measure the PT to a reduction in vitamin K–dependent coagulation factors.

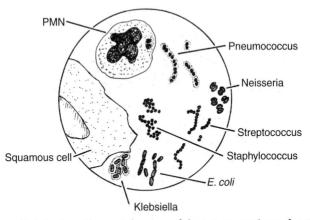

Figure E–1 Sputum Gram stain. A useful sputum specimen for the identification of a bacterial cause of pneumonia should have ≥25 polymorphonuclear cells (PMNs) and fewer than 10 squamous cells per low-power field.

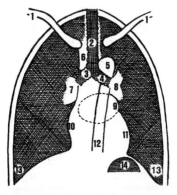

Figure E–2 Posteroanterior chest x-ray.

1. Clavicles
2. Trachea
3. Right mainstem bronchus
4. Left mainstem bronchus
5. Aortic knuckle
6. Superior vena cava
7. Right pulmonary artery
8. Left pulmonary artery
9. Left atrium
10. Right atrium
11. Left ventricle
12. Aortic stripe
13. Costophrenic angles
14. Gastric bubble

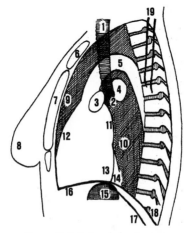

Figure E–3 Lateral chest x-ray.

1. Trachea
2. Left mainstem bronchus
3. Right pulmonary artery
4. Left pulmonary artery
5. Aortic arch
6. Manubrium
7. Sternum
8. Breast shadow
9. Retrosternal space
10. Retrocardiac space
11. Left atrium
12. Right ventricle
13. Left ventricle
14. Inferior vena cava
15. Gastric air bubble
16. Left hemidiaphragm
17. Right hemidiaphragm
18. Costophrenic angle
19. Scapular shadows

	Respiratory Tract Pathogens						Staphylo-cocci		Gram-Negative Rods				
	Streptococcus pyogenes	*Mycoplasma pneumoniae*	*Haemophilus influenzae*	*Legionella* species	*Chlamydia*	Oropharyngeal anaerobes	*Staphylococcus aureus*	Methicillin-resistant *S. aureus*	*Escherichia coli*	Coliform species	*Klebsiella*	*Pseudomonas aeruginosa*	*Bacillus fragilis*

Does the patient have a community-acquired pneumonia and not have a chronic medical condition?

MACROLIDE

Erythromycin
Azithromycin
Clarithromycin

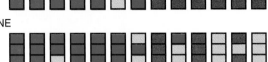

TETRACYCLINE

Doxycycline
Minocycline
Tetracycline

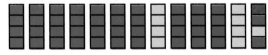

Does the patient have a pneumonia that has been acquired in the hospital or has the patient been exposed to antibiotics or have a chronic medical condition?

FLUOROQUINOLONE (RESPIRATORY)

Levofloxacin
Moxifloxacin
Gemifloxacin
Gatifloxacin

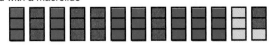

CEPHALOSPORIN (THIRD OR FOURTH GENERATION)
Should be used with a macrolide

Ceftriaxone
Cefotaxime
Ceftizoxime

Is there a risk that this infection is due to a multiple-resistant gram-negative organism or *Pseudomonas aeruginosa*? More than one agent is generally required.

CARBAPENEM

Imipenem/
cilastatin
Meropenem
Aztreonam

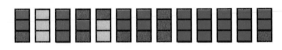

■ Effective　□ Varied sensitivity　■ Not effective　□ Not proven
Bold Drug of first choice based on cost, effectiveness, and experience with use.

Figure E–4 Selected antibacterials for common infections in the hospital.

	Respiratory Tract Pathogens						Staphylococci		Gram-Negative Rods				
	Streptococcus pyogenes	*Mycoplasma pnemoniae*	*Haemophilus influenzae*	*Legionella* species	*Chlamydia*	Oropharyngeal anaerobes	*Staphylococcus aureus*	Methicillin-resistant *S. aureus*	*Escherichia coli*	Coliform species	*Klebsiella*	*Pseudomonas aeruginosa*	*Bacillus fragilis*

AMINOGLYCOSIDE

Netilmicin
Gentamicin
Amikacin
Tobramycin

PENICILLIN

Piperacillin
Mezlocillin
Ticarcillin

CEPHALOSPORIN

Ceftazidime

Could this infection be due to a methicillin-resistant staphylococcus?

GLYCOPEPTIDE

Vancomycin
Teicoplanin
Rifampin

Is this an uncomplicated urinary tract infection?

PENICILLIN

Amoxicillin/clavulanate

CEPHALOSPORIN

Cefazolin
Cefalexin
Cefadroxil
Cefaclor
Cefuroxime

■ Effective   □ Varied sensitivity   ■ Not effective   □ Not proven
Bold Drug of first choice based on cost, effectiveness, and experience with use.

Figure E–4, cont'd

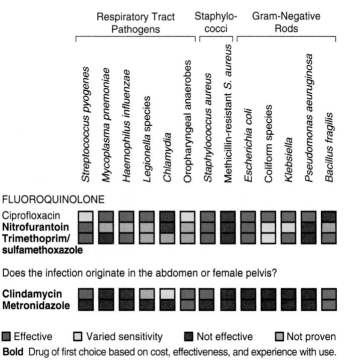

Figure E–4, cont'd For legend, see p. 428.

TABLE E–1 Intravenous Antibiotic Dose Adjustments Relative to Renal Function

Drug	Dose	Creatinine Clearance (hr)		
		>0.8 mL/sec >50 mL/min	0.8–0.4 mL/sec 50–25 mL/min	<0.4 mL/sec <25 mL/min
Acyclovir	5–10 mg/kg	8	12	24
Amikacin	5–7 mg/kg	24	48	Reduce dose
Ampicillin	1–2 g	6	6–12	12–24
Aztreonam/cilastatin	30–40 mg/kg	8	8–12	24
Cefazolin	1–2 g	8	12	12–24
Cefotaxime	1–2 g	8–12	12	12–24
Cefoxitin	1–2 g	8	12	12–24
Ceftazidime	1–2 g	8	12	12–24
Ceftizoxime	0.5 –4 g	8	12	12–24
Ceftriaxone	1–2 g	24	24	24
Ciprofloxacin	200–600 mg	12	12–24	24
Clindamycin	600 mg	8	8	8
Cloxacillin	250–1000 mg	4–6	4–6	4–6
Doxycycline	50–100 mg	12	24–36	48–96
Erythromycin	0.5–1 g	6	6	6
Gatifloxacin	400 mg	24	24–36	36–48
Gentamicin	5–7 mg/kg	24	48	Reduce dose
Imipenem/cilastatin	500 mg	6–8	8	12
Levofloxacin	250–500 mg	24	24–36	36–48

Continued

431

TABLE E-1 Intravenous Antibiotic Dose Adjustments Relative to Renal Function—cont'd

Drug	Dose	Creatinine Clearance (hr)		
		>0.8 mL/sec >50 mL/min	0.8–0.4 mL/sec 50–25 mL/min	<0.4 mL/sec <25 mL/min
Parenteral Therapy				
Meropenem	0.5–1 g	8	12	24
Metronidazole	500 mg	8	8–12	12
Mezlocillin	4–6 g	4–6	6–12	12
Netilmicin	16–20 mg/kg	24	48	Reduce dose
Penicillin G	Variable	4–6	8–12	12–18
Piperacillin	2–4 g	4–6	6–12	12
Piperacillin/tazobactam	2–4 g	4–6	6–12	12
Rifampin	600 mg	12	12	12
Teicoplanin	6 mg/kg	12	24–36	48–96
Tetracycline	250–500 mg	12	24–36	48–96
Ticarcillin/clavulanate	1–6 g	6	8	12–24
Tobramycin	5–7 mg/kg	24	48	Reduce dose
Vancomycin	15 mg/kg	12–72	2–10 days	Reduce dose

Appendix

SI Units Conversion Table

SI is the abbreviation for *le Système International d'Unites*. The SI is an outgrowth of the metric system and provides a uniform system of reporting laboratory data among nations. Most laboratory values in *On Call* are presented in SI units. Because some laboratories have not yet converted to this system of reporting, a conversion table for commonly measured laboratory parameters is provided.

Laboratory Test	Previous Reference Intervals	Previous Unit	Conversion Factor	SI Reference Intervals	SI Unit Symbol
Erythrocyte count					
Female	3.5–5.0	$10^6/mm^3$	1	3.5–5.0	$10^{12}/L$
Male	4.3–5.9	$10^6/mm^3$	1	4.3–5.9	$10^{12}/L$
Erythrocyte sedimentation rate (ESR)					
Female	0–30	mm/hr	1	0–30	mm/hr
Male	0–20	mm/hr	1	0–20	mm/hr
Hemoglobin					
Female	12.0–15.0	g/dL	10	120–150	g/L
Male	13.6–17.2	g/dL	10	136–172	g/L
Leukocyte count					
Number fraction (differential)		%	0.01		1
Platelet count	130–400	$10^3/mm^3$	1	130–400	$10^9/L$
Reticulocyte count	10,000–75,000	$/mm^3$	0.001	10–75	$10^9/L$
Number fraction	1–24	Number per 1000 RBCs	0.001	0.001–0.024	1
Albumin (serum)	0.1–2.4	%	0.001	0.001–0.024	1
	4.0–6.0	g/dL	10.0	40–60	g/L
Alkaline phosphatase	30–120	U/L	0.01667	0.5–2.0	μkat/L
Amylase (serum)	0–130	U/L	0.01667	0–2.17	μkat/L
Aspartate aminotransferase (AST)	0–35	U/L	0.01667	0–0.58	μkat/L
Bilirubin					
Total	0.1–1.0	mg/dL	17.10	2–18	μmol/L
Conjugated	0–0.2	mg/dL	17.10	0–4	μmol/L

Calcium (serum)				
Male	8.8–10.3	mg/dL	0.2495	2.20–2.58	mmol/L
Female (<50 yr)	8.8–10.0	mg/dL	0.2495	2.20–2.50	mmol/L
Female (>50 yr)	8.8–10.2	mg/dL	0.2495	2.20–2.56	mmol/L
Calcium ion (serum)	4.4–5.1	mEq/L	0.500	2.20–2.56	mmol/L
CO_2 content (= $HCO_3 + CO_2$)	2.00–2.30	mEq/L	0.500	1.00–1.15	mmol/L
CO (proportion of Hb that is $COHb$)	22–28	%	1.00	22–28	mmol/L
	<15	%	0.01	<0.15	1
Chloride (serum)	95–105	mEq/L	1.00	95–105	mmol/L
Cholesterol (plasma)					
<29 yr	<200	mg/dL	0.02586	<5.20	mmol/L
30–39 yr	<225	mg/dL	0.02586	<5.85	mmol/L
40–49 yr	<245	mg/dL	0.02586	<6.35	mmol/L
>50 yr	<265	mg/dL	0.02586	<6.85	mmol/L
Complement (serum)					
C3	70–160	mg/dL	0.01	0.7–1.6	g/L
C4	20–40	mg/dL	0.01	0.2–0.4	g/L
Creatine phosphokinase (CPK) (serum)	0–130	U/L	0.01667	0–2.16	µkat/L
MB fraction	>5 in MI	%	0.01	>0.05	1
Creatinine					
Serum	0.6–1.2	mg/dL	88.40	50–110	µmol/L
Urine	Variable	g/24 hr	8.840	Variable	mmol/d
Creatinine clearance	75–125	mL/min	0.01667	1.24–2.08	mL/sec
Digoxin (plasma)					
Therapeutic	0.5–2.2	ng/mL	1.281	0.6–2.8	nmol/L
	0.5–2.2	µg/L	1.281	0.6–2.8	nmol/L
Toxic	>2.5	ng/mL	1.281	>3.2	nmol/L

Continued

Laboratory Test	Previous Reference Intervals	Previous Unit	Conversion Factor	SI Reference Intervals	SI Unit Symbol
Electrophoresis, serum protein					
Albumin	60–65	%	0.01	0.60–0.65	1
Alpha-1 globulin	1.7–5.0	%	0.01	0.02–0.05	1
Alpha-2 globulin	6.7–12.5	%	0.01	0.07–0.13	1
Beta globulin	8.3–16.3	%	0.01	0.08–0.16	1
Gamma globulin	10.7–20.0	%	0.01	0.11–0.20	1
Albumin	3.6–5.2	g/dL	10.0	36–52	g/L
Alpha-1 globulin	0.1–0.4	g/dL	10.0	1–4	g/L
Alpha-2 globulin	0.4–1.0	g/dL	10.0	4–10	g/L
Beta gobulin	0.5–1.2	g/dL	10.0	5–12	g/L
Gamma globulin	0.6–1.6	g/dL	10.0	6–16	g/L
Ethanol (plasma)					
Legal limit (driving)	<80	mg/dL	0.2171	<17	mmol/L
Toxic	>100	mg/dL	0.2171	>22	mmol/L
Ferritin (serum)	18–300	ng/mL	1.00	18–300	µg/L
Fibrinogen (plasma)	200–400	mg/dL	0.01	2.0–4.0	g/L
Folate					
Serum	2–10	ng/mL	2.266	4–22	nmol/L
RBC	140–960	ng/mL	2.266	550–2200	nmol/L
Gamma-glutamyltransferase (GGT) (serum)	0–30	U/L	0.01667	0–0.50	µkat/L
Gases (arterial blood)					
Po₂	75–105	mm Hg (= Torr)	0.1333	10.0–14.0	kPa
Pco₂	33–44	mm Hg (= Torr)	0.1333	4.4–5.9	kPa

Test	Conventional Range	Conventional Units	Conversion Factor	SI Range	SI Units
Glucose					
Serum (fasting)	70–110	mg/dL	0.05551	3.9–6.1	nmol/L
Spinal fluid	50–80	mg/dL	0.05551	2.8–4.4	nmol/L
Haptoglobin (serum)	50–220	mg/dL	0.01	0.50–2.20	g/L
Hemoglobin (blood)					
Male	14.0–18.0	g/dL	10.0	140–180	g/L
Female	11.5–15.5	g/dL	10.0	115–155	g/L
Iron (serum)					
Male	80–180	µg/dL	0.1791	14–32	µmol/L
Female	60–160	µg/dL	0.1791	11–29	µmol/L
Iron binding capacity (serum)	250–460	µg/dL	0.1791	45–82	µmol/L
Lactate dehydrogenase (LDH) (serum)	50–150	U/L	0.01667	0.82–2.66	µkat/L
LD1	15–40	%	0.01	0.15–0.40	1
LD2	20–45	%	0.01	0.20–0.45	1
LD3	15–30	%	0.01	0.15–0.30	1
LD4	5–20	%	0.01	0.05–0.20	1
LD5	5–20	%	0.01	0.05–0.20	1
LD1	10–60	U/L	0.01667	0.16–1.00	µkat/L
LD2	20–70	U/L	0.01667	0.32–1.16	µkat/L
LD3	10–45	U/L	0.01667	0.22–0.76	µkat/L
LD4	5–30	U/L	0.01667	0.08–0.50	µkat/L
LD5	5–30	U/L	0.01667	0.02–0.50	µkat/L
Lipase (serum)	0–160	U/L	0.01667	0–2.66	µkat/L
Lithium ion (serum) (therapeutic)	0.50–1.50	mEq/L	1.00	0.50–1.50	mmol/L
		µg/L	0.001441		mmol/L
		mg/dL	1.441		mmol/L
Magnesium (serum)	1.8–3.0	mg/dL	0.4114	0.80–1.20	mmol/L
	1.6–2.4	mEq/L	0.500	0.80–1.20	mmol/L

Continued

Laboratory Test	Previous Reference Intervals	Previous Unit	Conversion Factor	SI Reference Intervals	SI Unit Symbol
Osmolality					
Plasma	280–300	mOsm/kg	1.00	280–300	mmol/kg
Urine	50–1200	mOsm/kg	1.00	50–1200	mmol/kg
Phosphate (serum)	2.5–5.0	mg/dL	0.3229	0.80–1.60	mmol/L
Potassium ion					
Serum	3.5–5.0	mEq/L	1.00	3.5–5.0	mmol/L
Urine (diet dependent)	25–100	mEq/24 hr	1.00	25–100	mmol/d
Protein, total					
Serum	6.0–8.0	g/dL	10.0	60–80	g/L
Urine	<150	mg/24 hr	0.001	<0.15	g/day
Sodium ion					
Serum	135–147	mEq/L	1.00	135–147	mmol/L
Urine	Diet dependent	mEq/24 hr	1.00	Diet dependent	mmol/day
Theophylline (plasma)					
Therapeutic	10.0–20.0	mg/L	5.550	55–110	μmol/L

Thyroid tests (serum)					
TSH	2–11	μU/mL	1.00	2–11	mU/L
T$_4$	4.0–11.0	μg/dL	12.87	51–142	nmol/L
TBG	12.0–28.0	μg/dL	12.87	150–360	nmol/L
Free T$_4$	0.8–2.8	ng/dL	12.87	10–36	pmol/L
T$_3$	75–220	ng/dL	0.01536	1.2–3.4	nmol/L
T$_3$ uptake	25–35	%	0.01	0.25–0.35	1
Transferrin (serum)	170–370	mg/dL	0.01	1.70–3.70	g/L
Triglycerides (plasma)	<160	mg/dL	0.01129	<1.80	mmol/L
Urate (as uric acid)					
Serum	2.0–7.0	mg/dL	59.48	120–420	μmol/L
Urine	Diet dependent	g/24 hr	5.948	Diet dependent	mmol/day
Urea (serum)	8–18	mg/dL	0.3570	3.0–6.5	mmol/L
Vitamin B$_{12}$ (plasma or serum)	200–1000	pg/mL	0.7378	150–750	pmol/L
		ng/dL	7.378		pmol/L

The On-Call Formulary

This formulary is a quick reference for information on medications that are commonly encountered or prescribed by the student or resident on call.

Antibacterial susceptibility guidelines and doses for patients are presented in Figure E–4. Drugs used in cardiopulmonary resuscitation are presented in table format on pages 385 to 416.

Doses listed are for adult patients with normal renal and hepatic function. Adverse effects in bold are those that most frequently limit the usefulness of the drug.

ACYCLOVIR (Zovirax) *Nucleoside analog*

Indications:	Herpes zoster.
Actions:	Inhibits viral replication by inhibiting DNA synthesis. A nucleoside analog related to guanosine.
Side effects:	Nausea, vomiting, diarrhea, headache, rash, paresthesias.
Comments:	Drug of choice for herpes zoster.
Dose:	800 mg PO q4hr, 4 or 5 times a day. 10 mg/kg IV q8hr. Reduce dose or dose frequency if creatinine clearance <25 mL/min.

ALLOPURINOL (Zyloprim) *Xanthine oxidase inhibitor*

Indications:	Gout, uric acid nephropathy, tumor lysis syndrome.
Actions:	Inhibits xanthine oxidase, thus reducing the oxidation of hypoxanthine and xanthine in the formation of uric acid. Has a similar action on some therapeutic drugs with a purine structure, including mercaptopurine and azathioprine, resulting in a decrease in their rate of metabolism.
Side effects:	Rash, fever, GI upset, hepatotoxicity.
Comments:	Aminophylline, mercaptopurine, and azathioprine levels may be increased by allopurinol. Attacks of acute gout may occur shortly after starting allopurinol.
Dose:	100–300 mg PO QD after meals. Up to 800 mg/day (in divided doses) may be required in severe cases. Reduce the dose in renal or hepatic insufficiency.

AMIKIN (see Aminoglycoside antibiotics)

AMINOGLYCOSIDE ANTIBIOTICS

Indications:	Moderate to severe gram-negative systemic infections. Usually used in combination with another antibiotic.

See Figure E–4 for usual bacterial sensitivities. Antibacterial sensitivities should always be done.

Actions: Interfere with the initiation of bacterial protein synthesis in susceptible organisms. Active against only aerobic gram-negative bacteria and staphylococci.

Side effects: Use limited because of **renal, cochlear, and vestibular toxicity.** Neuromuscular blockade can occur, particularly when used in association with other neuromuscular blocking drugs or anesthetics or if given rapidly IV or IP. Serum creatinine measurements should be made at the initiation of therapy and every 3 to 4 days during therapy.

Dose: Once-daily dosing has replaced more frequent dosing for most indications. When the aminoglycoside is used for synergy in enterococcal endocarditis and gram-positive infections, shorter dosing intervals may be required. Elderly patients should be given doses at the low end of the range.

Drug	Trade Name	Comments	Usual Dose for Systemic Infection (see Table E–2 for doses in renal impairment)
Amikacin	Amikin	Active against many gram-negative organisms resistant to other aminoglycosides	5–7 mg/kg once daily IV
Gentamicin	Garamycin		5–7 mg/kg once daily IV
Netilmicin	Netromycin	Active against many gram-negative organisms resistant to gentamicin May be less nephrotoxic than gentamicin	16–20 mg/kg once daily IV
Tobramycin	Nebcin, Tobrex	May be less nephrotoxic than gentamicin	5–7 mg/kg once daily IV

AMINOPHYLLINE (Phyllocontin)   *Bronchodilator*

Indications: Bronchospasm, but no longer considered a first-line agent because in adults it may not improve the bronchodilation achieved with the safer, aggressive use of inhaled bronchodilators.

Actions: Phosphodiesterase inhibitor resulting in smooth muscle relaxation and bronchodilation. Also, stimulates the respiratory center.

Side effects: Tachycardia, **ventricular ectopy,** nausea, vomiting, headaches, **seizures,** insomnia, nightmares.

Comments: Theophylline clearance is decreased by erythromycin, cimetidine, propranolol, allopurinol, and a number of other drugs.

Dose: Aminophylline loading dose is 5 mg/kg IV over 30 to 45 minutes, up to a maximum of 500 mg, followed by a maintenance dose of 0.5 to 0.7 mg/kg per hour. Maintenance doses in patients with CHF or liver disease and in the elderly should be reduced to 0.3 mg/kg per hour; smokers require a larger dose of 0.9 mg/kg per hour.

AMIODARONE HYDROCHLORIDE
FOR IV INFUSION   *Antiarrhythmic*

Indications: Ventricular tachycardia.

Actions: The initial acute effects are predominantly an AV intranodal conduction delay and an increase in nodal refractoriness due to calcium channel blockade.

Side effects: **Hypotension, bradycardia** due to excess AV block, cardiac arrest, cardiogenic shock.

Comments: Use with extreme caution in patients known to be predisposed to bradycardia or AV block.

Dose: 150-mg IV bolus in 100 mL 5% dextrose over 10 minutes, with a maintenance IV infusion of 540 mg over 18 hours (0.5 mg/min).

AMPHOTERICIN B (Fungizone)   *Antifungal*

Indications: Systemic fungal infections.

Actions: Binds to sterols in cell membranes, increasing their permeability with a loss of a variety of essential small molecules.

Side effects: Fever, chills, nausea, vomiting, diarrhea, hypotension, **nephrotoxicity,** hypokalemia, hypomagnesemia, thrombophlebitis.

Comments: Premedication with antipyretics, antihistamines, antiemetics, and corticosteroids may reduce some of the side effects.

Dose: Patients should receive a test dose of 1 mg IV in 100 mL D5W over 2 hours. If the test dose is tolerated, another dose of 10 mg can be given on the first day. The dose can then be increased by 5 mg every day until the desired dose of 0.5 mg/kg per day is reached. Infusion time should be 4 to 6 hours. Reduce the dose or dose frequency in renal impairment. Monitor renal function.

ANGIOTENSIN-CONVERTING ENZYME (ACE) INHIBITORS

Indications: Hypertension, CHF.

Actions: Inhibit the enzyme responsible for the conversion of angiotensin I to angiotensin II, resulting in vasodilatation in many vascular beds. Increases bradykinin and vasodilator prostaglandins.

Side effects: **Hypotension,** dysgeusia, **cough,** rash, angioedema, neutropenia, proteinuria, renal insufficiency. Cough is probably due to the accumulation of prostaglandins, kinins, or substance P. There is no apparent difference in the frequency of cough among the various ACE inhibitors.

Comments: May cause hyperkalemia if used in patients receiving potassium-sparing diuretics or potassium supplements.

Drug	Trade Name	Dose	Comments
Captopril	Capoten	6.25–25 mg PO BID or TID	Remains the standard ACE inhibitor and may carry a lower risk of renal insufficiency than the longer-acting drugs
Enalapril	Vasotec	2.5–40 mg PO once daily	Onset following IV injection is within
Enalaprilat	Enalaprilat	1.25–5 mg IV q6hr	15 min, with a
Lisinopril	Zestril, Prinivil	2.5–20 mg PO once daily	maximum effect in 1–4 hr

ANTACIDS

Indications: Symptomatic relief of pain and discomfort of peptic ulcer, reflux esophagitis; prophylaxis of stress ulcers.

Actions: Neutralize gastric acid. Alginic acid compound has a demulcent effect, providing a protective coating to the lower esophageal and gastric mucosa.

Drug	Trade Name	Side Effects	Dose
Aluminum hydroxide	Amphojel Basaljel	Constipation, nausea, hypophosphatemia, **aluminum toxicity in patients with renal failure**	30–60 mL PO q1–2hr during the acute phase; 30–60 mL PO q1–4hr PC and QHS for chronic therapy
Aluminum hydroxide/ magnesium hydroxide	Maalox Gelusil	Diarrhea, nausea, **hypermagnesemia in patients with renal failure**	30–60 mL PO q1–2hr during the acute phase; 30–60 mL PO q1–4hr PC and QHS for chronic therapy
	Mylanta	The addition of Mg attempts to counteract the influence of $Al(OH)_3$ to cause constipation	
Alginic acid compound	Gaviscon	Nausea, vomiting, eructation, flatulence **Contains sodium**	10–20 mL of liquid PO or 2–4 tablets chewed 1–4 times daily after meals and QHS; may be followed by a drink of water

ANTIDIARRHEAL DRUGS

Drug	Trade Name	Usual Adult Dose	Side Effects	Comments
Loperamide	Imodium	4 mg PO q4hr up to a maximum of 16 mg in 24 hr	Abdominal cramps, distention, dry mouth Toxic mega-colon in ulcerative colitis	Onset in 2–4 hr Less effective if given on a PRN basis
Diphenoxylate hydrochloride with atropine	Lomotil	5 mg PO 3 or 4 times/day	Abdominal cramps, distention, dry mouth, sedation, headache Toxic mega-colon in ulcerative colitis	Contains atropine Onset somewhat slower than loperamide
Bismuth subsalicylate	Pepto-Bismol	30 mL or 2 tablets PO q30min up to a maxi-mum of 8 doses/24 hr	Darkening of tongue and stools, tinnitus	Avoid in patients with salicylate sensitivity Onset in 0.5–2 hr

ANTIFIBRINOLYTICS

Indications: Prevention and treatment of bleeding due to excessive fibrinolysis.

Actions: Competitively inhibit the activation of plasminogen and, at high doses, noncompetitively inhibit plasmin.

Side effects: Nausea, vomiting, diarrhea. Increases risk of thromboembolic events. Dizziness, hypotension, particularly with IV administration. Rash.

Drug	Trade Name	Dose	Comments
Aminocaproic acid	Amicar	4–5 g IV over 1 hr, followed by maintenance infusion of 1–1.25 g/hr	Should be used only under specialist direction
Tranexamic acid	Cyklokapron	25 mg/kg PO 3–4 times/day 10 mg/kg IV 3–4 times/day Reduce the frequency of dosing if renal function is impaired	Used mostly to prevent rather than treat bleeding due to excessive fibrinolysis in hemophilia

ANTIFUNGAL AGENTS FOR ORAL/ESOPHAGEAL CANDIDIASIS

Indications:	Oral candidiasis can be treated with topical or systemic therapy. Local treatment is generally recommended to reduce the likelihood of the emergence of azole-resistant organisms. Esophageal candidiasis requires systemic therapy.
Actions:	Bind to sterols in cell membranes, increasing their permeability with the loss of a variety of essential small molecules.
Side effects:	Drugs for systemic therapy are all associated with frequent adverse effects, including **GI intolerance, hepatotoxicity,** rash, pruritus, and headaches, as well as many drug interactions.

Drug	Trade Name	Dose/ Preparation	Comments
Clotrimazole	Mycelex troche Lotrimin	One 10 mg troche 5 times daily	Not well tolerated—nausea, vomiting, bad taste
Nystatin	Mycostatin	4–6-mL suspension QID or 1–2 flavored pastilles 4–5 times/day	Not well tolerated—nausea, vomiting, bad taste
Fluconazole	Diflucan	100 mg PO daily Reduce dose or dose frequency in renal impairment	Drug of first choice for systemic therapy
Itraconazole	Sporanox	Solution 200 mg PO daily Experience limited in renal impairment	The solution (not the capsule formulation) is of equal efficacy as fluconazole; fluconazole-resistant cases may respond to itraconazole
Ketoconazole	Nizoril	200–400 mg PO daily	Causes gynecomastia in men; poorly absorbed, particularly with drugs that reduce gastric acidity

ANTINAUSEANT DRUGS

Drug	Trade Name	Usual Adult Dose	Side Effects	Comments
Metoclo-pramide	Maxeran Reglan	5–10 mg PO, IM, or IV	**Drowsiness,** lethargy	Stimulates gastric motility
Dimenhy-drinate	Dramamine Gravol	50 mg PO or 25 mg IM or IV q4–6 hr PRN	**Drowsiness,** dizziness, dry mouth, urinary retention	An antihistamine with anti-cholinergic effects

Continued

Continued

Drug	Trade Name	Usual Adult Dose	Side Effects	Comments
Diphenhy-dramine	Benadryl	25–50 mg PO, IM, or IV q6–8 hr PRN	**Drowsiness,** dizziness, dry mouth, urinary retention	An antihistamine with anti-cholinergic effects
Prochlor-perazine		5–10 mg IV or IM or 25 mg PR		
Prometh-azine	Phenergan	25–50 mg PO, IM, or PR q4–6hr PRN or 12.5–25 mg IV q4–6hr	**Drowsiness,** dizziness, dry mouth, urinary retention	An antihistamine with anti-cholinergic effects
Chlorpro-mazine	Largactil	For nausea with severe migraine, 0.1 mg/kg IV over 20 min; repeat after 15 min to a maximum of 37.5 mg	CNS depression, hypotension, **extrapyra-midal effects,** jaundice	Limit use to nausea accompanying severe migraine

ANTIPLATELET DRUGS

Indications: Thromboembolic arterial occlusions.

Actions: Thrombi are formed as a result of platelets adhering to damaged luminal surfaces of arteries. Platelets are activated by a variety of stimuli, including the prostacyclin-thromboxane pathways, and adhere to one another under the influence of fibrinogen and von Willebrand's factor to initiate clot formation. These factors bind to activated glycoprotein IIb/IIIa receptors on the platelet surface.

Some agents (e.g., aspirin, ridogrel) inhibit the prostacyclin-thromboxane pathways; some (ticlopidine, clopidogrel) interfere with platelet membrane function, inhibiting platelet aggregation; others (e.g., abciximab, tirofiban) act as antagonists at the glycoprotein IIb/IIIa binding sites. There is intense pharmaceutical development addressing other potential sites that influence platelet function, underlining the fact that an ideal agent is yet to be found.

Drug	Trade Name	Dose	Comments	Clinical Use
Inhibitors of the Prostacyclin-Thromboxane System				
Aspirin	Aspirin	Maximally effective at doses of 80–325 mg PO daily	Gold standard in the prevention of cerebrovascular disease and stroke because of its relative safety and very low cost	MI, unstable angina, stroke, transient ischemic attack
Dipyridamole	Persantine	75 mg PO QID		Used as an adjunct to warfarin to prevent prosthetic valve thrombosis
Platelet Membrane Active			Side effects include GI symptoms and rash	
Ticlopidinel	Ticlid	250 mg PO BID with food	Can be associated with fatal **agranulocytosis** May be slightly more effective than aspirin in preventing cerebrovascular events Onset of action is delayed—beneficial effect not seen until after 2 wk of therapy	Stroke/transient ischemic attack; acute coronary syndromes
Clopidogrel	Plavix	300 mg PO, then 75 mg PO daily	Used in combination with aspirin for acute coronary syndromes; onset of action is 2 hr	Acute coronary syndromes
Glycoprotein IIb/IIIa Receptor Antagonists			Inhibits platelet activation and aggregations Bleeding complications are increased with concomitant heparin therapy	

Continued

Continued

Drug	Trade Name	Dose	Comments	Clinical Use
Abciximab	ReoPro	0.25 mg/kg IV load, then 0.125 µg/kg/min IV (maximum 10 µg/min)	No dosage adjustment required in renal insufficiency	As an adjunct in interventional cardiology to prevent cardiac ischemic complications; not recommended for acute coronary syndromes
Eptifibatide	inte-grilin	180 µg/kg IV bolus, followed by infusion of 2 µg/kg/min	Dosage adjustment required in renal insufficiency	As an adjunct in inter-ventional cardiology to prevent cardiac ischemic complications; acute coronary syndromes
Tirofiban	Aggra-stat	0.4 µg/kg/min IV for 30 min, then 0.1 µg/kg/min IV	May cause reversible thrombo-cytopenia Dosage adjustment required in renal insufficiency	As an adjunct in interventional cardiology to prevent cardiac ischemic complications; acute coronary syndromes

ANTIPSYCHOTIC DRUGS

Indications: Antipsychotic drugs are used primarily in the treatment of schizophrenia; however, they are also useful in a variety of situations in general medicine. Though used to control behavioral problems in patients in the general hospital setting, they are considered second line because of their many potential side effects. A better choice for control of a combative patient is a benzodiazepine such as lorazepam (see Chapter 7). The newer atypical antipsychotics have not been shown to have any advantage over the two agents listed below in the conditions identified.

Actions: Block dopamine and serotonin receptors. Variable in their ability to block alpha-adrenergic, H_1, and cholinergic receptors.

Side effects: Sedation, anticholinergic effects, postural hypotension, drug-induced parkinsonism, akathisia, tardive dyskinesia.

Drug	Trade Name	Uses Outside of Psychiatry	Dose	Comments
Chlorpro-mazine	Largactil	Severe nausea of migraine Behavioral disturbance associated with amphet-amine overdose Hiccoughs	0.1 mg/kg IV over 20 min 1.0 mg/kg IM	Use associated with hypotension, particularly in the elderly, because of its alpha-adrenergic blocking effect; this effect may be useful to lower the elevated BP in amphetamine overdose
Haloperidol	Haldol	Agent of second choice (after lorazepam) to control a combative patient	1–10 mg IM	Less hypotension but more marked extrapyramidal effects than chlorpromazine

ANTIRETROVIRAL DRUGS

The current standard of care is to use antiretroviral drugs in combination. Current initial treatment regimens (known as highly active antiretroviral therapy, or HAART) usually include two NRTIs with a PI or an NNRTI.

Nucleoside/Nucleotide Reverse Transcriptase Inhibitors (NRTIs)

Actions: Bind to the reverse transcriptase enzyme and prevent conversion of the viral genome to double-stranded DNA.

Drug	Trade Name	Dose	Side Effects
Abacavir	Ziagen	300 mg PO BID	Nausea, vomiting, lethargy, fatigue **Hypersensitivity, fever, rash, GI symptoms**
Didanosine (ddI)	Videx	>50 kg, 400 mg PO daily; <50 kg, 250 mg daily, on an empty stomach	**Pancreatitis**, peripheral neuropathy, **diarrhea, hepatitis**
Lamivudine (3TC)	Epivir	150 mg PO BID	**Neutropenia**, GI symptoms
Stavudine (d4T)	Zerit	>60 kg, 40 mg PO BID; <60 kg, 15–30 mg PO BID	**Peripheral neuropathy, pancreatitis**
Zalcitabine (3TC)	Hivid	0.75 mg PO TID	Aphthous stomatitis, pancreatitis, rash, peripheral neuropathy

Continued

Continued

Drug	Trade Name	Dose	Side Effects
Zidovudine (AZT)	Retrovir	200 mg PO TID or 300 mg PO BID	Anemia, myopathy, GI symptoms, headache, **lactic acidosis**

Non–Nucleoside Reverse Transcriptase Inhibitors (NNRTIs)

Actions: Bind to the reverse transcriptase enzyme and prevent conversion of the viral genome to double-stranded DNA.

Drug	Trade Name	Dose	Side Effects
Delavirdine	Rescriptor	400 mg PO TID	**Rash**, elevated liver enzymes
Efavirenz	Sustiva	600 mg PO daily	**Dreams, hallucinations,** headaches, rash
Nevirapine	Viramune	200 mg PO daily, increasing to 200 mg PO BID after 2 wk	**Rash**, nausea, fever, elevated liver enzymes

Protease Inhibitors (PIs)

Actions: Prevent the production of viral proteins from precursor polypeptides, resulting in the production of immature, noninfectious viral particles.

Drug	Trade Name	Dose	Side Effects
Indinavir	Crixivan	800 mg PO q8hr on an empty stomach	Diarrhea, **hyperglycemia,** hemolytic anemia, **renal calculi,** lipodystrophy
Nelfinavir	Viracept	750 mg PO TID or 1250 mg PO BID with food	Diarrhea, **hyperglycemia,** rash, elevated liver enzymes, lipodystrophy
Ritonivir	Norvir	300 mg PO BID, increasing gradually to 600 mg PO BID with food	Elevated lipid levels, GI symptoms, **hyperglycemia,** elevated liver enzymes, **lipodystrophy**
Saquinavir	Invirase Fortovase	600 mg PO q8hr 1200 mg PO q8hr	Rash, GI symptoms, **lipodystrophy, hyperglycemia**

BENZTROPINE MESYLATE   *Anticholinergic (antimuscarinic)*

Indications: Drug-induced extrapyramidal reactions. A drug of choice for terminating acute dystonic reactions. Useful in the symptomatic treatment of Parkinson's disease.

Actions:	An anticholinergic (antimuscarinic) agent with antihistaminic and local anesthetic properties.
Side effects:	**Tachycardia, dizziness,** dry mouth, mydriasis, urinary hesitancy/retention.
Comments:	Onset of effect is 2 to 3 minutes after IM or IV injection or 1 to 2 hours after an oral dose. Effects may persist for 24 hours or longer.
Dose:	1 to 2 mg PO, IM, or IV for acute dystonic reactions. If symptoms return, the dose can be repeated.

BETA-ADRENERGIC BLOCKERS

Indications:	Angina pectoris, post-MI, treatment of SVTs, hypertension, thyrotoxicosis, heart failure.
	Cardioselective agents are useful in patients with peripheral vascular disease to avoid peripheral beta block and unopposed alpha activity, further reducing peripheral perfusion.
	Esmolol is useful in any situation in which a short duration of action is desired (e.g., aortic dissection).
	Nadolol is less lipid soluble than propranolol and may be associated with fewer CNS side effects (e.g., nightmares).
Actions:	Competitive antagonism of beta-adrenergic receptors in the vascular smooth muscle and the heart, as well as bronchial smooth muscle.
Side effects:	**Hypotension, bradycardia,** bronchospasm, nausea, fatigue, nightmares.
Comments:	It is usually useful to start with a small dose and increase as required, because there is considerable individual variability in response.

Drug	Trade Name	Usual Dose
Noncardioselective		
Propranolol	Inderal	10–80 mg PO BID to QID
		Aortic dissection: 0.1 mg/kg by slow IV push, divided into 3 equal doses at 2- to 3-min intervals; repeat after 2 min if necessary; do not exceed 1 mg/min
Nadolol	Corgard	10–40 mg PO daily
Esmolol	Brevibloc	0.5 mg/kg/min IV loading dose over 1 min, followed by infusion of 0.05 mg/kg/min (maximum 0.3 mg/kg/min)
Cardioselective		
Acebutolol	Monitan, Sectral	100–200 mg PO BID
Atenolol	Tenormin	25–50 mg PO
		Hypertensive emergencies: 100 mg PO
		SVTs: 5 mg IV over 5 min at 10-min intervals, to a total of 15 mg
Metoprolol	Betaloc	50–200 mg PO BID for hypertension, angina, migraine prophylaxis
		1–2 mg/min IV up to 5 mg by direct injection; repeat PRN at 2–5-min intervals, up to a total of 15 mg

BISACODYL (Dulcolax) *Laxative*

Indications:	Constipation.
Actions:	Stimulates peristalsis.
Side effects:	Abdominal cramps, rectal bleeding.
Comments:	Onset PO in 6 to 10 hours; onset PR in 15 to 60 minutes. Avoid in pregnancy, MI. May worsen **orthostatic hypotension, weakness, and incoordination in the elderly.**
Dose:	10 to15 mg PO QHS PRN; 10 mg suppository PR PRN.

BISMUTH SUBSALICYLATE (Pepto-Bismol) *Antibacterial, anti-inflammatory*

Indications:	Peptic ulcer disease, diarrhea.
Actions:	Acts locally at the ulcer site to promote healing of gastric and duodenal ulcers; has antibacterial activity, including against *Helicobacter pylori*. Neutralizes bacterial toxins and is useful in traveler's diarrhea. Salicylate is thought to provide an anti-inflammatory action.
Side effects:	Darkening of the tongue and stools, tinnitus.
Comments:	Avoid in patients with **salicylate sensitivity.** Used in combination with an antibiotic in the eradication of *H. pylori*.
Dose:	2 tablets or 30 mL PO QID; for diarrhea, 2 tablets every 30 minutes, to a maximum of eight doses per day.

CALCITONIN SALMON (Salcatonin, Caltine) *Hypercalcemia treatment*

Indications:	Hypercalcemia of neoplastic disease, multiple myeloma, primary hyperparathyroidism.
Actions:	Decreases bone resorption, thus inhibiting the release of calcium. Increases the renal loss of calcium.
Side effects:	**Anaphylaxis,** GI symptoms, local inflammation at injection site.
Comments:	Onset in 15 minutes, peak at 4 hours, duration 8 to 24 hours.
Dose:	4 IU/kg every 12 hours SC or IM. May be increased to 8 IU/kg if response is not satisfactory.

CALCIUM CHANNEL BLOCKERS

Indications:	Angina pectoris, coronary spasm, hypertension, hypertensive crisis, treatment of SVTs, left ventricular diastolic dysfunction.
Actions:	Inhibit calcium influx through cell membranes. Nifedipine and nimodipine are more selective than diltiazem and verapamil for vascular sites, with less effect on myocardial contractility, automaticity, and conduction.
Side effects:	**Hypotension,** flushing, dizziness, constipation, headaches, **peripheral edema.** The edema is due to vasodilatation and does not respond to diuretics.
Comments:	Absorption is highly variable. The absorption of nifedipine and nimodipine is enhanced by grapefruit juice (flavinoids inhibit cytochrome P450).

Drug	Trade Name	Dose	Comments
Diltiazem	Cardizem	30–90 mg PO QID IV administration should take place only in monitored patients 0.25 mg/kg IV (usual dose 15–25 mg) may be given over 2 min for rate control or to "break" an SVT	Causes less reduction in cardiac contractility than verapamil
Verapamil	Isoptin, Calan	80–120 mg PO TID IV administration should take place only in monitored patients 2.5–5 mg IV may be given over 1–2 min for rate control or to "break" an SVT; this dose may be repeated	Calcium gluconate 1–2 g IV may reverse the negative inotropic and hypotensive effects but not the AV block of verapamil and diltiazem
Nifedipine	Adalat, Procardia	Hypertensive crisis: 5–10 mg PO For chronic management of hypertension, the long-acting preparation is preferable, e.g., nifedipine PA (or CC, CR, LA) 30–90 mg/day PO	Nifedipine has a greater effect than verapamil and diltiazem on peripheral vasculature
Nimodipine	Nimotop	Subarachnoid hemorrhage: 60–90 mg PO q4hr 1 mg/hr IV via continuous infusion, increasing PRN to 2–3 mg/hr	Combined nimodipine and surgical therapy appears to provide better results than surgery alone, particularly in patients presenting with mild to moderate neurologic deficits

CALCIUM GLUCONATE   *Calcium supplement*

Indications: Symptomatic hypocalcemia, hyperkalemia; adjunct in CPR protocol.

Actions: Replace Ca^{2+} in deficiency states. Decreases cardiac automaticity, raises resting potential of cardiac cells.

Side effects: Administration of Ca^{2+} to patients on digoxin may precipitate ventricular dysrhythmias due to the combined effects of digoxin and Ca^{2+}.

Comments: 500 mg of calcium gluconate = 2.3 mmol Ca^{2+}. 10% solution contains 0.45 mmol Ca^{2+}/mL.

Dose: 1 to 15 g PO daily for control of hypocalcemia. For more immediate effects, 5 to 10 mL of a 10% solution IV in 100 mL of D5W over 30 minutes. In severe hyperkalemia or in cases of tetany or laryngeal stridor associated with hypocalcemia, the same dose can be given directly IV over 2 minutes.

CAPSAICIN   *Substance P depletor*

Indications: Postherpetic neuralgia.
Actions: Releases and depletes substance P from sensory neurons, rendering the skin insensitive to pain.
Side effects: An extract of jalapeño (Mexican red) peppers that stings and burns on application.
Comments: Burns mucous membranes, so care must be taken to wash hands after applying.
Dose: Available as a 0.025% or 0.075% cream in a petrolatum base. Apply 3 to 5 times daily.

CARBAPENEM ANTIBIOTICS

Indications: Systemic infections due to multiple resistant gram-negative coliforms, bacteroides. In *Pseudomonas* infections, should be combined with an aminoglycoside.
Actions: Bind to penicillin-binding proteins of cell walls of susceptible bacteria, causing impaired cell wall synthesis and cell lysis.
Side effects: Nausea, diarrhea, vomiting, eosinophilia, rash, seizures. Local reactions at infusion sites, including phlebitis.
Comments: Should be reserved for use in severe systemic infections due to mixed organisms resistant to antibacterials with a narrower spectrum of activity. Cilastatin has no antibacterial action but prevents the metabolism of carbapenem by dehydropeptidase in the proximal renal tubular cells and therefore decreases the rate of excretion.
                 Not associated with anaphylactic reactions to penicillin.

Drug	Trade Name	Dose (see Table E–1 for doses in renal impairment)
Aztreonam/ cilastatin	Azactam	90–120 mg/kg/day IV or IM in divided doses q6 or 8 hr
Imipenem/ cilastatin	Primaxin	250–1000 mg IV q8hr to a maximum dose of 50 mg/kg or 4 g, whichever is lower
		Do not administer as a direct IV injection
Meropenem	Merrem	500–1000 mg PO or IV q8hr
		Reduce dose or dose frequency in renal impairment

CEPHALOSPORINS

Indications: In spite of the number of cephalosporins, used alone, they are rarely the first choice for the empirical treatment of bacterial infections in hospitalized patients. Combined with other agents, they can be useful in a number of severe infections:
                 Sepsis due to *Escherichia coli*, indole-positive *Proteus*, and *Providencia stuartii* (third-generation cephalosporin with an aminoglycoside)
                 Meningitis, epiglottitis, or other serious infection due to *Haemophilus influenzae* (third-generation cephalosporin with vancomycin with or without rifampin)

Hospital-acquired pneumonia (third-generation cephalosporin with a macrolide or a fluoroquinolone)

Klebsiella pneumoniae pneumonia (third-generation cephalosporin with an aminoglycoside)

Actions: Like other beta-lactam antibiotics, cephalosporins bind to bacterial cell membrane penicillin-binding proteins, thus inhibiting cell wall synthesis and causing cell lysis. They were originally divided into "generations" based on their in vitro activities against gram-negative organisms. With the expanding of this spectrum through successive generations, activity against gram-positive aerobes is weakened.

Side effects: **Diarrhea, allergic reactions,** false-positive glycosuria clinitest results.

About 8% of patients allergic to penicillins will have an allergic reaction to first- and second-generation cephalosporins; the overall incidence of allergic reactions to cephalosporins is 4%. This is less likely with third-generation drugs, probably because of the interference with binding caused by the bulky side chains.

Comments: Cephalosporins, particularly the third- and fourth-generation parental preparations, are expensive.

Dose: Doses and dose intervals vary among products and may have to be altered in the presence of renal impairment (see Table E–1).

Drug	Trade Name	Oral Preparation	Parenteral Preparation
First Generation			
Cefazolin	Ancef, Kefzol		Yes
Cephalexin	Keflex and others	Yes	
Cefadroxil	Duricef	Yes	
Second Generation			
Cefoxitin	Mefoxin		Yes
Cefaclor	Ceclor		Yes
Cefuroxime	Zinacef, Kefurox,	Yes	
Cefuroxime axetil	Ceftin		
Third Generation			
Ceftriaxone	Rocephin		Yes
Cefotaxime	Claforan		Yes
Ceftizoxime	Ceftizox		Yes
Third–Fourth Generation			
Ceftazidime	Fortaz, Ceptaz, Tazicef, Tazidime		Yes

CHLORAL HYDRATE (Noctec and others)   *Hypnotic*

Indications:	Insomnia.
Actions:	Depression of CNS activity.
Side effects:	Gastric irritation, rash.
Comments:	Do not use in patients with liver or kidney disease.
Dose:	0.5 to 1 g PO or PR.

CHLORPROPAMIDE (Diabinese, Chloranase)   *Oral hypoglycemic*

Indications:	Type 2 diabetes mellitus.
Actions:	Sulfonylurea stimulates insulin secretion and increases the effect of insulin on the liver to increase gluconeogenesis and on muscle to increase glucose utilization.
Side effects:	**Hypoglycemia,** rash, blood dyscrasias, jaundice, hyponatremia, edema.
Comments:	Has a long duration of action (20 to 60 hours) and is cleared largely by the kidneys. Hypoglycemic reactions may be prolonged in the elderly and in patients with renal impairment.
Dose:	100 to 500 mg/day PO in 1 or 2 doses.

CITROVORUM FACTOR (leucovorin)   *Folic acid derivative*

Indications:	Folate deficiency. Enhances the cytotoxicity of 5-fluorouracil. Diminishes the effect of methotrexate.
Actions:	A metabolite of folic acid required as a coenzyme for nucleic acid synthesis.
Side effects:	Hypersensitivity.
Comments:	Should not be used to treat vitamin B_{12} deficiency anemia, because the anemia may respond while neurologic sequelae progress.
Dose:	1 mg PO daily in folate deficiency.

CLINDAMYCIN (Dalacin)   *Antibiotic*

Indications:	Serious anaerobic infections due to organisms arising in the abdomen or pelvis.
Actions:	Inhibits protein synthesis in susceptible bacteria.
Side effects:	GI symptoms, rash, hypersensitivity reactions, **pseudomembranous enterocolitis.**
Comments:	Parenteral doses are associated with local reactions.
Dose:	150 to 450 mg PO every 6 to 8 hours. 600 to 3000 mg IV in 2 to 4 divided doses.

DAPSONE (DDS, Avlosulfone)   *Anti-infective*

Indications:	Leprosy, dermatitis herpetiformis, *Pneumocystis carinii* pneumonia.
Actions:	A sulfone that, like the sulfonamides, competes with paraaminobenzoic acid for incorporation into folic acid.
Side effects:	**Hemolysis, anemia, widespread allergic rash, fever.**

Comments:	Most often used in prevention but can be added to trimethoprim-sulfamethoxazole in the treatment of *Pneumocystis carinii* pneumonia. Absorption may be interfered with if used with ddI.
Dose:	100 mg PO daily. Reduce dose in renal impairment.

DEMECLOCYCLINE (Declomycin) *Tetracycline*

Indications:	Occasionally useful in patients with chronic SIADH. Not useful as an antibiotic because of its renal effects.
Actions:	A tetracycline antibiotic that interferes with the kidney's ability to produce a concentrated urine.
Side effects:	Epigastric burning, nausea, vomiting, **phototoxicity**, polyuria and polydipsia.
Comments:	Less useful as an antibacterial than doxycycline or minocycline because of its incomplete absorption and its renal effects.
Dose:	300 to 600 mg PO twice daily.

DESMOPRESSIN (DDAVP injection) *Hemostasis agent*

Indications:	To maintain hemostasis in patients with hemophilia A and factor VIII levels greater than 5% or with mild to moderate von Willebrand's disease (Type I).
Actions:	A synthetic analog of antidiuretic hormone with identical actions on water reabsorption in the renal tubule. Has an additional action to release factor VIII complex and plasminogen activator from endothelial cell storage sites. This action peaks in 1 hour and lasts 8 to 12 hours. It may also have a direct effect on the vessel wall, decreasing bleeding at an injury site.
Side effects:	Facial flushing, tachycardia, mild hypotension, water retention, headaches, nausea, abdominal pain, **allergic reactions.**
Comments:	Should not be used in hemophilia B because it has no effect on factor IX. Should not be used in severe type I or type IIB von Willebrand's disease because a response is less likely and severe thrombocytopenia may develop.
Dose:	10.0 g/m^2 (maximum dose 20 g) by slow IV infusion.

DIGOXIN (Lanoxin) *Digitalis glycoside*

Indications:	SVT, CHF.
Actions:	Slows AV conduction; increases the force of cardiac contraction; Na$^+$-K$^+$-ATPase inhibitor.
Side effects:	**Dysrhythmias,** nausea, vomiting, neuropsychiatric disturbances.
Comments:	80% renally excreted, so dose must be reduced in patients with renal impairment and in the elderly. Avoid hypokalemia, which can predispose to digitalis-induced arrhythmias.

Dose: IV: 0.125 to 0.5 mg every 6 hours to a total of 1 mg; then
               0.125 to 0.25 mg/day.
               PO: 0.125 to 0.5 mg every 6 hours to a total of 1.5 mg; then
               0.125 to 0.25 mg/day. Higher doses may be required to
               control SVTs.

DIURETICS

Thiazides and Related Drugs

Indications: Edema, cardiac failure, hypertension.
Actions: Block Na^+ and Cl^- reabsorption in the cortical diluting
               segment of the loop of Henle.
Side effects: Electrolyte depletion, hyperuricemia, hyperglycemia, hyper-
               calcemia, pancreatitis, jaundice.

Drug	Trade Name	Usual Dose	Comments
Hydrochloro-thiazide	Hydro-DIURIL	12.5–50 mg PO daily	Despite the long list of side effects, generally well tolerated
Metolazone	Zaroxolyn	2.5–10 mg PO daily	Longer acting than chlorothiazide
Chlorthalidone	Hygroton	6.25–25 mg PO daily	Duration of action >24 hr

Aldosterone Antagonists

Indications: Edema, ascites, hypertension, hyperaldosteronism.
Actions: Block the action of aldosterone on the renal tubules, result-
               ing in a loss of sodium and water.
Side effects: Hyponatremia, **hyperkalemia**, gynecomastia, confusion,
               headache.

Drug	Trade Name	Usual Dose	Comments
Spironolactone	Aldactone	25–200 mg PO daily	Most effective in hyperaldosteronism; higher doses are required in primary hyperaldosteronism. In hypertension, equipotent as thiazides but associated with more side effects

Loop Diuretics

Indications: Cardiac failure.
Actions: Inhibitor of Na^+ and Cl^- reabsorption in the ascending loop
               of Henle.

Side effects:	Electrolyte depletion, hyperuricemia, hyperglycemia, anorexia, nausea, vomiting, diarrhea, hearing loss.		

Drug	Trade Name	Usual Dose	Comments
Furosemide	Lasix	40 mg PO or IV	Loop diuretics are well and promptly absorbed from the GI tract
Bumetanide	Bumex	0.5–1 mg PO or IV	No advantage over furosemide and usually more expensive

FERROUS SULFATE   *Iron supplement*

Indications:	Iron deficiency.
Actions:	Replaces iron stores.
Side effects:	**Constipation,** nausea, diarrhea, abdominal cramps.
Comments:	Stools may turn black but do not have the typical tarry appearance of melena.
Dose:	325 mg/day PO TID.

FIBRINOLYTIC AGENTS

Indications:	Acute MI, DVT, pulmonary embolism, acute nonhemorrhagic stroke, acute peripheral arterial catheters and occlusion of indwelling catheters. No single agent is officially approved for use in all conditions. The choice of agent should be based on the results of ongoing trials.
Actions:	Catalyze the conversion of plasminogen to the naturally occurring fibrinolytic agent plasmin. Plasmin lyses the clot by breaking down the fibrin and fibrinogen.
Side effects:	All agents carry an approximately equal risk of bleeding complications, including intracranial and retroperitoneal hemorrhage, pericardial bleeding, GU and GI bleeding, epistaxis, ecchymoses, gingival bleeding, and bleeding from puncture sites. Streptokinase and anisoylated plasminogen streptokinase activator complex carry the additional risk of allergic reactions and resistance to the effects with repeat administration.

Drug	Trade Name	Action	Comments	Dose in Myocardial Infarction	Doses in Other Conditions
Streptokinase		Binds to free circulating plasminogen to form a complex that converts additional plasminogen to plasmin	The least expensive agent Plasma half-life of principal fraction 80 min	1.5 million IU in 50 mL D5W over 60 min IV	Peripheral arterial occlusion: 5000–10,000 IU /hr intra-arterially
Alteplase	tPA, Activase	Binds to fibrin and activates plasminogen to form plasmin Is said to be clot specific but has a similar influence on circulating plasminogen as does streptokinase	The fibrinolytic agent with which there is the most experience	15 mg IV, followed by 0.75 mg/kg (up to 50 mg) over 30 min, then 0.5 mg/kg (up to 35 mg) over 60 min to a total of 100 mg	Pulmonary thromboembolism: 15 mg IV, followed by 50 mg IV over 30 min, then 35 mg over the next hour Stroke: 0.9 mg/kg over 60 min, with 10% of the dose given IV over the first minute Peripheral arterial occlusion: 0.05–0.1 mg/kg/hr intra-arterially
Reteplase	rPA, Retavase	Binds to fibrin, but less tightly than alteplase, allowing it to diffuse more freely through the clot	Half-life about 11–19 min	10 IU IV over 2 min, with a second 10 IU IV in 30 min	Peripheral arterial occlusion: 0.5 IU/hr intra-arterially
Anisoylated plasminogen streptokinase activator complex	APSAC	A complex of streptokinase and plasminogen that catalyzes the conversion of plasminogen to plasmin	Plasma half-life 40–90 min	30 IU IV over 2–5 min	

FLUMAZENIL *Benzodiazepine antagonist*

Indications:	Reversal of benzodiazepine sedation.
Actions:	Competitive antagonism of benzodiazepine receptors.
Side effects:	Seizures, nausea, dizziness, agitation, pain at injection site.
Comments:	Onset of reversal within minutes. Contraindicated in patients with cyclic antidepressant overdose (risk of precipitating seizures).
Dose:	0.2 mg IV over 15 seconds. Wait 1 minute. If ineffective, this can be followed by additional doses of 0.2 mg IV every 60 seconds to a maximum dose of 1 mg. If the patient becomes resedated, this regimen can be repeated again in 20 minutes. No more than 3 mg total dose should be given in 1 hour.

FLUOROQUINOLONES

Indications:	Rarely indicated as drugs to be used empirically in hospitalized patients, except for the treatment of community-acquired pneumonia (levofloxacin) or in an individual free of chronic disease with an uncomplicated urinary tract infection (ciprofloxacin). A drug of first choice in infections due to *Salmonella typhi* and *Shigella*. Used as an agent of first choice with or without rifampin in *Legionella* infections.
Actions:	A class of agents modeled after nalidixic acid (a nonfluorinated quinolone) that inhibits bacterial gyrase, an enzyme responsible for developing double-stranded DNA.
Side effects:	GI symptoms, depression, allergic reactions, nephropathy, **photosensitivity** reactions (can be particularly serious with levofloxacin, norfloxacin, and sparfloxacin), **QT interval prolongation** (particularly with gatifloxacin, moxifloxacin, and sparfloxacin), seizures (ciprofloxacin).
Comments:	The emergence of bacterial resistance to the fluoroquinolones is a serious concern, suggesting that their use should be limited. Multiple drug interactions have been reported.

Drug	Trade Name	Route	Dose (reduce dose or dose frequency if creatinine clearance <30 mL/min; see Table E–1 for IV dose adjustments in renal impairment)
Ciprofloxacin	Cipro, Ciloxan	PO, IV	PO: 100–750 mg q12hr IV: 400–1200 mg/day in 2–3 divided doses The oral dose is well absorbed, equal in efficacy to the IV dose, and much less costly; 750 mg PO is equivalent to 400 mg IV
Gatifloxacin	Tequin	PO, IV	PO/IV: 400 mg once daily
Levofloxacin	Levaquin	PO, IV	PO/IV: 250–500 mg q24hr
Norfloxacin	Noroxin	PO	PO: 400 mg q12hr
Moxifloxacin	Avelox	PO	PO: 400 mg once daily
Sparfloxacin	Zagam	PO	PO: 400 mg first day, then 200 mg daily

GLUCOCORTICOIDS

Indications: Glucocorticoids are used principally to take advantage of their anti-inflammatory effect.

The choice among the parenteral preparations is influenced mostly by the experience with the particular agents rather than because important differences have been shown among them.

Actions: Inhibition of the recruitment of leukocytes and monocyte-macrophages in response to a variety of stimuli, with the subsequent inhibition of these cells to release a number of substances that mediate increased vascular permeability, vasodilatation, and contraction of various nonvascular smooth muscles, including bronchial smooth muscle.

In short-term use or longer-term inhalational use, the other glucocorticoid effects are negligible.

Comments: Relative anti-inflammatory potency: dexamethasone 0.75 mg = hydrocortisone 20 mg = methylprednisolone 4 mg = prednisolone 5 mg. Note that the initial doses that follow are not entirely rational and reflect these agents' wide range of safety in short-term use.

Glucocorticoids are efficiently absorbed from the oral route.

Drug	Trade Name	Side Effects	Comments	Initial Dose
Dexametha-sone	Decadron	Headache, nausea, vomiting, hypersensitivity reactions	No mineralo-corticoid effects	Bacterial meningitis: 10 mg PO or starting with the first dose of antibiotics
Hydrocorti-sone Cortisol	Solu-Cortef	Na⁺ retention, potassium loss		Anaphylactic shock or acute asthma: 500 mg PO or IV
Methyl-pred-nisolone	Medrol	Na⁺ retention, potassium loss		Acute asthma: 128 mg PO (eight 16-mg tablets) or 125 mg IV
Prednisone		Na⁺ retention, potassium loss		Acute asthma: 40–60 mg PO
Beclometha-sone	Beclovent Vanceril	Oral and pharyngeal candidiasis, laryngeal myopathy	Has **no role** in the acute treatment of asthma Combination products of these two agents are available	Chronic asthma: 2 inhalations BID to QID; may be more effective if inhaled 3–5 min after an inhaled bron-chodilator

GLYCOPEPTIDE ANTIBIOTICS

Indications:	Serious infections due to beta-lactam–resistant gram-positive organisms and infections due to gram-positive organisms in patients with a severe allergy to beta-lactam antibiotics. Also useful prophylactically in patients at high risk of endocarditis and in life-threatening antibiotic-associated colitis.
Actions:	Suppresses RNA synthesis in susceptible bacteria.
Comments:	Use of vancomycin and teicoplanin should be restricted to reduce the likelihood of the development of resistance in enterococci and staphylococci.

Drug	Trade Name	Comments	Side Effects	Dose (see Table E–1 for dose adjustments in renal impairment)
Rifampin	Rifampicin	Useful in mycobacterial infections and in prophylaxis of meningococcal infections IV preparation is restricted in availability	Hypersensitivity, rash, urticaria, confusion, GI symptoms, **nephrotoxicity**	Staphylococcal infections: 20 mg/kg/day PO in 1 or 2 divided doses
Teicoplanin	Targocid	Effective against methicillin-resistant staphylococci Marginally less toxic than vancomycin	Histamine release related to rate of infusion ("red-man syndrome"), chills, fever, **ototoxicity, nephrotoxicity,** phlebitis at infusion site	12 mg/kg/day IV in 1 or 2 divided doses
Vancomycin	Vancocin	Effective against methicillin-resistant staphylococci *Clostridium difficile* infections	Histamine release related to rate of infusion ("red man syndrome"), chills, fever, **ototoxicity, nephrotoxicity,** neutropenia, phlebitis at infusion site	30 mg/kg/day IV in 2–4 divided doses 125–500 mg PO q6hr

H₂-RECEPTOR ANTAGONISTS

Indications:	Peptic ulcer disease, gastroesophageal reflux.
Actions:	Bind to H_2 receptors, blocking gastric acid production.

Side effects: Diarrhea, headache, dizziness.
Comments: All have similar effects, except that cimetidine reduces the
                  microsomal enzyme metabolism of drugs, including oral
                  anticoagulants, phenytoin, and theophylline.

Drug	Trade Name	Oral Dose for Peptic Ulcer Disease	IV/IM Dose for Conditions Due to Excess Gastric Acid	Side Effects
Cimetidine	Tagamet	800–1200 mg HS or in divided doses QID or BID	300 mg IV or IM q6–8hr	Gynecomastia, impotence, **confusion**, diarrhea, leukopenia, thrombocytopenia, increase in serum creatinine
Famotidine	Pepcid	40 mg HS or 20 mg BID	20 mg IV q12hr	Headache, dizziness, constipation, diarrhea
Nizatidine	Axid	300 mg HS or 150 mg BID	Not applicable	Sweating, urticaria, somnolence, elevation of hepatic enzymes
Ranitidine	Zantac	300 mg HS or 150 mg BID	50 mg IV q8hr	Jaundice, gynecomastia, headache, confusion, leukopenia

HEPARIN

Indications: Prophylaxis and treatment of DVT, pulmonary embolism,
                  embolic cerebrovascular accident; adjunct in the treat-
                  ment of unstable angina.
Actions: Enhances the activity of antithrombin III. The heparin–
                  antithrombin III complexes inactivate several coagulation
                  enzymes, particularly thrombin and factor Xa.
Side effects: **Hemorrhage, thrombocytopenia.**
Comments: Monitor aPTT closely when using IV heparin.
Dose: For treatment of DVT or pulmonary embolism, 100 U/kg
                  IV bolus (usual dose 5000 to 10,000 U IV), followed
                  by a maintenance infusion of 100 to 1600 U/hr, using
                  the lower range for patients with a higher risk of
                  bleeding.
                  For prophylaxis, 5000 U SC every 8 hours.

HEPARINS—LOW MOLECULAR WEIGHT

Indications:	Prophylaxis and treatment of DVT, unstable angina, MI, pulmonary embolism.
Actions:	Catalyze antithrombin to neutralize several procoagulant enzymes, including thrombin, factor IIa, and factor Xa.
Side effects:	**Hemorrhage**, thrombocytopenia (although less than standard heparin).
Comments:	Compared with standard heparin, have less plasma protein binding, are almost completely excreted by the renal route, and have a longer half-life. The dose is more predictable, and the kinetics are not dose dependent. The aPTT is not predictably prolonged and should not be measured to monitor the dose.
	Newer antithrombotics related to the low-molecular-weight heparins include danaparoid and fondaparinux. Danaparoid is a mixture of nonheparin glycosaminoglycans derived from porcine mucosa, with an action similar to low-molecular-weight heparins. Fondaparinux is a synthetic agent that selectively inhibits factor Xa.

Recommended Doses of LMWH in the Treatment of Pulmonary Embolism

Product	Dose
Dalteparin (Fragmin)	200 IU/kg by deep SC injection once daily For patients with an increased risk of bleeding, 100 IU/kg q12hr or 100 IU/kg by continuous IV infusion over 12 hr
Enoxaparin (Lovenox)	1.5 mg/kg by deep SC injection once daily or 1 mg/kg SC q12hr Dose should not exceed 180 mg daily
Nadroparin (Fräxiparine)	171 IU/kg by deep SC injection once daily or 86 IU/kg SC q12hr Dose should not exceed 17,000 IU daily
Tinzaparin (Innohep)	175 IU/kg by deep SC injection once daily

Recommended Doses of LMWH and Related Antithrombotics in the Prevention and Treatment of Deep Vein Thrombosis

Product	Treatment Dose	Prophylaxis Dose
Dalteparin	200 IU/kg by deep injection SC once daily For patients with an increased risk of bleeding, 100 IU/kg q12hr or 100 IU by continuous IV infusion over 12 hours.	2500–5000 IU SC once daily
Enoxaparin	1.5 mg/kg by deep SC injection once daily or 1 mg/kg SC q12hr Dose should not exceed 180 mg daily	30 mg SC BID
Nadroparin	171 IU/kg by deep SC injection once daily or 86 IU/kg SC q12hr Dose should not exceed 17,000 IU daily	2850 IU SC once daily

Continued

Recommended Doses of LMWH and Related Antithrombotics in the Prevention and Treatment of Deep Vein Thrombosis—cont'd

Product	Treatment Dose	Prophylaxis Dose
Tinzaparin	175 IU/kg by deep SC injection once daily	50–75 IU/kg SC once daily
Other Antithrombotics		
Danaparoid (Orgaran)	2250 IU IV bolus, followed by 400 IU/hr for 4 hr, then 300 IU/hr for 4 hr, then 150–200 IU/hr	750 IU SC BID
Fondaparinux (Arixtra)	Currently indicated only for prophylaxis	2.5 mg SC once daily

HYDRALAZINE (Apresoline)   *Arteriolar vasodilator*

Indications:	Hypertension.
Actions:	Arteriolar vasodilator.
Side effects:	**Tachycardia, SLE reaction** at higher doses (>200 mg/day).
Comments:	Very limited effect on veins, so little postural hypotension.
Dose:	10 to 25 mg PO every 6 hours.

INSULIN   *Hypoglycemic*

Indications:	Diabetes mellitus.
Actions:	Enhances hepatic glycogen storage, enhances the entry of glucose into cells, inhibits the breakdown of protein and fat. Enhances the entry of K^+ into cells.
Side effects:	Hypoglycemia, local skin reactions, lipohypertrophy.
Comments:	Less immunogenicity with human insulin than with insulin from animal sources.
Dose:	Extremely variable.

Insulin	Onset	Peak	Effective Duration
Rapid Acting			
Insulin lispro (analog)	10–30 min	30 min–2.5 hr	3–4 hr
Insulin aspart (analog)	15 min	30–60 min	1–3 hr
Short Acting			
Regular (soluble)	30–60 min	2–3 hr	3–6 hr
Intermediate Acting			
NPH (isophane)	2–4 hr	4–10 hr	10–16 hr
Lente (insulin zinc suspension)	2–4 hr	4–12 hr	12–18 hr

Continued

Continued

Insulin	Onset	Peak	Effective Duration
Long Acting			
Ultralente (extended insulin zinc suspension)	6–10 hr	10–16 hr	18–20 hr
Insulin glargine (analog)	2–4 hr	Peakless	24 hr
Combinations			
50% NPH, 50% regular	30–60 min	Dual	10–16 hr
70% NPH, 30% regular	30–60 min	Dual	10–16 hr
75% NPL, 25% lispro	<15 min	Dual	10–16 hr

ISOSORBIDE DINITRATE (Isordil, Sorbitrate)   *Vasodilator*

Indications:	Angina pectoris, CHF.
Actions:	Venous, coronary, and arteriolar vasodilator.
Side effects:	Headache, **hypotension**, flushing.
Comments:	Nitrate tolerance may develop with prolonged, continuous administration.
Dose:	5 to 30 mg PO four times a day.

LABETALOL (Trandate, Normodyne)   *Alpha-1 and beta blocker*

Indications:	Hypertensive emergencies.
Actions:	Alpha-1 blocking action is predominant in acute use but is accompanied by nonspecific beta blockade.
Side effects:	**Postural hypotension**, bronchospasm, jaundice, bradycardia, negative inotropic effect.
Comments:	Effect is largely due to alpha-1-adrenergic blocking activity. Contraindications are the same as for "pure" beta blockers.
Dose:	For a hypertensive emergency, 20 mg IV every 10 to 15 minutes, followed by incremental doses (e.g., 20, 20, 40, 40 mg) as needed. Alternatively, an infusion beginning at 2 mg/min and titrating to BP response may be given, with a maximum daily dose of 2400 mg. Labetalol 200 mg PO can be given as an interim measure if the IV preparation is not immediately available.

LEVODOPA-CARBIDOPA (Sinemet)   *Dopamine agonist*

Indications:	Parkinson's disease.
Actions:	Levodopa is converted to dopamine in the basal ganglia. Carbidopa inhibits the peripheral destruction of levodopa.
Side effects:	Anorexia, nausea, vomiting, abdominal pain, dysrhythmias, **behavioral changes, orthostatic hypotension**, involuntary movements.
Comments:	Side effects are common.
Dose:	Begin with 1 tablet 100 mg levodopa/10 mg carbidopa PO BID, increasing the dose until the desired response is obtained, with a maximum dose of 8 tablets (800 mg/80 mg) per day.

LIDOCAINE (Xylocaine)   *Class IB antiarrhythmic*

Indications: Prophylaxis and treatment of ventricular tachycardia.

Actions: Lengthens the effective refractory period in the ventricular conducting system. Decreases ventricular automaticity.

Side effects: Nausea, vomiting, hypotension, confusion, seizures, perioral paresthesias.

Comments: Lower maintenance doses are required in the elderly and in patients with CHF, liver disease, and hypotension.

Dose: For ventricular tachycardia and fibrillation, 1 to 1.5 mg/kg IV. For refractory ventricular fibrillation, may give an additional 0.5 to 0.75 mg/kg IV push; repeat in 5 to 10 minutes to a maximum total dose of 3 mg/kg. This can be followed by a maintenance dose of 1 to 4 mg/min IV.

MACROLIDE ANTIBIOTICS

Indications: Community-acquired pneumonia.

Actions: Inhibit bacterial growth by inhibiting protein synthesis. Macrolide antibiotics are bacteriostatic. They have been in widespread human and animal use and have been used as growth promoters in animals for food production for half a century.

Side effects: The major adverse effects are **GI symptoms** such as nausea, vomiting, abdominal cramps, and diarrhea. High IV doses of clarithromycin and erythromycin are associated with **hearing loss** and **QT prolongation.** Allergic reactions, eosinophilia, hepatotoxicity, taste disturbance, and headache are less frequent adverse effects.

Drug	Trade Name	Common Uses	Comments	Dose
Erythromycin	Numerous	Community-acquired respiratory infections	GI side effects are more likely with erythromycin, largely through the stimulation of motility Less expensive	1–2 g PO daily in divided doses, usually q6hr Reduce dose or dose frequency if creatinine clearance <25 mL/min 1–2 g IV daily by continuous infusion or in divided doses q6–8hr diluted in 250 mL of saline over 60 min

Continued

Continued

Drug	Trade Name	Common Uses	Comments	Dose
Azithromycin	Zithromax	Community-acquired respiratory infections *Mycobacterium intracellulare*	Has greater activity against some GU pathogens: *Chlamydia trachomatis, U. urealyticum, Neisseria gonorrhoeae, Treponema pallidum*	500 mg PO daily on an empty stomach
Clarithromycin	Biaxin	Community-acquired respiratory infections *Mycobacterium intracellulare*	Has greater activity against *Haemophilus influenzae, M. catarrhalis, Helicobacter pylori*	500 mg PO q12hr with or without food Reduce dose or dose frequency if creatinine clearance <30 mL/min

METRONIDAZOLE (Flagyl) *Antibiotic*

Indications:	Systemic infections due to *Bacteroides fragilis*, amebiasis, *Trichomonas* vaginal infections. Used in combination with amoxicillin in *Helicobacter pylori* and *Clostridium difficile* infections.
Actions:	Binds to DNA, inhibiting DNA repair and synthesis. Bactericidal.
Side effects:	Chest pain, palpitations, metallic taste, hypersensitivity, **vertigo, disorientation.**
Comments:	Approximately 80% absorbed, so the oral route is preferred to reduce costs.
Dose:	For *Helicobacter pylori*, 500 mg PO twice daily with amoxicillin 1 g twice daily.
	For *Clostridium difficile* infections, 500 mg every 6 hours.
	For systemic anaerobic infections, 15 mg/kg IV, followed by 7.5 mg/kg PO or IV every 6 hours.

NALOXONE HYDROCHLORIDE (Narcan) *Narcotic antagonist*

Indications:	Narcotic antagonism.
Actions:	Competitive antagonist at all three classes of narcotic receptors.
Side effects:	Nausea, vomiting; **may precipitate withdrawal in narcotic addicts.**
Comments:	Effect is shorter than that of many narcotics.
Dose:	0.2 to 2 mg IV, IM, or SC every 5 minutes to a maximum dose of 10 mg.

NITROFURANTOIN (numerous)   *Urinary tract anti-infective*

Indications:	Uncomplicated urinary tract infections.
Actions:	Active against *Escherichia coli* and other gram-negative coliforms. Action unknown.
Side effects:	**GI symptoms** are relatively common; rare allergic reactions; dizziness.
Comments:	Well absorbed orally; absorption is increased with food.
Dose:	Regular-release, 50 to 100 mg PO four times daily. Slow-release product, 100 mg PO twice daily.
	A single larger dose (200 mg) given once may be as effective as longer-term therapy.

NITROGLYCERIN   *Vasodilator*

Indications:	Angina pectoris, CHF.
Actions:	Venous, coronary, and arteriolar vasodilator.
Side effects:	**Headache, hypotension,** flushing.
Comments:	Nitrate tolerance may develop with prolonged, continuous administration.
Dose:	Sublingual: 0.3 to 0.6 mg.
	Lingual aerosol: 1 or 2 doses sprayed on or under the tongue every 3 to 5 minutes to a maximum of 3 times/15 min.
	Transdermal patch: 0.2 mg/hr, increasing to 0.8 mg/hr. Patch should be left on for 10 to 12 hours, then off for 12 to 14 hours to avoid tolerance.
	Transdermal ointment: 0.5 to 4 inches every 4 to 8 hours. Rotate sites. Leave off for at least 6 hours/day to avoid tolerance.
	Oral sustained release: 2 to 9 mg two to three times a day.

OCTREOTIDE ACETATE (Sandostatin)   *Somatostatin analog*

Indications:	Used mainly in the carcinoid syndrome and in tumors secreting vasoactive intestinal peptide. Also used in bleeding esophageal varices.
Actions:	Suppresses the secretion of serotonin, pancreatic peptides, gastrin, vasoactive intestinal peptide, insulin, glucagon, secretin, and motilin. Reduces collateral splanchnic blood flow.
Side effects:	Abdominal pain, transient hypoglycemia and hyperglycemia. May decrease glomerular filtration rate and increase intestinal transit time.
Comments:	Expensive.
Dose:	For bleeding esophageal varices: 50 µg IV bolus, followed by 50 µg/min IV infusion.

PENICILLINS—NARROW SPECTRUM

Indications:	Infections due to many gram-positive bacteria, including non–beta-lactamase–producing *Staphylococcus aureus* and *Staphylococcus epidermidis, Streptococcus pyogenes, Peptostreptococcus, Streptococcus pneumoniae, Bacillus anthracis, Clostridium tetani, Enterococcus.*
Actions:	Bind to specific protein sites in the bacterial cell wall, inhibiting cell wall synthesis. Not stable against beta-lactamase.
Side effects:	Diarrhea, nausea, skin rash, **allergic reactions, anaphylaxis** (0.04%).

Drug	Trade Name	Usual Dose (reduce dose or dose frequency if creatinine clearance <30 mL/min)	Comments
Penicillin G Benzylpenicillin	Crystapen Megacillin	500,000–1 million units PO 3–6 times daily 10 million–20 million units IM or IV daily in divided doses	The most effective penicillin if organisms are sensitive; unfortunately, in the hospital, many infections are due to resistant organisms
Penicillin V Phenoxymethyl-penicillin	Numerous	250–500 mg PO q6–8hr	The preferred narrow-spectrum penicillin for oral use

PENICILLINS—BROAD SPECTRUM

Indications: Infections due to *Enterococcus faecalis, Listeria monocytogenes, Proteus mirabilis, Borrelia burgdorferi* (Lyme disease), *Helicobacter pylori*. Prophylaxis against infective endocarditis after GU procedures.

Actions: An antibacterial spectrum that includes some gram-negative bacteria. Bind to specific protein sites in the bacterial cell wall, inhibiting cell wall synthesis. Not stable against beta-lactamase.

Side effects: Diarrhea, nausea, skin rash, allergic reactions.

Drug	Trade Name	Dose (reduce dose or dose frequency if creatinine clearance <30 mL/min)	Comments
Ampicillin	Ampicin	Prophylaxis in GU procedures: 2 g IV or IM with gentamicin 1.5 mg/kg IV or IM immediately before catheterization or cystoscopy, followed by ampicillin 1 g IV or IM 6 hr later Usual dose: 250–500 mg PO or IV q6hr Higher doses, 150–200 mg/kg/day IV or IM, are required in severe infections	Less well absorbed orally than amoxicillin but available as a parenteral preparation
Amoxicillin	Amoxil	Usual dose: 250–500 mg PO q8hr For severe infections, doses up to 6 g/day may be required	Much better absorbed than ampicillin; not available as a parenteral preparation

Continued

Continued

Drug	Trade Name	Dose (reduce dose or dose frequency if creatinine clearance <25 mL/min)	Comments
Amoxicillin/ clavulanate		*Helicobacter pylori* infection: 1 g amoxicillin with metronidazole 500 mg PO BID Usual dose: 250 mg amoxicillin/125 mg clavulanic acid PO q8hr Severe infections: 500 mg/ 125 mg PO q8hr Do not substitute two 250/ 125 mg tablets to achieve this dose level; the increased amount of clavulanic acid is associated with more GI side effects	Much better absorbed than ampicillin; not available as a parenteral preparation Clavulanate inhibits penicillinase, extending the antibacterial spectrum

PENICILLIN—BROAD-SPECTRUM ANTIPSEUDOMONAL

Indications: This group of penicillins is active against a variety of gram-negative bacilli, including *Pseudomonas aeruginosa*. However, it is inactivated by beta-lactamase. Piperacillin and ticarcillin are available in a form combined with a penicillinase inhibitor, which extends the antibacterial spectrum to beta-lactamase–producing bacteria.

Actions: The antibacterial spectrum of penicillin has been expanded with the development of a number of semisynthetic derivatives. They bind to specific protein sites in the bacterial cell wall, inhibiting cell wall synthesis. Unfortunately, with this advance, most new penicillins have lost some of their activity against other bacteria.

Side effects: **Allergic reactions, impaired platelet aggregation and bleeding tendencies,** eosinophilia, thrombocytopenia, neutropenia, thrombophlebitis at infusion sites.

Comments: In moderate or severe gram-negative infections, these penicillins are usually used empirically with an aminoglycoside.

Drug	Trade Name	Dose (see Table E–1 for dose adjustments in renal impairment)	Comments
Mezlocillin	Mezlin	18–24 g/day IM or IV in 4–6 divided doses	Adverse effects include anemia

Continued

Continued

Drug	Trade Name	Dose (see Table E–1 for dose adjustments in renal impairment)	Comments
Piperacillin	Piperacil	6–18 g/day IV in 4–6 divided doses	Adverse effects include GI symptoms, diarrhea
Piperacillin/ tazobactam	Tazocin		
Ticarcillin	Tipcart	4–24 g/day IM or IV in 4–6 divided doses	IM dose is painful; can be mixed with lidocaine 1% (without adrenalin) by deep injection with no more than 2 g/injection
Ticarcillin/ clavulanate	Timentin		

PENTAMIDINE (Pentacarinat) *Antibiotic*

Indications:	*Pneumocystis carinii* pneumonia.
Actions:	Interferes with DNA replication.
Side effects:	**Hypotension, nephrotoxicity, hypoglycemia, hypersensitivity.**
Comments:	Injectable pentamidine is associated with side effects in 60% of patients.
	Aerosolized pentamidine is well tolerated except for cough, especially in patients who smoke or have asthma.
Dose:	4 mg/kg per day in 50 to 250 mL D5W given IV over 2 hours. For prophylaxis, 300 mg every 4 weeks by Respirgard II nebulizer.

PHENAZOPYRIDINE (Pyridium) *Urinary analgesic*

Indications:	Urethritis, cystitis.
Actions:	Analgesic effect on inflamed urinary tract mucosa.
Side effects:	Orange discoloration of urine, nausea.
Comments:	Has no antibacterial effect. Avoid in renal impairment.
Dose:	200 mg PO three times a day after meals.

PHENTOLAMINE (Rogitine) *Alpha-adrenergic blocker*

Indications:	Catecholamine crisis in pheochromocytoma.
Actions:	Competitively blocks the effects of epinephrine and norepinephrine at alpha-1- and alpha-2-adrenergic receptors. Causes arteriolar and slight venular vasodilatation, with a compensatory increase in heart rate and contractility.
Side effects:	**Hypotension, tachycardia, angina, cerebral ischemia,** GI symptoms.
Comments:	Use with extreme caution in patients with cardiac or cerebrovascular disease.
Dose:	For emergency control of hypertension, 2.5 to 5 mg IV, best given by infusion at a rate of 5 to 10 µg/kg per minute.

PHENYTOIN (Dilantin)   *Anticonvulsant, antiepileptic*

Indications:	Seizure disorders.
Actions:	Anticonvulsant. Reduces Na^+ transport across cerebral cell membranes.
Side effects:	**Hypotension, cardiac dysrhythmias, ataxia,** nystagmus, dysarthria, hepatotoxicity, gingival hypertrophy, hirsutism, megaloblastic anemia, lymphadenopathy, fever, rash.
Comments:	At therapeutic doses, the drug is metabolized in the liver at zero order (a fixed, absolute amount per unit time). Relatively small changes in dose can cause major changes in serum concentrations over the long term.
Dose:	For status epilepticus, 18 mg/kg loading dose IV in NS at a rate of 25 to 50 mg/min. For epilepsy, 300 mg/day.

PHYTONADIONE (Vitamin K_1)   *Vitamin K*

Indications:	Vitamin K deficiency, reversal of warfarin effect.
Actions:	Essential for hepatic synthesis of factors II, VII, IX, and X.
Side effects:	Hematoma formation with SC or IM administration.
Comments:	Avoid IV administration because of **hypotension** and **anaphylaxis.** Serious hemorrhage due to excessive warfarin is better treated with fresh frozen plasma.
Dose:	2.5 to 10 mg PO, SC, or IM.

PLICAMYCIN (Mithracin)   *Parathyroid hormone inhibitor*
 Antitumor antibiotic

Indications:	Hypercalcemia due to neoplasms.
Actions:	Lowers calcium by blocking parathyroid hormone action on osteoclasts.
Side effects:	Nausea and vomiting, nephrotoxicity, local reactions due to extravasation, facial flushing.
Comments:	**A toxic agent of restricted availability.** Onset of effect is within hours, with a peak effect at 72 hours. Duration of a single injection is 7 to 10 days.
Dose:	25 µg/kg per day, with repeat doses given no sooner than 48 hours.

POTASSIUM   *Potassium supplement*

Indications:	Hypokalemia.
Actions:	Potassium supplement.
Side effects:	Nausea, vomiting, diarrhea, abdominal discomfort, hyperkalemia.
Comments:	Danger of **hyperkalemia in patients with renal impairment** and those on ACE inhibitors.
Dose:	Micro-K Extencaps: 8 mmol K^+. Micro-K 10 Extencaps: 10 mmol K^+. Slow-K: 8 mmol K^+. Kay Ciel Elixir: 20 mmol/15 mL. Prevention: 24 to 40 mmol/day. Treatment: 60 to 120 mmol/day or more.

PRIMAQUINE   *Antimalarial*

Indications:	Malaria, *Pneumocystis carinii* pneumonia.
Actions:	Unknown.

| Side effects: | GI symptoms, **methemoglobinemia, leukopenia, hemolytic anemia in patients with glucose-6-phosphate deficiency.** |
| Dose: | Used in combination with clindamycin in the treatment of *Pneumocystis* pneumonia at a dose of 15 to 30 mg/day PO with clindamycin 600 to 900 mg IV or clindamycin 300 to 400 mg PO every 6 to 8 hours. |

PROCAINAMIDE (Pronestyl, Procan) *Class Ia antiarrhythmic*

Indications:	Atrial and ventricular tachydysrhythmias.
Actions:	Reduces the maximum rate of depolarization in atrial and ventricular conducting tissue.
Side effects:	**Hypotension,** anorexia, nausea, vomiting, heart block, proarrhythmia, rash, fever, SLE-like syndrome, arthralgias.
Comments:	Similar to quinidine, except that it does not have an atropinic effect. Cross-allergy to procaine.
Dose:	1 g PO loading dose, followed by 250 to 500 mg PO every 3 hours; delayed-release preparations can be given every 6 hours.
	For life-threatening tachydysrhythmia, 20 mg/min IV infusion until the arrhythmia has been suppressed, hypotension occurs, the QRS widens by >50%, or a total dose of 17 mg/kg has been given. This can be followed by a maintenance infusion of 1 to 4 mg/min. Alternatively, for refractory VF/VT, 100 mg IV push doses every 5 minutes to a maximum dose of 1 g.

PROTAMINE SULFATE *Heparin antagonist*

Indications:	Reversal of heparin anticoagulation.
Actions:	Binds to and inactivates heparin.
Side effects:	**Hypotension, bradycardia,** flushing.
Comments:	Overdosage may paradoxically result in worsening hemorrhage, because protamine possesses anticoagulant activity.
Dose:	1 mg/100 units of heparin IV, slowly, based on an estimation of the circulating heparin. Do not give more than 50 mg in a 10-minute period.

PROTON PUMP INHIBITORS

Indications:	Gastroesophageal reflux disease, peptic ulcer, NSAID-induced gastropathy.
Actions:	Inhibition of gastric proton pumps, thus inhibiting basal and stimulated gastric acid secretion.
Side effects:	Headache, diarrhea, abdominal pain, nausea.
Comments:	Generally well tolerated. **Many interactions** when coadministered with other drugs (e.g., phenytoin, warfarin, ketoconazole, diazepam).

Drug	Trade Name	Dose
Esomeprazole	Nexium	20 mg PO daily
Lansoprazole	Zoton	15 mg PO daily
Omeprazole	Losec, Prilosec	20 mg PO daily
Pantoprazole	Protium, Protonix	40 mg PO daily
Rabeprazole	Pariet	20 mg PO daily

QUININE SULFATE   *Antimalarial*

Indications: Nocturnal leg cramps.
Actions: Unknown.
Side effects: Nausea, **visual disturbances, hemolytic anemia,** thrombo-
                  cytopenia.
Comments: Side effects are unusual at this dose, which is one tenth that
                  used in malaria.
Dose: 200 to 300 mg PO at bedtime as needed.

SALBUTAMOL
(Ventolin, Proventil)   *Beta-2 agonist*

Indications: Bronchospasm.
Actions: Beta-2-adrenergic agonist.
Side effects: Headache, dizziness, nausea, **tremor, palpitations.**
Comments: Larger doses cause tachycardia.
Dose: 2.5 to 5 mg in 3 mL NS by nebulizer every 4 hours as
                  needed. In severe bronchospasm, may be required every
                  3 to 5 minutes initially.

SODIUM POLYSTYRENE
SULFONATE (Kayexalate)   *Cation exchange resin*

Indications: Hyperkalemia.
Actions: Nonabsorbable cation exchange resin.
Side effects: Nausea, vomiting, gastric irritation, sodium retention.
Comments: 20 mmol of Na^+ is exchanged for 20 mmol of K^+ for each
                  15 g PO. Mg^{2+} and Ca^{2+} may also be exchanged.
Dose: 15 to 30 g in 50 to 100 mL of 20% sorbitol PO every 3 to 4
                  hours, or 50 g in 200 mL of 20% sorbitol or D20W PR by
                  retention enema for 30 to 60 minutes every 6 hours as
                  needed.

SUMATRIPTAN SUCCINATE (Imitrex)   *5-Hydroxytryptamine antagonist*

Indications: Intermittent treatment of migraine.
Actions: Selective 5-hydroxytryptamine–like receptor agonist. Causes
                  vasoconstriction, particularly of the dilated carotid arterial
                  circulation in migraine.
Side effects: Can cause **coronary artery spasm.** Contraindicated in coro-
                  nary artery disease; concomitant use of ergot alkaloids;
                  uncontrolled hypertension; use of MAOIs, SSRIs, or
                  lithium; and hemiplegic migraine. Flushing, dizziness,
                  feelings of heat, pressure, malaise, fatigue, drowsiness,
                  nausea, vomiting.
Comments: SC injection accompanied by local pain. Peak effects after
                  SC dose in 15 minutes; after PO dose, in 0.5 to 5 hours.
Dose: 100 mg PO. Do not repeat if first dose has no effect. If
                  successful, recrudescences can be treated with further
                  doses, not to exceed 300 mg PO in 24 hours.
                  6 mg SC.

TETRACYCLINES

Action: Inhibit bacterial growth by inhibiting protein synthesis.
                  Tetracyclines are bacteriostatic. They have been in wide-
                  spread human and animal use and have been used as

growth promoters in animals for food production for half a century.

Comments: Resistance has limited their effectiveness in both gram-positive and gram-negative bacterial infections. Resistance to one tetracycline usually implies resistance to the others. They should not be used in pregnancy or in children younger than 8 years because they can inhibit bone growth and discolor developing teeth.

Drug	Trade Name	Common Uses	Side Effects	Usual Dose
Doxycy-cline	Vibramycin	Community-acquired pneumonia, Rocky Mountain spotted fever, relapsing fever, *Chlamydia* infections	Epigastric burning, nausea, vomiting, photosensitivity	100 mg PO q12hr; minimally affected by food 100–200 mg IV daily in 1 or 2 infusions Reduce dose if creatinine clearance <30 mL/min
Minocy-cline	Minocin	Community-acquired pneumonia	GI symptoms, rash, hypersensitivity, drug-induced SLE	100 mg PO q12hr Reduce dose if creatinine clearance <30 mL/min
Tetracy-cline	Achromycin	Community-acquired pneumonia, Lyme disease, acne	GI symptoms, photosensitivity; thrombophlebitis associated with IV use	250–500 mg PO q6hr on an empty stomach 250–500 mg IV q12hr Avoid in renal impairment

THIAMINE (Vitamin B$_1$)   *Vitamin B$_1$*

Indications: Thiamine deficiency, prophylaxis of Wernicke's encephalopathy.
Actions: Vitamin B$_1$ replacement.
Side effects: IV administration may result in hypotension or, rarely, anaphylactic shock. Well absorbed orally.
Comments: Consider the oral route even in "emergencies."
Dose: 100 mg/day PO, IM, or IV for 3 days. For the IV route, give slowly over 5 minutes.

TRIMETHOPRIM-SULFAMETHOXAZOLE, CO-TRIMOXAZOLE
(Bactrim)   *Sulfonamide, folate antagonist*

Indications: Uncomplicated urinary tract infections. Drug of first choice for *Pneumocystis carinii* infections. Shigellosis.

Actions:	The sulfonamide inhibits the incorporation of paraaminobenzoic acid (PABA) into folic acid, and trimethoprim inhibits dihydroreductase, thus reducing the prodution of tetrafolic acid.
Side effects:	GI symptoms, rash, **hypersensitivity reactions,** eosinophilia, anemia.
Dose:	TMP 160/SMX 800 (2 regular-strength tablets) every 12 hours PO.
	15 to 20 mg/kg trimethoprim with 25 to 50 mg/kg of sulfamethoxazole every 12 hours IV. Reduce dose or dose frequency if creatinine clearance <30 mL/min.

VASOPRESSIN (Pitressin, Pressyn) *Antidiuretic agent*

Indications:	Principal use is to replace endogenous antidiuretic hormone in deficiency states. Used in bleeding esophageal varices.
Actions:	Increases water reabsorption by the renal tubules. Causes contraction of smooth muscle of the GI tract and all parts of the vascular bed, with a lesser effect on large veins. Reduces portal pressure.
Side effects:	Water intoxication, nausea, cramps, myocardial ischemia.
Comments:	**Care must be taken to control water balance.**
Dose:	100 units in 250 mL of D5W at the rate of 0.4 unit/min (60 mL/hr).

WARFARIN (Coumadin) *Oral anticoagulant*

Indications:	Prophylaxis and treatment of DVT, pulmonary embolism, embolic cerebrovascular accident.
Actions:	Inhibits vitamin K–dependent clotting factors.
Side effects:	Hemorrhage, nausea, vomiting, skin necrosis, fever, rash.
Comments:	Individualize dosage to maintain PT in the desired range. Many drugs interact to increase or decrease the effect of warfarin: always look up new medications before starting them in patients on warfarin to see whether they interact. Fresh frozen plasma is the treatment of choice to rapidly reverse the effect of warfarin. An alternative is vitamin K.
Dose:	Give 10 mg daily for 2 days; then give an estimated maintenance dose of 5 to 7.5 mg/day, modified according to the PT or INR.

Index

Note: Page numbers followed by f refer to figures; t refer to tables; b refer to boxes.